PHYTOTHERAPY ESSENTIALS:

Healthy Children

Optimising Children's Health with Herbs

PHYTOTHERAPY ESSENTIALS:

Healthy Children

Optimising Children's Health with Herbs

BY ROB SANTICH

Adjunct lecturer
School of Health
University of New England
NSW Australia

& KERRY BONE

Associate Professor
School of Health
University of New England
NSW Australia

PHYTOTHERAPY PRESS

First Edition May 2008

Copyright © Rob Santich & Kerry Bone May 2008

Published by Phytotherapy Press,
PO Box 661, Warwick, Queensland 4370
Tel +61 7 4661 9653
www.herbaleducation.com.au

ISBN 978-0-646-48616-1

Design and layout by Sue Hamlet,
Fledge Design Studio, Warwick, Queensland

Printed by Colourwise, Brisbane, Queensland on 100% recycled paper

This book is written for professional prescribing and should not be
taken as a guide to self treatment.

Preface

As the father of four children, who at the time of writing are now 25, 22, 18 and 8 years of age, I have seen and treated all of their childhood illnesses. The most serious of these was whooping cough. These first-hand experiences represented a steep learning curve. My undergraduate studies did not include herbal paediatrics and at the time there were no specialised texts on the subject. Those books that did mention the herbal treatment of children seemed to me to be terribly cautious, recommending only the gentlest of herbs. This contrasted starkly with the approach taken by the medical profession. There were no apparent reservations with prescribing newborn babies and children the harshest of drugs.

In my early years of practice the majority of my patients were children, built mainly through referrals from my wife who was and still is a preschool teacher. Over the years I have seen many chronic paediatric health problems completely resolved with the appropriate use of herbal medicines. So when Kerry Bone proposed the idea of coauthoring a book on herbs for children, I thought this would be an excellent opportunity to share these clinical experiences in print as a contribution to the further development of herbal paediatrics. This book represents our endeavours to not only produce an evidence-based practical guide for the herbal clinician, but also a work based on many years of clinical experience.

Rob Santich

Avalon, Australia 2008

In my clinical practice I consult with a wide range of patients. Living in a small country town, I treat the townsfolk as well as people from the land who often travel long distances to see me. I see men and women, young and old and many people whose families are relatively new to Australia and who come with a cultural background of phytotherapy. I find working with children can be very challenging but at the same time immensely rewarding. One factor that has an enormous influence on treatment outcome is the parents' efforts with children's compliance and I do salute them for their persistence in this area. I have seen some wonderful outcomes with young patients and I hope that this book will assist other practitioners to obtain similar results.

Kerry Bone

Warwick, Australia, 2008

BOTH AUTHORS WOULD LIKE to express many thanks to Patricia Bone, Vicki Matthews and Sue Hamlet for their invaluable assistance with the development and publication of this work. Thanks also to Amanda Williams for her suggestions for the title.

Rob Santich also wishes to thank his children Joel, Mitchel, Ella & Grace for being his greatest teachers; his wife Lynda for support and infinite patience; herbal teachers Denis Stewart and Kerry Bone for their inspiration and passion; and Oglala Lakota mentors and friends, Tommy Crow, Orville Reddest and John Around Him for helping clarify his path in life.

Table of Contents

CHAPTER ONE

Basic Principles

THE SPECIAL NEEDS OF CHILDREN are recognised across all levels of social structure: children are not miniature adults. Any potential benefits and risks of herbal therapy in children will differ from those in adults, therefore the principles that govern herbal practice should also differ. With these important considerations in mind, the objective of this book is to provide healthcare professionals with an evidence-based and up-to-date guide to the herbal treatment of common infant and childhood conditions.

This introductory chapter will cover a number of basic issues, such as the factors influencing bioavailability in children, dose and dosage forms and ensuring good compliance. It finishes with an overview of the key safety issues.

One of the most important issues in paediatric herbal therapeutics is indeed the question of safety. At present, for obvious ethical reasons, there is little direct information from a paediatric setting to address this issue. Herbal clinicians therefore have no choice but to rely largely on safety data from adult studies. In addition, this book draws on the extensive clinical experience of the authors in treating children, and above all is guided by common sense, a consideration which is often absent from the herbal safety debate.

Bioavailability of Herbs in Children

The following is a review of the physiological factors specific to infants and children that may affect phytochemical metabolism and hence the bioavailability of herbal treatments.

Route of Administration

Several methods can be used to administer herbs to children, however most common is the oral administration of herbal teas or extracts. The immaturity of the child's digestive tract means that gastrointestinal absorption may differ from an adult. It is likely that most herbal extracts are absorbed in a similar manner to drugs, either by simple passive diffusion or by carrier-mediated active transport. With simple diffusion, influencing factors include pH, the presence or type of gastric contents, gastrointestinal (GI) time and GI motility.[1] In other words, the length of time a medication is in contact with the gastrointestinal mucosa will directly affect its absorption.

Gastric emptying time depends on postnatal age, with emptying times of up to 6 to 8 hours reported in extreme cases.[2] It can also be influenced by the position of breast feeding, with right lateral and upright feeding encouraging more favourable emptying times.[3] In contrast, intestinal transit time appears to be shorter in young children.[4,5] Taken together, these considerations suggest that erratic patterns of absorption may be an issue with some children, which could lead to inadequate bioavailability and hence clinical activity. Many common paediatric disorders such as diarrhoea and hyperperistalsis may also diminish absorption.[1] Eventually, by the age of 10 to 12 years, the child's GI tract resembles that of an adult. However, at this age other difficulties arise which can impact absorption, such as noncompliant behaviour, poor nutrition and unpredictable dietary habits.[1]

Neonates and infants also demonstrate an immaturity in the secretion and activity of their bile and pancreatic fluid during the first few months of life that results in impaired fat digestion.[2] This immaturity is evidenced by the reduced absorption of the fat-soluble vitamins D and E, probably arising from an inadequate bile acid pool in the ileum.[2] A low lipase environment, coupled with the minimal bile acid production, may also contribute to difficulties in absorbing lipid-soluble phytochemicals.

Herbal baths are also a traditional method for treating neonates and infants.[6] This means of administering herbal extracts, whether they be infusions, decoctions or alcoholic extracts added to bath water, is supported by a number of considerations. Neonates and infants have a larger skin surface area relative to their body weight than an adult. Coupled with reduced epidermal and stratum corneum thickness, this leads to a more efficient transdermal absorption.[7,8]

Body Composition and Hepatic Function

The bodies of neonates and infants have different relative percentages of water and lipids than older children and adults.[2,9,10] At birth there is a greater percentage of body water and less body lipids. This increases the volume in which any water-soluble phytochemicals are distributed (hence diluting their levels in tissue) and can also contribute to decreased retention of lipid-soluble phytochemicals.[10]

Liver growth continues after birth until it reaches its mature size. The liver constitutes 5% of the body weight at birth, but only 2% in the adult.[11] The neonate has less than 20% of the number of hepatocytes of an adult liver. The neonatal liver also has a decreased capacity to metabolise, detoxify and excrete xenobiotics, which include both pharmaceutical drugs and plant phytochemicals.[12] There are decreased levels of many cytochrome P450 (phase I) and phase II enzymes. For example, the development of physiological jaundice in a neonate is probably due to a reduced capacity for glucuronide conjugation.

Although the foetal liver can process many xenobiotics, the neonate has a prolonged half-life for the metabolism of most drugs. However, significant and rapid maturation of this capacity occurs in the first year of life.[12] For example, the phase II enzyme N-acetyltransferase 2 mediates the transformation of a large number of drugs and chemicals. Before 15 months of age about 50% of infants are slow acetylators, but by the age of 3 years this enzyme is fully expressed.[12]

Metabolism by Intestinal Flora

The role of gut flora in phytochemical metabolism, particularly in terms of the metabolism of glycosides, is well-recognised and has been extensively reviewed elsewhere. Readers not familiar with this subject or in need of a refresher are referred to that body of work.[13]

The foetal intestine is sterile and bathed in swallowed amniotic fluid.[14] At birth, gut colonisation begins with the bacteria that are derived from the mother during delivery. Microbes from the vaginal canal and the perineal area enter the mouth and the stomach of vaginally-delivered infants. Within a few minutes after birth, the gastric flora of the newborn child reflects the cervical flora of the mother.[15,16] Environmental factors such as the level of hygiene or antibiotics administered to either the mother or neonate can contribute to a modification of this type of transmission.[17] By the end of the first postnatal week, the diet represents the most important influence on microflora composition. Exclusive breast feeding promotes the growth of bifidobacteria that play a role in resisting pathogenic bacteria and are associated with a healthy neonate stool flora.[18] The intestinal microflora in breastfed infants is composed almost exclusively of bifidobacterium, with few coliforms. A change in the composition of the microflora occurs at weaning, due to *Escherichia coli* and other bacteria present in food.[18] This leads to a significant decrease in lactobacilli and an increase in putrefactive bacteria.[17]

The change in the microflora at weaning is important for the hydrolysis of plant glycosides, with the increasing activity of bacterial enzymes such as β-glucosidase.[17] Based on this information, an infant's capacity to hydrolyse glycosides will increase following weaning and will follow a developmental pattern with increasing age. The metabolism of plant glycosides by gut flora can be an important step in their absorption or therapeutic activation.[13]

Dose and Dosage Forms

The above considerations make the calculation of an appropriate and safe herbal dose for a neonate or infant a relatively imprecise affair. This is especially so for the neonate and infant less than 12 months, where considerable care and caution should be exercised. Nonetheless, there are various methods used to calculate dosages for children that are widely used. These have been reviewed elsewhere.[19] Only two methods will be proposed in this work: a method for older children based on body weight, which takes into account the faster metabolism of children, and a method for young infants based on age.

Compared to adults, children have a higher resting energy expenditure per kilogram(kg) body weight or per kg of lean body mass. This declines steadily with years of growth.[20,21] The higher rate of energy expenditure is necessary for growth and development. Hence it makes sense to apply a dosage calculation that accounts for these factors. The recommended equation is as follows:

(1.5 x weight in kg + 10) yields the percentage of the adult dose.

Expressed in terms of pounds (lb), the formula is:

$$\frac{(1.5 \text{ x weight in lb})}{2.2} + 10$$

For example if a child weighs 20 kg (44 lbs), then that child should receive (1.5 x 20) + 10, or 40% of the adult dose.[18]

In the case of a multi-ingredient liquid herbal formula, the prescription is constructed as one would for an adult, using the recommended weekly doses. Then the standard dose (for example 5 mL three times a day (TDS)) can be subjected to the above calculation. In the case of tablets, the adult daily dose can be subjected to the same calculation to find the daily dose for the child.

As noted above, applying a different rule for young infants is often more prudent. The rule is as follows and applies to infants up to 2 years:[19]

$$\frac{\text{Age in months}}{150} \times \text{adult dose} = \text{child's dose}$$

The Alcohol Issue

The use of ethanolic extracts in herbal paediatrics remains a controversial issue, with concerns expressed that alcoholic extracts are inappropriate to use for neonates and infants. This does appear to have some basis in terms of their capacity to clear ethanol, especially for infants less than 12 months of age. The CYP2E1 isoenzyme involved in the metabolism of small molecules such as ethanol rises steadily after birth to reach 40% of adult values through the first year of life. Adult values are reached between the ages of 1 to 10 years, thus displaying a great deal of individual variability.[22,23] Alcohol dehydrogenase (ADH), the rate-limiting enzyme responsible for the biotransformation of ethanol, also exhibits an age-related developmental increase in activity.[2] However, by 12 to 30 months ADH activity is equal to or greater than that found in adults.[24]

The question regarding the safety of alcohol is really one of dose. By way of example (and using the first calculation method described above), a child weighing 10 kg is prescribed *Matricaria recutita* (chamomile) 1:2 extract in 60% ethanol for colic. The adult dose for chamomile 1:2 is 20 to 40 mL per week, or in terms of the standard dose, 1 to 2 mL three times a day (TDS).[19] To establish an appropriate dose for this child, the following calculation is applied: 1.5 x 10 kg + 10 = 25. This is the percentage of the adult dose to use, which can be represented as the factor 0.25. Taking the maximum adult standard dose of 2 mL, this makes the child's dose 2 mL x 0.25, which is 0.5 mL. To calculate the amount of ethanol in this 0.5mL dose, multiply 0.5 by 0.6 (representing the 60% ethanol) to give 0.3 mL. This represents a very low amount of ethanol, and rarely seems to cause any problems, even in very young infants.

Because of the controversy that clouds the use of alcoholic extracts for infants, it has been suggested that glycetracts or glycerites (extracts made with glycerol and water) may be the answer. However, it is important not to overrate the value of such extracts.[13] Glycerol is a poor solvent for most phytochemicals and glycetracts are less stable than alcoholic extracts. In a comparison of the therapeutic effect of an alcoholic versus a non-alcoholic galenical preparation, it was demonstrated that an alcoholic extract had greater efficacy. The dose of the alcohol-free preparation needed to be adjusted to a much higher level to obtain the same clinical effect.[25]

If alcohol is a concern, a more practical way of administering a concentrated herbal dose is to use a tablet. If the child cannot swallow tablets, then a crushed tablet (or part thereof) can be used, mixed with a suitable vehicle such as a small quantity of fruit concentrate or honey as appropriate.

A commonly suggested practice when using alcoholic extracts is to remove the alcohol by adding freshly boiled water to the standard dose. However, if a small proportion of boiling water is added to a small dose of herbal medicine, the resulting average temperature will only be approximately 60° to 70°C. Since ethanol evaporates at around 78°C, this will not be sufficient to cause significant evaporation. Hence this commonly recommended practice has no rational basis. Moreover, a mixture of ethanol and water forms an azeotrope that boils at approximately 80°C, evaporating equal proportions of alcohol and water.[26] To effectively drive off ethanol, sustained heating at 80°C for at least 5 minutes would be necessary. This could damage the activity of some herbs.

Taste and Compliance Issues

Poor adherence to treatment is a recognised problem in paediatrics.[27] Estimates of non-adherence or non-compliance for conventional medicines range from 25% to 60%, reaching a peak during adolescence with increasing personal independence.[27,28] The issue of taste can present a significant added challenge to the herbal clinician, which can be even more difficult if the child has not been previously exposed to herbal liquids. Most children are averse to take anything that is not immediately orally pleasing and will reject perceived nasty tastes. The masking of a bitter tasting herb can be a major formulation challenge that is not easily solved. What is absolutely necessary is the cooperation and determination of the parent or caregiver in persuading the child to take his or her herbs. Behavioural modification strategies such as an appropriate reward can increase compliance. Additionally, most modern families live extremely busy lives. It is therefore important to ensure that protocols are simple and are compatible with such demands.

One of the oldest solutions for masking the unpleasant taste of a herbal liquid is to use a sweetening agent. There are several alternatives available. For example honey or maple syrup can be blended with a herbal formulation or added to the standard dose. The use of glycetracts is another convenient method of sweetening a mixture, with the glycetract of marshmallow root most often used for this purpose. Good quality glycetracts for herbs that are often indicated in common paediatric conditions are also available, such as Echinacea. However, as noted earlier, glycetracts should not be relied upon to do most of the therapeutic work. There are also various flavouring mixes available that can be added to a formula at a level of 15 to 20%.

If all these techniques fail to achieve compliance, the following innovative method has proven useful. The parent or caregiver prepares a jelly (jello) and pours the mixture into an ice cube tray with small compartments. The standard dose is then placed in each compartment. The standard dose readily diffuses through the jelly before it sets, therefore there is no need to blend the mixture. The tray is then placed in a refrigerator to set. The child is given one jelly cube as each dose, which can then be followed by water, fruit juice or an appropriate reward.

The age at which a child can effectively swallow tablets or capsules is an important safety consideration in order to avoid inadvertent inhalation or choking. There is little information in the literature, however it is generally acknowledged that tablets are acceptable for children of school age.[29] This depends of course on the tablet size and shape, and since herbal tablets are generally larger than conventional drugs, it is likely that they can only be swallowed by children above the age of 9 or 10 years. It may also be necessary to reduce the size of the tablet with the use of a tablet cutter once the dosage calculation is applied.

In order to increase compliance, tablets can be substituted for liquids in younger children. But first the tablets must be crushed and mixed with either honey or a suitable conserve and administered on a teaspoon. This method of administering tablets is in fact suitable for children of all ages. If the dosage form is a capsule then the contents of the capsule (or part thereof) can be emptied and mixed with an appropriate vehicle.

Administering Herbs to Breastfed Infants

A common suggestion for treating breastfed neonates is to have the mother consume the herbal extracts in the belief that therapeutic doses will pass into the breast milk. Although there appears to be some documentation of this practice in at least one traditional herbal medicine system,[30] there is a general lack of guidance concerning the doses a nursing mother would need to take for an adequate phytochemical transfer. This is coupled with an almost complete lack of pharmacokinetic studies that would inform such a practice. It should also be noted that this practice is not used in conventional medicine.

The transfer of most phytochemicals and drugs into breast milk is usually by passive diffusion and the overall rate and extent of transfer is influenced by numerous factors. These include the stage of lactation, chemical characteristics of the drug or phytochemical, the concentration the drug or phytochemical reaches in the blood and the composition of the milk (water, lipid and protein content and pH).[31,32,33] Some weak bases can preferentially enter breast milk as a result of the pH gradient that exists between blood (pH = 7.4) and breast milk (pH = 8.0).[32] The balance between the herbal dose and the elimination rate in the mother will ultimately determine the maternal blood and milk levels.[31]

Colostrum is secreted for the first 2 to 3 days after birth. At this stage of lactation the epithelial cells lining the alveoli have open junctions allowing both small and large molecules (like proteins) to be easily transferred by a process termed paracellular diffusion. Here the concentration in maternal blood essentially controls drug or phytochemical transfer into colostrum.[31] Milk secretion commences around day 3 or 4 after birth and at this stage the gaps between the epithelial cells close. The major pathway for the passive diffusion of drugs or phytochemicals then must be transcellular.[31] Mature milk of relatively stable composition is produced 2 to 3 weeks after birth; the major components are ions, proteins and lipids.[31] The lipid fraction of the milk is important, as lipid-soluble chemicals may dissolve in the lipid droplets as they form in the alveolar epithelial cells and thereby be cosecreted.

In terms of what is currently known about the transfer of phytochemicals in breast milk, only a handful of studies exist. The pharmacokinetics of rhein, an anthraquinone found in both rhubarb root and senna, has been investigated. Several pharmacokinetic studies on healthy volunteers have demonstrated that rhein appears in the blood and shows a rapid rise after oral ingestion, followed by a slow decline.[34,35] Further to this, the excretion of rhein (from senna) into breast milk was investigated in 100 breast milk samples from 20 postpartum women. Following daily doses of 5 g of a senna laxative (containing 15 mg of rhein) for 3 days, the rhein concentration in milk samples from every lactation during the post-dose 24 hours was measured. Values varied between 0 and 27 ng/mL, with values below 10 ng/mL found in 94% of samples. Based on median values, only 0.007% of the rhein intake was excreted into breast milk and none of the breastfed infants had an abnormal stool consistency.[36] Rhein is highly water soluble and slightly acidic,[37] properties that would perhaps act against each other in the transfer to breast milk.

Based on this example, it is unlikely that the normally recommended doses of most herbal medicines taken by the mother will have any therapeutic effect in the infant. Any observed effects are more likely due to other factors such as an unrelated spontaneous recovery. Hence, until more information becomes available, it is recommended that herbal doses intended for a breastfed child are always directly administered to the child.

In terms of treating breastfed infants with herbal medicines, the following method has demonstrated good compliance. The appropriate dose of the herbal extract is blended with 5 mL of expressed breast milk or infant formula. The resultant mixture is then drawn into a syringe and applied with steady pressure to the back of the infant's mouth. It may take several applications to deliver the full 5 mL. The infant is then placed on the breast to feed, or given a bottle of water or infant formula.

The corollary issues of the safety of herbs during pregnancy and lactation are not a focus of this book. These complex issues have been extensively reviewed elsewhere and the reader is referred to that text.[38]

Further Considerations

There is an observable difference in the rate of recovery from illness between infancy and adulthood. In general, an infant has a greater rate of spontaneous recovery from an acute illness than an adult.[39,40] In other words it is not uncommon for infants to become rapidly ill due to the immaturity of their immune systems and (with the exception of virulent pathogens) recover within a few days. The herbal clinician's goal in these cases is to promote and enhance this innate self-healing capacity. Arguably the most effective strategy for an acute infection is therefore the use of the diaphoretic and immune-enhancing remedies.

As a result of the higher energy expenditure, infancy is generally characterised as being warm or hot in nature. Have you ever noticed how difficult it can be to place warm clothes on children in winter? In addition, many of the conditions experienced during infancy are acute infections that are "hot" in nature. This emphasises the importance of the ultimately cooling remedies in paediatrics, especially diaphoretics. The bitter tasting herbs will also exert a cooling effect. However the clinician must here keep in mind the compliance issue with children and take the recommended steps for taste correction.

Aside from oral herbal medicines, other methods of administration are appropriate for children. Suppositories formulated under sterile conditions at appropriate doses can provide a dosage form that avoids an unpleasant taste and bypasses the first pass effect of the liver, being absorbed into the bloodstream via the rectal mucosa. The vaporisation or atomisation of essential oils into the sick room for the treatment of respiratory tract infections provides direct antimicrobial and anticatarrhal activities, complementing any diaphoretic and immune-enhancing herbal treatments. Topical preparations of various forms are appropriate for many conditions from nappy (diaper) rash to middle ear infections. These useful supplementary dosage forms will be considered, where appropriate, in subsequent chapters.

Efficacy and Safety Information

As a general rule infants and children can be administered the same herbs as adults, albeit at lower dosages. However there are some qualifications. Powerful laxatives such as senna and strong tasting herbs such as wormwood, ginger and garlic should be used with caution.[39] Potentially toxic herbs such as Tylophora and Phytolacca (poke root) are best avoided. However, the reader will note that there are case histories in this text where poke root has been used in older children. Certain herbal actions such as diaphoretic, immune-enhancing, antimicrobial and spasmolytic (both gut and respiratory) appear prominently in herbal paediatrics because of the specific needs of children.

Modern herbal clinicians rely on two primary sources for the evidence that validates and informs their practice: scientific and traditional. Reliable published traditional evidence comes from texts such as Ellingwood[41] and Felter and Lloyd.[42] It is clear that these Eclectic physicians were skilled and heroic paediatric prescribers, using potent herbs such as aconite, belladonna, gelsemium and poke root. Most of these remedies listed are no longer recommended for children because of their potential toxicity.[43] Other sources of traditional information include the documented practice of herbalism in the United Kingdom and the rest of Europe.[44,45]

A less Eurocentric context exists in traditional communities in Australia, with the world's longest surviving paediatric practice among the Aborigine people. Currently more than 100 surviving Language Groups preserve their paediatric herbal traditions within the context of a complete medical system. Much of this practice takes place in some of earth's most inhospitable and waterless environments. This herbal tradition utilises a comprehensive materia medica which treats infants and nurtures children into adolescence in a harsh environment.[46,47]

Several scientific articles have been published in peer review journals that discuss herbal use in paediatrics in terms of efficacy, safety, toxicity and adverse reactions. It is clearly evident that herbal medicine, and complementary and alternative medicine (CAM) therapies in general, are popular treatment choices for many parents and caregivers.[48,49,50] An often cited reason for this choice is the perception that such remedies are free of serious side effects. However, a more comprehensive analysis of the reasons parents/caregivers choose naturopathic medicine for their children has recently been published.[51] This cross-sectional survey received 92 responses from parents/caregivers of children aged from 0 to 15 years consulting naturopathic doctors from three states in Canada. Five primary reasons for choosing naturopathic medicine were identified by qualitative analysis. Parents wanted a system of care that looked beyond the physical symptoms of disease to the source of the problem and furthermore offered treatments that resolved the underlying causes rather than masking the symptoms. They expressed the desire for a system that treated the whole person and emphasised wellness with a proactive and preventative approach. A choice of care that was in the best interests of the child was a focus of many parents. Parents also raised concerns in relation to the side effects of drugs and wanted safer alternatives. Moreover they wanted reliable information in order to make a choice on the course of treatment and believed they received that from naturopathic doctors. Parents also felt that naturopathic medicine met the specific needs of the child, because conventional medicine was ineffective in treating the child's condition. Finally a perceived benefit of naturopathic medicine came from many parents, having themselves experienced a positive outcome with the approach.

In terms of adverse reaction reports for CAM therapies, herbal medicines are most often implicated. A recent publication from the WHO Monitoring Center incorporated some 8,985 case reports of adverse reactions associated with herbal medicines between 1968 to 1997.[52] Approximately 100 of these reports concerned children and adolescents between the ages of 10 to 20 years.[53] The bulk of these reports were anecdotal, with systematic investigations rarely undertaken. Hence causality is uncertain.[50] Experts agree that the most commonly documented reason for toxic or adverse reactions is the presence of adulterants.[38,50,53] This concern clearly highlights the importance of using herbal preparations of the highest quality. A complete review of this subject can be found elsewhere.[38]

By way of contrast, a recently published US study found a total of 1,087 adverse drug reactions to conventional drugs over a 10-year period among hospitalised paediatric patients.[54] An Italian study found that the incidence of adverse drug reactions was 15.1 cases per 1,000 children.[55] Both figures clearly exceed the frequency of adverse herbal reactions documented in the WHO study.

In terms of efficacy data, it is true to say that there is a deficiency of randomised controlled trials of herbal medicines in children. However this is not to say there are none. Those many trials that have been published will be reviewed in the appropriate chapters of this text.

Specific Herbal Safety Information for Children

The following recommendations have been based on traditional evidence for safe use in children, scientific investigations and a knowledge of the relevant phytochemical constituents found in the herb. They have largely been collated from a specialised herbal safety text.[38]

HERB	SAFETY INFORMATION
Andrographis	Considered safe for children based on several lines of evidence. No adverse events were reported in a 3-month study using oral Andrographis extract for the prevention of the common cold. Andrographis is traditionally used in Ayurvedic medicine to treat bowel complaints in infants and children.
Arnica	For topical use only.
Astragalus	No specific information available, but adverse effects are not expected.
Bacopa	Considered safe for children based on several lines of evidence. Bacopa is used in children in Ayurvedic medicine and has been used in three clinical trials involving children.
Barberry & Indian barberry	Berberine has been used to treat diarrhoea and giardiasis in children, suggesting that berberine-containing plants may be used. However the use of these herbs is contraindicated in neonatal jaundice.
Bearberry	Treatment is not recommended for children under the age of 12 years.
Bilberry fruit	Considered safe based on the favourable clinical results and tolerability of a concentrated bilberry powder for infants with acute diarrhoea.
Bittersweet	No safety information available. Use is not recommended due to the saponin content and the possibility of gastric irritation.
Black cohosh	No safety information available. However the herb is noted by Eclectic physicians as being of benefit in the treatment of fever in children.
Black haw	No specific information available, but adverse effects are not expected.
Black walnut hulls	No safety information available.
Bladderwrack	No safety information available.
Blue cohosh	A number of reports exist of poisoning in children attracted to the blue fruits.

HERB	SAFETY INFORMATION
Blue flag	Used to treat infantile eczema. However no specific safety information is available, but adverse effects are not expected if appropriate doses are used.
Boldo	Best avoided due to the potential toxic properties of Boldo.
Boswellia	No specific information available, but adverse effects are not expected.
Buchu	No specific information available, but adverse effects are not expected.
Bugleweed & gypsywort	No safety information available, but due to antithyroid activity caution is advised.
Bupleurum	No safety information available.
Burdock root	No specific information available, but adverse effects are not expected.
Butcher's broom	No safety information available.
Calendula	No specific information available, but adverse effects are not expected.
Californian poppy	No specific information available, but adverse effects are not expected. Used traditionally as a sedative and analgesic in children.
Cascara	It is inappropriate to provide stimulant laxatives to children under 10 years of age.
Cat's claw	Use in children under 3 years of age is said to be contraindicated in Europe due to a lack of clinical data rather that evidence of adverse effects.
Celery seed	No safety information available.
Chamomile, German	Considered benign when taken by children.
Chaparral	No safety information available.
Chaste tree	No safety information available.
Chickweed	No specific information available, but adverse effects are not expected, other than allergy.
Clivers	No specific information available, but adverse effects are not expected.
Codonopsis	No specific information available, but adverse effects are not expected.
Corn silk	No specific information available, but adverse effects are not expected. Eclectic physicians used corn silk in bladder disorders of children.

HERB	SAFETY INFORMATION
Couch grass	No specific information available, but adverse effects are not expected.
Cramp bark	No specific information available, but adverse effects are not expected.
Cranberry	Adverse effects are not expected if taken at the recommended doses.
Cranesbill	No specific information available, but adverse effects are not expected if taken within the recommended doses.
Crataeva	No specific information available, but adverse effects are not expected.
Damiana	No specific information available, however a slimming tea is used in Mexico that is also served to children.
Devil's claw	No specific information available, but adverse effects are not expected.
Dong quai	No specific information available, but adverse effects are not expected.
Echinacea	Adverse effects are not expected. Echinacea has been used in clinical investigations for both otitis media and upper respiratory tract infections in children from 2 to 11 years of age.
Elder flower	No safety information available.
Elecampane	No safety information available.
Ephedra	Only to be used in children over 6 years of age. The dose should not deliver in excess of 0.5 mg/kg of total alkaloids in a single dose or more than 2.0 mg/kg per daily dose.
Euphorbia	No specific information available, but adverse effects are not expected, if taken within the recommended dosage range. Used to treat diarrhoea and dysentery in children and in Ayurvedic medicine for a variety of childhood disorders.
Evening primrose oil	Adverse effects are not expected. Evening primrose oil and its key constituent gamma linolenic acid have been administered to children in clinical trials.
Eyebright	No specific information available, but adverse effects are not expected.
False unicorn root	No safety information available.
Fennel	Apart from the rare case of allergic reaction, no adverse effects are expected. Fennel has been administered to infants in clinical trials.
Fenugreek	No specific information available, but adverse effects are not expected.
Feverfew	No safety information available.

HERB	SAFETY INFORMATION
Fringe tree	No adverse effects are expected. Eclectic physicians recommended fringe tree as a gentle and effective treatment for infantile jaundice.
Garlic	No specific information available, but adverse effects are not expected, other than possible mild gastrointestinal discomfort. Garlic should not be administered to children younger that 3 years.
Gentian	No specific information available, but adverse effects are not expected apart from a reaction to the strong bitter taste.
Ginger	Generally considered safe for children. The pungent taste may cause compliance issues.
Ginkgo	No side effects were observed in infants from 2 to 7 months old with hypoxic-ischaemic encephalopathy treated with standardised Ginkgo leaf extracts for 2 months. Reports of poisoning in children after the ingestion of the seeds.
Ginseng, Korean	No specific information available, but adverse effects are not expected.
Globe artichoke	No specific information available, but adverse effects are not expected.
Goat's rue	No safety information available.
Golden rod	No specific information available, but adverse effects are not expected.
Golden seal	Berberine has been used to treat diarrhoea and giardiasis in children, suggesting that berberine-containing plants such as golden seal may be used. However their use is contraindicated in neonatal jaundice.
Gotu kola	Adverse effects are not expected. Gotu kola dried leaf has been clinically evaluated as a mental tonic for mentally disabled children and a leaf concentrate used as a nutritional porridge for preschool children.
Greater celandine	No safety information available, but prolonged use is unsuitable in children.
Grindelia	No specific information available, but adverse effects are not expected.
Gymnema	No specific information available, but adverse effects are not expected.
Hawthorn leaf & flower	No specific information available, but adverse effects are not expected.
Hops	No specific information available, but adverse effects are not expected.

HERB	SAFETY INFORMATION
Horsechestnut	Poisoning in children due to the ingestion of the seeds or infusions prepared from the leaves and twigs have been reported, including fatalities. However analysis of human exposures to *Aesculus spp.* which included 1527 children aged between 0 to 5 years reported nontoxic effects in the majority of cases. Cases of toxicity may have resulted from ingestion of the seed capsule.
Horsetail	No safety information available.
Hydrangea	No specific information available, but adverse effects are not expected.
Jamaica dogwood	No safety information available.
Kava	The Australian Therapeutic Goods Administration recommends that kava-containing medicines should not be taken by children under 12 years of age. In Polynesia kava has been used traditionally in children for general debility, stomach disorders and for fretting.
Lavender	No specific information available, but adverse effects are not expected.
Lemon balm	No specific information available, but adverse effects are not expected.
Licorice	As children often consume licorice confectionery, care should be taken to avoid excessive exposure. The use of licorice as a flavouring agent in herbal medicines should be moderated.
Lime flowers	No safety information available.
Marshmallow	No specific information available, but adverse effects are not expected.
Meadowsweet	Clinicians should be aware of the possibility of Reye's syndrome, an acute sepsis-like illness encountered exclusively in children below 15 years of age. The cause is unknown, although antiviral agents and salicylate derivatives have been implicated. However, it is unknown whether the salicylates in meadowsweet are capable of causing this reaction.
Motherwort	No safety information available.
Mullein	No specific information available, but adverse effects are not expected.
Myrrh	No specific information available, but adverse effects are not expected.
Nettle leaf & root	No specific information available, but adverse effects are not expected.
Oregon grape	Berberine has been used to treat diarrhoea and giardiasis in children, suggesting that berberine-containing plants may be used. However their use is contraindicated in neonatal jaundice.

HERB	SAFETY INFORMATION
Pasque flower	No safety information available.
Passionflower	No specific information available, but adverse effects are not expected.
Pau d'arco	Information provided to the Brazilian Ministry of Health in 1967 indicated that purple pau d'arco was suitable to administer to children.
Pennyroyal	No specific information available, but its use is not advised.
Peppermint	No adverse effects are expected from the use of galenical peppermint leaf preparations. The direct application of peppermint essential oil preparations to the nasal area or chest of babies and small children must be avoided because of the risk of laryngeal and bronchial spasm.
Poke root	No information is available for poke root, but recommended dosage should be adhered to and adjusted accordingly.
Prickly ash	No specific information available, but adverse effects are not expected.
Raspberry leaf	No specific information available, but adverse effects are not expected if taken within the recommended dosage.
Rehmannia	No adverse effects are expected if taken within the recommended dosage.
Rosemary	No safety information available.
Sage	No adverse effects are expected if taken within the recommended dosage.
Saw palmetto	No specific information available, but adverse effects are not expected.
Schisandra	A 90% ethanolic tincture and an extract have been successfully used to treat infantile diarrhoea.
Senna	It is inappropriate to provide stimulant laxatives to children under 10 years of age. Using senna preparations in infants and young children is associated with nappy (diaper) rash, skin blisters in the perianal area and skin sloughing.
Shatavari	Used in South-East Asia as a nutrient tonic in children.
Shepherd's purse	No specific information available, but adverse effects are not expected.
Siberian ginseng	No specific information available, but adverse effects are not expected.
Skullcap	Adverse effects are not expected if taken within the recommended dosage. Eclectic physicians recommended skullcap infusion to calm the teething child.

HERB	SAFETY INFORMATION
St John's wort	Has been trialled successfully for the treatment of depression and psychovegetative disturbances in 101 children under 12 years old. Tolerability was good and no adverse events were reported.
St Mary's thistle	Adverse effects are not expected. Children administered silymarin for 30 days showed no clinical or biochemical adverse effects.
Tansy	No information is available, but caution is advised. Used traditionally to treat worm infestation in children.
Thuja	No specific information available, but use should be restricted to recommended dosage.
Thyme	No safety information available.
Turmeric	No specific information available, but adverse effects are not expected.
Tylophora	No safety information available. Best avoided in children.
Valerian	No safety information available. However it is recommended that Valerian be avoided in children under 3 years of age.
White horehound	No specific information available, but adverse effects are not expected.
Wild cherry	No specific information available, but adverse effects are not expected.
Wild lettuce	No safety information available.
Willow bark	Clinicians should be aware of the possibility of Reye's syndrome, an acute sepsis-like illness encountered exclusively in children below 15 years of age. The cause is unknown, although antiviral agents and salicylate derivatives have been implicated. However, it is unknown whether the salicylates in willow bark are capable of causing this reaction.
Withania	Adverse events were not reported in a clinical trial using oral Withania in children for 60 days. Withania is traditionally used in Ayurvedic medicine to treat failure to thrive in children.
Wormwood	No safety information available. Best avoided in children.
Yarrow	No specific information available, but adverse effects are not expected.
Yellow dock	No specific information available, but adverse effects are not expected.
Zizyphus seed	No specific information available, but adverse effects are not expected.

References

1   Suggs DM. *J Am Nurse Pract* 2000;**12**(6): 236-239
2   Benedetti MS, Baltes EL *Fund Clin Pharmacol* 2003;**17**(3): 281-299
3   Villanueva-Meyer J, Swischuk LE, Cesani F et al. *J Nuc Med* 1996;**37**(8): 1356-1358
4   Gilman JT. *Clin Pharmacokinet* 1990; **19**(1): 1-10
5   Pedersen S, Steffensen G. *J Pediatr* 1987; **110**(6): 953-959
6   McIntyre A. *Herbal Treatment of Children.* Elsevier Butterworth Heinemann, Edinburgh, 2005, pp. 11-12.
7   Routledge PA. *J Antimicrob Chemother* 1994; **34**(A): 19-24
8   Keans GL, Abdel-Rahman SM, Alander SW et al. *NEJM* 2003; **349**(12): 1157-1167
9   Ginsberg G, Hattis D, Miller R, Sonawane B. *Pediatrics* 2004; **113**(4): 973-982
10 Stephenson T. *Br J Clin Pharmacol* 2005; **59**(6): 670-673
11 de Zwartt LL, Haenen HE, Versantvoort CH et al. *Regul Toxicol Pharmacol* 2004; **39**(3): 282-309
12 Pineiro-Carrero VM, Pineiro EO. *Pediatrics* 2004; **113**(4): 1097-1106
13 Mills S, Bone K. *Principles and Practice of Phytotherapy: Modern Herbal Medicine.* Churchill Livingstone, Edinburgh, 2000, p.123.
14 Fanaro S, Chierici R, Guerrini P, Vigi V. *Acta Paediatr* 2003; **441**(92): 48-55
15 Brook I, Barrett CT, Brinkman CR et al. *Pediatrics* 1979; **63**(3): 451-455
16 Orrhage K, Nord CE. *Acta Paediatr* 1999; **88**(430): 47-57
17 Benedetti MS, Whormsley R, Baltes EL. *Expert Opin Metab Toxicol* 2005; **1**(3): 447-471
18 Tortora CJ, Funke BR, Case CL. *Microbiology: An Introduction* 7th Ed. Benjamin Cummings, USA, pp. 407-410.
19 Bone K. *A Clinical Guide to Blending Liquid Herbs.* . Churchill Livingstone, Edinburgh, 2003.
20 Weinsier RL, Schutz Y, Bracco D. *Am J Clin Nutr* 1992; **55**(4): 790-794
21 Hsu A, Heshka S, Janumala I et al. *Am J Clin Nutr* 2003; **77**(6): 1506-1511
22 Oesterheld JR. *J Child Adolescent Psychopharmacol* 1998; **8**(3): 161-174
23 Hakkola J, Tanaka E, Pelkonen O. *Pharmacol Toxicol* 1998; **82**(5): 209-217
24 Kearns GL. *Curr Opinion Ped* 1995; **7**(2): 220-223
25 Industry News. *Zeitschrift fur Phytotherapie* 1997; **18**: 296
26 Verbal Communication. Dr R Lehmann, General Manager Research & Development, MediHerb, 2007.
27 Costello I, Wong ICK, Nunn AJ. *Child:Care Health Development* 2004; **30**(6): 647-665
28 Hampson SE, Skinner TC, Hart J et al. *Health Technol Assess* 2001; **5**(10): 1-79
29 Nunn T, Williams J. *Br J Clin Pharmacol* 2005; **59**(6): 674-676
30 Gutmanis J. *Kahuna La'au Lapa'au-The Practice of Hawaiian Herbal Medicine.* Island Heritage, Aiea, Hawaii, 1995.
31 Ilett KF, Kristensen JH. *Expert Opin Drug Saf* 2005; **4**(4): 745-768
32 Clewell RA, Gearhart JM. *Environ Health Pers* 2002; **110**(6): A333-A337
33 Spigset O, Hagg S. *CNS Drugs* 1998; **9**(2): 111-134
34 Zhu W, Wang XM, Zhang L et al. *Am J Chin Med* 2005; **33**(6): 839-850
35 Zhu W, Zhang L, Wang XM et al. *Zhongguo Zhong Yao Za Zhi* 2005; **30**(18): 1458-1461
36 Faber P, Strenge-Hesse A. *Pharmacology* 1988; **36**(1): 212-220
37 Wichtl M. *Herbal Drugs and Phytopharmaceuticals.* Medpharm, Stuttgart, 2004.
38 Mills S, Bone K. *The Essential Guide to Herbal Safety.* Churchill Livingstone, Edinburgh, 2005.
39 Weiss RF, Fintelmann V. *Herbal Medicine* 2nd Ed. Thieme, Stuttgart, 2000.
40 Schilcher H. *Phytotherapy in Paediatrics.* Medpharm, Stuttgart, 1997.
41 Ellingwood F, Lloyd JU. *American Materia Medica, Therapeutics and Pharmacognosy.* 11th Edn. Naturopathic Medical Series: Botanical Volume 2. First published 1898, reprinted Eclectic Medical Publications, Portland, 1983.
42 Felter HW, Lloyd JU. King's American Dispensatory. 18th Edn, 3rd revision, Volumes 1 & 2. First published 1905, reprinted Eclectic Medical Publications, Portland, 1983.
43 Winston D. *J Am Herbalists Guild* 2004: 5(1): 59-64
44 British Herbal Medicine Association. British Herbal Compendium, Volume 1. BHMA, Bournemouth, 1992.
45 British Herbal Medicine Association. British Herbal Compendium, Volume 2. BHMA, Bournemouth, 2006.
46 Pearn J. *J Paediatr Child Health* 2005; **41**(5-6): 284-290
47 Peile AR. *Body and Soul: An Aboriginal View.* Hesperian Press, Carlisle WA, 1997
48 Hrastinger A, Dietz B, Bauer R et al. *J Ped* 2005; **146**(3): 311-317
49 Lim A, Cranswick N, Skull S et al. *J Paediatr Child Health* 2005; **41**(8): 424-427
50 Ernst E. *Clin Pediatr* 2003; **42**(3): 193-196
51 Leung B. *Townsend Letter* 2007; Feb/March: 104-106
52 Farah MH, Edwards R. *Pharmacoepidemiol Drug Safety* 2000; **9**(2): 105-112
53 Ernst E. *Eur J Pediatr* 2003; **162**(2): 72-80
54 Le J, Nguyen T, Law AV et al. *Pediatrics* 2006; **118**(2): 555-562
55 Menniti-Ippolito F, Raschetti R, Da Cas R et al. *Lancet* 2000; **355**(9215): 1613-1614

CHAPTER TWO

Common Disorders of the Neonate

Introduction

AN IMPORTANT CHARACTERISTIC of the physiology of the neonate is the relative instability of the various hormonal and neurological control systems. This results from the immaturity of the various organ systems, coupled with the adjustments necessary for a new life in the outside world.[1,2] The infant's gastrointestinal system is quite immature and most digestive processes function poorly until approximately 3 months of age.[1,2] As a consequence, the most commonly encountered problem is gastro-oesophageal reflux.[3] Colic is also relatively common.

Susceptibility to infectious diseases is an important consideration in the care of the neonate. The development of the immune system begins in the embryo, continues through foetal life and is not complete until several years after birth. At birth the neonate emerges from a protective, germ-free environment and hence lacks antigenic experience.[4] However, the infant inherits a strong head start from the maternal antibodies diffusing through the placenta. Once born, the baby does not at first form significant amounts of antibodies. By the end of the first month of life gamma globulin levels can fall to less than half of those at birth, with a corresponding depletion in immunity. Despite this decrease, there is usually sufficient protective cover from the remaining antibodies against many major childhood infections.[1,2] Thereafter, the baby's immune system begins to form antibodies and the gamma globulin levels return to normal by 12 to 20 months.[1]

Cellular and innate immunity are also immature, as evidenced by the unique susceptibility of the neonate to certain viral, fungal, protozoal and bacterial infections. This immaturity is directly related to low levels and an under-functioning of the various immune cells.[5] For example, the most important immune cell directed against bacterial infection in the neonate is the neutrophil.[5] When infection and inflammation occur, circulating neutrophils accumulate and adhere to blood vessel epithelial cells at the site involved. They must deform in order to migrate into tissues.[6] In neonates neutrophils have a reduced ability to adhere to tissues and deform. Consequently fewer cells reach the site of any infection or inflammation.[5,7] Another consistent observation is a decreased chemotaxis of neutrophils: neonates have a lower ability to produce chemoattractants and their neutrophils are less responsive to these chemotactic stimuli.[5,7] For those cells that do reach the site of infection and inflammation, there are further challenges. Neonates produce fewer opsonins such as fibronectin, immunoglobulins and complement.[8] Since opsonisation renders bacteria and other cells more susceptible to phagocytosis,[1,2] neonate neutrophils have an impaired phagocytic capacity.[5,7,8] The net result is that newborns have a limited ability to protect themselves against bacterial pathogens.

The relationship between breast feeding and infant immunity is well recognised. A study from the 1930's involving more than 20,000 mothers and infants investigated the incidence of infectious disease in infants with respect to feeding mode. Infants receiving their mothers' milk were found to have a lower risk of diarrhoeal disease, respiratory infections, otitis media and other infectious diseases.[9] These findings have by and large been replicated in subsequent studies.[10,11,12] In fact, the evidence points to an overwhelming affirmation of the nutritional and immunological value of breast milk.

Nappy (Diaper) Dermatitis

Nappy dermatitis (ND) or diaper dermatitis is one of the most common skin conditions in infants. It is primarily a contact irritant dermatitis and is typically a reaction to more than one irritant.[13,14] The onset is usually between 3 weeks and 2 years of age, with the highest prevalence between 9 and 12 months.[15] Up to one third of infants may exhibit clinical symptoms of ND at any given time and the course typically waxes and wanes.[16,17]

Aetiological Factors

Friction and Wetness

Friction is the primary predisposing factor in ND, as indicated by the areas affected. Friction between the skin and the nappy leads to physical damage of the stratum corneum which is exacerbated by any wetness. This makes the skin fragile and more prone to frictional damage, creating a vicious cycle.[18]

Urine and Faeces

Prolonged exposure to urine and faeces in the nappy also contributes to the development of ND. In the presence of urine the skin becomes overly hydrated, which increases its permeability to potential irritants.[13,18] For many years it was thought that ammonia resulting from bacterial action on urine was the primary irritant. However, it is now clear that this is not the case. Recent research indicates that urine pH is the most important factor. Alkaline urine is not directly harmful to the skin, its interaction with faecal matter is the problem. Ureases produced by faecal bacteria interact with urine and increase the pH. This rise in pH increases the activities of faecal proteases and lipases, which then act as the major skin irritants.[13,18] Such research provides a rational explanation for the observation that infants fed pasteurised cows milk formula appear to be more prone to ND than breast-fed infants: it has been observed that the faeces of the former group are more heavily colonised by urease-producing bacteria.[19]

Secondary Infection

Evidence suggests that microbes such as *Candida albicans* do not play a direct role in the development of ND. However, the reduction in the protective function of the dermal barrier by the factors discussed above makes the skin more prone to secondary infection by yeast or bacteria.[13,18]

Exacerbating Factors

Antibiotic use for respiratory tract infections has been shown to increase the incidence of ND. This appears to correlate with a significantly increased presence of *Candida albicans* in the rectum and skin of these infants.[18]

Poor skin care and infrequent nappy changes will lower an infant's resistance to irritant dermatitis. The excessive use of liquid soaps and talcum powder are common problems in inappropriate skin care.[18]

Diarrhoea and the subsequent production of looser faeces will expose the skin to greater amounts of residual digestive enzymes such as proteases and lipases.[18]

Several nutrient deficiencies have also been associated with intractable ND such as zinc and biotin.[18]

Treatment Strategy

The primary strategy in the treatment of ND is to minimise the exposure of the skin to urine, faeces, moisture and friction. Therefore the frequency of nappy changes is an important consideration. Ideally the nappy should be changed as soon as possible after soiling. The baby should be bathed at least once a day and preferably twice a day while the rash remains. A thorough history of the child's cleansing routines should be obtained and any cleaning products screened for potential irritants. The child's diet may also be a contributing factor, with pasteurised milk and dairy products being known exacerbating factors.[18,19]

The practice of applying barrier creams in the nappy area following cleansing has been well established for many years. This is an opportunity to include herbal treatments. The objective should be to provide vulnerary and (if necessary) antimicrobial activities, as well as protection from wetting and friction.[14]

In this regard Calendula is probably superior to chamomile for the topical treatment of ND,[20] since it has demonstrated positive effects for the treatment of irritant and radiation-induced dermatitis.[21,22] However, a postmarketing surveillance study has found some value from combining both Calendula and chamomile extracts for ND. Eighty-two infants aged between 3 days and 48 months with uncomplicated ND were randomly assigned to receive either a zinc oxide cream or a cream consisting of zinc oxide and extracts of Calendula and chamomile. Efficacy, safety and satisfaction were judged by the parents throughout the treatment and by paediatricians at the end of the 7-day treatment period. The efficacy rating for both creams was found to be satisfactory, with no statistical difference between the groups. However, 78% of paediatricians responded that they would prescribe the Calendula/chamomile cream again.[23] Perhaps the results might have been more dramatic if the quality of the herbs had been optimised.

A high quality Calendula cream can be readily prepared by blending a low alcohol 1:2 extract of Calendula at a concentration of 5 to 10% into a suitable cream base. Chamomile 1:2 can be added at the same concentration. If *Candida albicans* is present, then tea tree (*Melaleuca alternifolia*) essential oil (TTO) at a concentration of no more than 2% can be included. The preparation can be applied after bathing and nappy changes. Several *in vitro* studies support the use of TTO preparations for superficial *C. albicans* skin infections.[24,25] TTO has also demonstrated efficacy for fluconazole-refractory oropharyngeal candidiasis in AIDS patients and in canine pruritic dermatitis.[26,27]

It should be noted that the topical use of TTO in children has come under the spotlight in recent times. A case report proposed a possible link between the topical application of products containing lavender and tea tree oil and prepubertal gynaecomastia.[28] The report described three boys aged 4, 10 and 7 who presented with gynaecomastia, but were otherwise in good health with normal serum concentrations of endogenous steroids. Investigation of the possible common factors between the boys revealed that the 4-year-old had been using a healing balm containing lavender oil, the 10-year-old a hair gel and a shampoo containing both lavender and tea tree oils and the 7-year-old a lavender-scented soap and skin lotion. A series of *in vitro* studies on human breast cancer cells exposed to lavender and tea tree oils found that both oils stimulated oestrogen-related genes and downregulated androgen-related genes. The conclusion was that both oils were oestrogenic and therefore the likely cause of the gynaecomastia. The boys were advised to stop using the essential oil products and the gynaecomastia resolved after several months. However, cause and effect was not adequately demonstrated (especially for TTO) and further studies are needed. In the meantime it would be prudent to advise only short-term use of both oils in infants.

In cases where the infant suffers from oral *Candida albicans*, an appropriate dose of propolis tincture (see Chapter 1) diluted with a little pure water can be applied to the oral cavity. Propolis at low concentrations has demonstrated antifungal activity against a range of superficial mycoses including *C. albicans*.[29] Furthermore, clinical work found a 5% propolis solution demonstrated efficacy in chronic vaginitis. The researchers concluded that propolis is a viable alternative treatment for chronic vaginal infection.[30] If the clinician has concerns about bee-related allergy or the ethanol content of propolis tinctures, extracts of Calendula and thyme can be combined and used in the same way.[31] Clinical experience of the authors has also shown that the hydrosol of tea tree is an effective oral application. Here the oral cavity is simply irrigated with the undiluted hydrosol. The hydrosol is also useful as a wash for the nappy area.

Treatment for Uncomplicated ND

Calendula	1:2	2.5 mL	25% alcohol
Natural cream base		50 g	

Blend ingredients to an even consistency. The cream is applied 3 times a day following nappy/diaper changes.

Case History

The mother of a 3-week-old male infant requested an alternative treatment for ND. The mother was using disposable nappies and changing them frequently. The infant's nappy area was inflamed and obviously irritated. The following cream was prepared:

Calendula	1:2	2.5 mL	25% alcohol
Essential oil of Lavender		2 drops	
Natural cream base		50 g	

The cream had an almost instantaneous effect, with a marked reduction in inflammation and irritation within the first day of treatment. At the time of writing the mother continues to use the cream at every nappy change as a barrier cream. This procedure has held the ND at bay. (This is my grandson, Jack. RS)

Infantile Seborrhoeic Dermatitis

Commonly known as cradle cap, infantile seborrhoeic dermatitis (ISD) usually presents as thick, greasy scales on the vertex of the scalp.[32] The condition is relatively common in early childhood. According to one Australian study involving 1,116 participants, ISD was present in 10% of boys and 9.5% of girls. The highest incidence occurred in the first 3 months of life and had decreased substantially by 12 months of age.[33]

Although several different pathogenic mechanisms have been proposed, the condition has been inadequately described. Organisms of the *Malassezia* genus or the yeast *Pityrosporum ovale* are associated with adult seborrhoeic dermatitis, however it is less clear whether this is the case for ISD.[34] An altered fatty acid metabolism with a transient impairment of the enzyme delta-6-desaturase might be a possible cause.[35] Similar to atopic dermatitis, this theory involves a proposed deficiency in the production of the metabolites of linoleic acid, in particular gamma linolenic acid (GLA). Supporting evidence for this hypothesis comes from the results of a clinical study involving 48 infants suffering severe cradle cap. It was found that the topical application of borage oil 5 mL BD, containing 25% GLA, resulted in a significant improvement after only 2 weeks. Improvement was observed not just in the areas where the borage oil was directly applied, but also in other areas.[35] Another hypothesis suggests that an over-production of a lipid-rich sebum contributes to the scaly buildup and possibly creates an ideal environment for the proliferation of the implicated micro-organisms.[33,34]

Treatment Strategy

A folk medicine treatment for cradle cap is the application of olive oil. As olive oil does not contain GLA, it probably works via other means to that described above. Olive oil application can be unpopular with mothers as it leaves the wraps and bedclothes stained with oil. An effective alternative strategy is the addition of high GLA oils such as borage oil, evening primrose oil or blackcurrant seed oil to a suitable cream base. One or two capsules are pierced with a sterile tool and blended with 50g of cream and applied 3 times per day. The clinical experience of the authors has demonstrated that a good quality natural cream base on its own is also an effective application. *Viola tricolour* (heartsease) has been traditionally used as a topical application to reduce pruritis in ISD.[36] A cream containing an extract of *V. tricolour* at approximately 5% concentration with 1 to 2 evening primrose oil capsules blended into 50g of cream base addresses both the presumed GLA deficiency and the irritation. Antipruritic alternatives to heartsease would include licorice extract, chickweed or chamomile.

Treatment for ISD

Evening primrose oil	1 or 2 capsules
Natural cream base	50 g
Licorice extract high in glycyrrhizin (optional)	1 mL of 1:1

Pierce the capsules with a sterile instrument and blend evenly with a suitable cream base. Apply to affected areas 3 times a day.

Infantile Colic

The most commonly accepted definition of infantile colic (IC) is the Wessel criteria which uses the "rule of three": crying for more than three hours per day, for more than three days per week, for more than three weeks. This definition should be applied to an infant who is well fed and otherwise healthy.[37] A systematic review of community-based studies on the incidence of IC found rates of between 5 and 25%, depending on the definition of colic and the study design.[38] Infantile colic typically begins at 2 weeks and usually resolves by 4 months of age. Crying appears to be concentrated in the late afternoon and evening, occurs in prolonged bouts and is unpredictable and spontaneous. The child cannot be soothed, even by feeding.[37]

Aetiology

IC is a poorly understood multifactorial disorder where gastrointestinal, psychosocial and neurodevelopmental issues have been proposed as causative factors.

Gastrointestinal involvement is clearly implicated in IC. The physical reactions of the infant, such as the leg position and facial grimacing certainly convey an impression that the pain is emanating from the abdominal area.[37] However, various medical writers appear to downplay the significance of gastrointestinal disturbances in IC. They cite as evidence a dated radiographic imaging study which demonstrated that infants experiencing colic have a normal gastric outline with no signs of spasm.[37,39,40] In contrast, herbal spasmolytics have been shown to be effective in several clinical studies (see below).

The association between food allergy and IC is a controversial one. There is little doubt that commercial pasteurised and homogenised cows milk and cows milk formulas can be problematic for many infants.[41,42] It appears that these products can induce intestinal hyperperistalsis by increasing several gut hormones, including s-motilin.[43] Furthermore, a sensitisation to pasteurised cows milk protein appears to be a factor in up to a third of infants with colic.[44] Maternal consumption of commercial pasteurised and homogenised cows milk is strongly associated with IC for breastfed infants.[44,45] What is lacking from this debate is an investigation of the benefit of raw milk from grass-fed cows farmed under organic conditions and milked in accordance with strict hygienic procedures. The clinical experience of one author (RS) has repeatedly demonstrated that problems are often resolved (with the aid of a little herbal medicine of course) when organic, hygienic, raw cows milk is consumed. For those readers who wish to explore this important issue, it has been reviewed elsewhere.[46] Other components of the maternal diet such as cruciferous vegetables, onions and chocolate are also associated with colic in exclusively breastfed infants.[47] Another food often given to infants is fruit juice. It has been suggested that IC is associated with sugar malabsorption from juices containing sorbitol and with a high fructose to glucose ratio, such as apple juice.[48]

The emotional state of the mother during pregnancy can influence the risk of colic. Studies have demonstrated that general psychosocial distress and trait anxiety during pregnancy are associated with IC.[49,50,51,52]

Another popular theory is the neurodevelopmental perspective. Colicky infants cry for longer periods of time and are more difficult to soothe once crying has begun. This, coupled with the fact that most infants outgrow colic, has lead to a conclusion these infants do not as yet have the capacity to regulate crying once it has begun. It is proposed that this pattern is due to the immaturity of the nervous system and is best viewed as a manifestation of normal emotional development.[53]

The Herbal Evidence

A time-honoured folk remedy for the treatment of colic is gripe water. Its use still appears to be common, at least in Sheffield UK, according to a survey of 200 Sheffield mothers. The survey found that 64% of mothers gave gripe water to their babies during the first month of life.[54] The original formula developed in 1851 contained alcohol, dill seed oil, water and bicarbonate and has spawned many imitations.[55]

The clinical investigation of herbal formulations for colic began in the early 1990s when a placebo-controlled study on 68 colicky infants was published. The blend evaluated was a proprietary herbal tea consisting of chamomile, vervain, licorice, fennel and lemon balm with natural flavours and glucose. After 7 days, improvements in colic scores were significantly higher for the herbal group than for the placebo group (1.7 ± 0.3 vs 0.7 ± 0.5), demonstrating the efficacy of the colic treatment over placebo.[56] There were several limitations to this study, including the short duration, subjective measurement of colic symptoms by parents and the comparatively large doses of liquid ingested (mean value 32 mL/kg/day). In terms of the administered herbal dose, it must be reiterated that this was a herbal tea and therefore a dilute preparation compared to tinctures or fluid extracts.

Research on this topic remained quiet until 2003, when results of a randomised, placebo-controlled study of the efficacy of emulsified fennel seed oil in 125 colicky infants were released. Using the Wessel criteria for evaluation, the research demonstrated that colic was eliminated in 65% of the infants in the active group and in only 23.7% of the control group (p < 0.01).[57] Then in 2005 a double blind, placebo-controlled trial of standardised extracts of chamomile, fennel and lemon balm in colicky infants was published. Diagnosis of the 88 infants was again by the Wessel criteria, with the daily crying times recorded by the parents over one week. Responders were defined as those infants for whom the crying time was reduced by 50% compared to the pretrial observation period. A reduction was observed for 85.4% of infants in the active group compared to 48.9% for placebo.[58]

Hence three clinical evaluations of herbal treatments with gut spasmolytic activity as a common theme have demonstrated significant efficacy. These studies also indirectly support the revered status of gripe water in folk medicine, since dill is a well-known herbal spasmolytic, with similar properties in this regard to the fennel used in the trials.

Treatment Strategy

The treatment strategy for IC is based around gentle nervines and spasmolytics. The following herbal formulation can be recommended:

Chamomile	1:2	20 mL
Fennel	1:2	20 mL
Lemon balm	1:2	20 mL
	Total	60 mL

Calculate the dose according to the guidelines for infants in Chapter 1 (using 5 mL as the adult dose) and administer this three times a day in water or juice. If necessary, also follow the Chapter 1 recommendations to increase compliance.

Case History

A mother presented with a 2-month-old female infant with a 5-week history of colic. The colicky episodes mostly occurred during the early evening, but occasionally at other times, and the infant could not be comforted. The infant was breast-fed and the maternal diet did not contain any of the known problematic foods. However this was the mother's first child and she reported a high level of stress and fatigue, but had sufficient milk.

The child was prescribed the following formulation:

Chamomile	1:2	25 mL
Fennel	1:2	25 mL
	Total	50 mL

Dose: 8 drops blended into 10 mL of breast milk and administered with a syringe three times a day.

The mother was prescribed the following:

Withania	1:2	100 mL

Dose: 2.5 mL with water three times a day

At follow-up 2 weeks later, the mother reported less fatigue and stress and the colicky episodes had reduced significantly. A further 2 weeks of treatment resulted in a resolution of the infant's colicky symptoms. The mother continued taking the Withania.

Gastro-oesophageal Reflux

Gastro-oesophageal reflux (GOR) is a physiological phenomenon occurring occasionally in all humans, especially during the postprandial period.[59] A cross-sectional survey of the Chicago area found that regurgitation occurs daily in almost 70% of 4-month-old infants and that approximately 25% of their parents consider regurgitation as a problem.[60] Emesis and regurgitation are the most common symptoms of gastro-oesophageal reflux disease in an infant. However, they can also be manifestations of several other disorders such as enteric infections, metabolic disorders and especially food allergies.[59] There appears to be no difference in the frequency of uncomplicated reflux between exclusively breastfed and formula-fed infants.[61] The high frequency of regurgitation in infants is associated with a transient immaturity of the digestive process, especially involving the oesophagus and stomach. Features of this immature system include a short abdominal oesophagus, an increased number of non-propagational oesophageal contractions and an increased number of transient lower oesophageal sphincter relaxations associated with delayed gastric emptying.[62]

Treatment Strategy

Antacids are often used as a conventional treatment for GOR.[62] A similar approach can be used in herbal therapeutics, albeit with much gentler agents. Clinical observation by the authors has demonstrated the effectiveness of meadowsweet 1:2 prescribed at an appropriate dose after feeding and diluted with breast milk or formula. The spasmolytic and carminative herbs recommended for the treatment of IC are best avoided in uncomplicated regurgitation, as many contain essential oils known to relax sphincters.[63] One exception is chamomile, which can be tried as an alternative to the meadowsweet. Mucilage in the form of slippery elm tea is a useful adjunct to the extracts. It can be used undiluted in 5 mL doses after feeding. Both meadowsweet and slippery elm will help to calm the excessive activity of the stomach and aid in synchronising its activity with the oesophageal sphincter.

Treatment for GOR

Meadowsweet   1:2

Calculate dose according to the guidelines for infants in Chapter 1, based on an adult dose of 2 mL. To be taken with water or juice.

Slippery elm tea, 5 mL to be taken with the meadowsweet three times a day after feeds.

Alternatively Gastric Mucosal Support tablets (see Appendix 1), or similar formulations, would be safe to use. About 1/4 to 1/8 of a tablet can be finely crushed and mixed well with the slippery elm tea or breast milk and given after feeds.

Diarrhoea

There are numerous factors that can cause diarrhoea in infants, including teething, antibiotic use, food allergy and infection.[31,64,65] As diarrhoea and the associated fluid loss is a potentially serious condition, an accurate diagnosis is essential. A 2-year prospective study of diarrhoeal illness in children from 0 to 36 months of age found that there were 465 sporadic cases and 170 outbreak-associated cases. Of these events, only 20% were associated with enteric pathogens.[66] In both developing and developed nations the major cause of acute diarrhoea is rotavirus.[67,68,69] However there are several other enteric viruses that can affect infants in the first year of life. These include the Norwalk virus and other human caliciviruses, astroviruses and enteric adenoviruses.[67,68,69] Enteric bacterial pathogens are also important causes of diarrhoeal disease, particularly in developing nations. The range of bacteria implicated include *Campylobacter jejuni*, *Salmonella spp.*, *Shigella spp.*, *Escherichia coli*, *Yersinia enterocolitica*, *Clostridium difficile*, *Vibrio cholerae*, *Aeromonas hydrophilia* and *Plesiomonas shigelloides*.[67,68,69] Parasitic infection can also cause diarrhoea and the two most common causes are *Giardia lamblia* and *Cryptosporidium parvum*.[69]

A Review of the Evidence

Many years ago Dr Christopher recommended the use of a tea prepared from tormentil root (*Potentilla tormentilla*) in the treatment of diarrhoea.[70] Interestingly, this approach was recently evaluated in 40 children with ages ranging from 3 months to 7 years suffering from rotavirus diarrhoea. The results of this randomised, double blind, placebo-controlled trial indicated that tormentil root extract significantly reduced the duration of rotavirus diarrhoea and the requirement for rehydration solutions, compared to placebo. The dose used was 3 drops three times daily of a 1:10 tincture (40% ethanol) for every year of the child's age.[71] Tormentil root is rich in tannins and one of the most notable effects of tannins in the gut is their dramatic effect on diarrhoea.[63] Tannins exert an astringent effect to check hypersecretion and also inhibit the viability of the infectious organism.[63] Given that tormentil extracts can be difficult to purchase outside Europe, a more than adequate tannin-containing antidiarrhoeal substitute is cranesbill root. Cat's claw, green tea and hawthorn are also good sources of gentle tannins, as is meadowsweet. Cat's claw will also provide immune support.

Further evidence on the value of tannins was provided by a recent *in vivo* and *in vitro* study using either green or black tea extracts on *Escherichia coli*-induced intestinal fluid loss. Both extracts produced a significant inhibition of disturbances in fluid and electrolyte balance brought about by *E. coli*.[72]

The alkaloid berberine is found in medicinal plants such as golden seal, barberry and Indian barberry. Berberine has been studied both for its antidiarrhoeal activity and antimicrobial activity against those organisms associated with bacterial diarrhoea, such as *Vibrio cholerae* and *E. coli*. A randomised, controlled trial of 165 patients with acute diarrhoea caused by either *V. cholerae* or *E. coli* demonstrated that berberine sulphate as a single dose (400 mg) caused a significant reduction in stool volume (compared to controls) in the *E. coli* group and a slight reduction in the cholera group. No side effects were noted, with the researchers indicating that the treatment was safe and effective for *E. coli*-associated diarrhoea.[73] *In vitro* studies demonstrate that berberine inhibits the growth of *V. cholerae* and *E. coli*. In the case of *E. coli*, berberine also inhibits the bacterial adhesion to mucosal surfaces.[63] (Note that alkaloids such as berberine are not compatible with tannins. Hence tannin-containing herbs must be administered at separate times to berberine-containing herbs.)

From a traditional perspective, Wiess and Fintelmann state that bilberry fruit is the most important antidiarrhoeal herb in paediatrics.[20] There is an obvious compliance advantage in terms of taste for prescribing bilberry 1:1 at an appropriate dose for uncomplicated infantile diarrhoea (see below). Immune support with Echinacea, Andrographis or cat's claw is also indicated.

Treatment of Diarrhoea

The treatment of infantile diarrhoea involves the use of astringent, antimicrobial and immune modulating remedies. The strong taste of the remedies may lead to poor compliance, particularly if the infant is feeling nauseous. If this is the case, the suggestions in Chapter 1 on compliance issues may prove useful. Otherwise, suitably well crushed tablets, given as fractional doses according to the guidelines in Chapter 1, can be recommended.

An example liquid formulation is:

Cranesbill or Cat's claw	1:2	30 mL
Bilberry	1:1	40 mL
Echinacea root blend	1:2	30 mL
	Total	100 mL

Calculate dose according to the guidelines for infants in Chapter 1, using 5 mL as the adult dose. To be taken with water or juice. As diarrhoea is an acute condition, the dose may need to be administered 4 or 5 times a day. Berberine-containing herbs such as golden seal can be administered at separate times, but with caution in young infants.

An alternative to the above liquid formulation is Echinacea Formula tablets (acute adult dose 6 per day) and Golden Seal tablets (acute adult dose 6 per day).

Calculate the infant's tablet dose according to the formula for infants in Chapter 1. For example, if the infant is 12 months old then the daily dose of each is ½ a tablet, best administered as ¼ tablet twice a day. Begin with one ¼ tablet dose per day of each (see the note below regarding immune herbs) and if there is no adverse reaction increase to the two doses. The tablets must be well crushed and mixed with breast milk or a suitable base (not honey). See Appendix 1 for the suggested formulations for these tablets.

Immune Support for the Neonate

This important issue is discussed in Chapter 3. However, it can be noted here that most immune supporting herbs, including Echinacea, are suitable for neonates, especially during the common cold or infectious diarrhoea. The major consideration is to be cautious with the dose used, beginning at the lowest end of the dosage scale.

References

1   Guyton AC, Hall JE. *Textbook of Medical Physiology* 10th Ed. Saunders, Philadelphia 2000.
2   Porth CM. *Pathophysiology* 7th Ed. Lippincott Williams & Wilkins. Philadelphia 2005.
3   Suwandhi E, Ton MN, Scharz SM. *Pediatric Annals* 2006; **35**(4): 259-266
4   Gasparoni A, Ciardelli L, Avanzini A et al. *Biol Neonate* 2003; **84**(4): 297-303
5   McKenney WM. *Crit Care Nurse* 2001; **21**(6): 35-47
6   Tortora GJ, Grabowski SR. *Principles of Anatomy and Physiology* 10th Ed. John Wiley & Sons, New York.
7   Carr R. *Br J Haematology* 2000; **110**(1): 18-28
8   Petrova A, Mehta R. *Ind J Pediatr* 2007; **74**(2): 185-191
9   Newburg DS, Ruiz-Palacios GM, Morrow AL. *Ann Rev Nutri* 2005; **25**: 37-58
10   Barriga C, Pombero I, Duran J et al. *Rev Esp Fisiol* 1995; **51**(4): 213-218
11   Pabst HF, Spady DW, Pilarski LM et al. *Acta Paediatr* 1997; **86**(12): 1291-1297
12   Bonuch KA, Freeman K, Trombley M. *Ach Pediatr Adolesc Med* 2006; **160**(9): 953-960
13   Shin HT. *Dermatologic Ther* 2005; **18**(2): 124-135
14   Atherton DJ. *Curr Med Res Opin* 2004; **20**(5): 645-649
15   Jordan WE, Lawson KD, Berg RW et al. *Pediatr Dermatol* 1986; **3**(3): 198-207
16   Ward DB, Fleischer AB, Feldman SR et al. *Pediatr Adolesc Med* 2000; **154**(9): 943-946
17   Akin F, Spraker M, Aly R et al. *Pediatr Dermatol* 2001; **18**(4): 282-290
18   Atherton DJ. *JEADV* 2001; **15**(Suppl 1): 1-4
19   Yoshioka H, Iseki K, Fujita K. *Pediatrics* 1983; **72**(3): 317-321
20   Weiss RF, Fintelmann V. *Herbal Medicine* 2nd Ed. Thieme, Stuttgart, 2000.
21   Fuchs SM, Schliemann-Willers S, Fischer TW, Elsner P. *Skin Pharmacol Physiol* 2005; **18**(4): 195-200
22   Pommier P, Gomez F, Sunyach MP et al. *J Clin Oncol* 2004; **22**(8): 1447-1453
23   Guala A, Oberle D, Ramos M. *J Altern Complement Med* 2007; **13**(1): 16-18
24   Hammer KA, Carson CF, Riley TV. *J Antimicrob Chemother* 1998; **42**(5): 591-595
25   Banes-Marshall L, Cawley P, Phillips CA. *Br J Biomed Sci* 2001; **58**(3): 139-145.
26   Vazquez JA, Zawawi AA. *HIV Clin Trials* 2002; **3**(5): 379-385
27   Reichling J, Fitzi J, Hellman K et al. *Dtsch Tierarztl Wochenschr* 2004; **111**(10): 408-414
28   Henley DV, Lipson N, Korach KS, Bloch CA. *NEJM* 2007; **356**(5): 479-485
29   Silici S, Koc NA, Ayangil D et al. *J Pharmacol Sci* 2005; **99**(1): 33-44
30   Imhof M, Lipovac M, Kurz C et al. *Int J Gynaecol Obstet* 2005; **89**(2): 127-132
31   McIntyre A. *Herbal Treatment of Children.* Elsevier Butterworth Heinemann, Edinburgh, 2005, p. 139.
32   Schwartz RA, Janusz CA, Janninger CK. *Am Fam Phys* 2006; **74**(1): 125-130
33   Foley P, Zuo Y, Plunkett A et al. *Arch Dermatol* 2003; **139**(3): 318-322
34   Valia R. *Ind J Dermatol Venereol Leprol* 2006; **72**(4): 253-254
35   Tollesson A, Frithz A, Stenlund K. *Pediatr Dermatol* 1997; **14**(6): 423-425
36   Weiss RF, Fintelmann V. *Herbal Medicine* 2nd Ed. Thieme, Stuttgart, 2000.
37   Roberts DM, Ostapchuk M, O'Brien JG. *Am Fam Phys* 2004; **70**(4): 735-740
38   Lucassen PL, Assendelft WJ, van Eijk JT et al. *Arch Dis Child* 2001; **84**(5): 398-403
39   Harley LM. *Clin Pediatr* 1969; **8**(3): 138-141
40   Hyman PE, Milla PJ, Benninga MA et al. *Gastrointestinology* 2006; **130**(5): 1519-1526
41   Lothe L, Lindberg T. *Pediatrics* 1989; **83**(2): 262-266
42   Hill DJ, Hosking CS, Heine RG. *Ann Med* 1999; **31**(4): 272-281
43   Lothe L, Ivarsson SA, Lindberg T. *Acta Paediatr Scand* 1987; **76**(2): 316-320
44   Jakobsson I, Lindberg T. *Pediatrics* 1983; **71**(2): 268-271
45   Clyne PS, Kulczycki A. *Pediatrics* 1991; **87**(4): 439-444
46   Schmid R. *The Untold Story of Milk.* NewTrends Publishing, Washington DC 2003.
47   Lust KD, Brown JE, Thomas W. *J Am Diet Assoc* 1996; **96**(1): 46-48
48   Duro D, Rising R, Cedillo M, Lifshitz F. *Pediatrics* 2002; **109**(5): 797-805
49   Rautava P, Helenius H, Lehtonen L. *BMJ* 1993; **307**(6904): 600-604

50   Sondergaard C, Olsen J, Friis-Hasche E et al. *Acta Paediatr* 2003; **92**(7): 811-816

51   Canivet C, Ostergren PO, Jakobsson I, Hagander B. *Int J Behav Med* 2004; **11**(1): 37-47

52   Canivet CA, Ostergren PO, Rosen AS et al. *Scand J Public Health* 2005; **33**(1): 26-34

53   Barr RG. *Pediatrics* 1998; **102**(5 Suppl E): 1282-1286

54   Illingworth C, Timmins J. *Health Visit* 1990; **63**(11): 378

55   Blumenthal I. *J R Soc Med I* 2000; **93**(4): 172-174

56   Weizman Z, Alkrinawi S, Goldfarb D, Bitran C. *J Pediatr* 1993; **122**(4): 650-652

57   Alexandrovich I, Rakovitskaya O, Kolmo E, et al. *Altern Ther Health Med* 2003; **9**(4): 58-61

58   Savino F, Cresi F, Castagno E at al. *Phytother Res* 2005; **19**(4): 335-340

59   Vandenplas Y, Hegar B. *J Gastroent Hepatol* 2000; **15**(6): 593-603

60   Nelson SP, Chen EH, Syniar GM et al. *Arch Pediatr Adolesc Med* 1997; **151**(6): 569-572

61   Hill DJ, Heine RG, Cameron DJS et al. *J Pediatr* 1999; **135**(1): 118-121

62   Cezard JP. *Digestion* 2004; **69**(1): 3-8

63   Mills S, Bone K. *Principles and Practice of Phytotherapy: Modern Herbal Medicine.* Churchill Livingstone, Edinburgh, 2000, p.29.

64   Johnston BC, Supina AL, Vohra S. *CMAJ* 2006; **175**(4): 377-383

65   Kotloff KL, Losonsky GA, Morris JG et al. *Pediatrics* 1989; **84**(2): 219-225

66   Bartlett AV, Moore M, Gary GW et al. *J Pediatr* 1985; **107**(4): 495-502

67   Thapar N, Sanderson IR. *Lancet* 2004; **363**(9409): 641-653

68   Alam NH, Ashraf H. *Pediatr Drugs* 2003; **5**(3): 151-165

69   Szajewska H, Mrukowicz JZ. *Pediatr Drugs* 2005; **7**(2): 111-122

70   Christopher JR. *Childhood Diseases,* Christopher Publications, Springville, Utah, 1978

71   Subbotina MD, Timchenko VN, Vorobyov MM et al. *Pediatr Infect Dis J* 2003; **22**(8): 706-711

72   Bruins MJ, Cermak R, Kiers JL et al. *J Pediatr Gastroenterol Nutr* 2006; **43**(4): 459-469

73   Rabbani GH, Butler T, Knight J et al. *J Infect Dis* 1987; **155**(5): 979-984

CHAPTER THREE

Common Childhood Infections and Fever Management

THIS CHAPTER CONTAINS A DISCUSSION of the important role of herbs in fever management and includes a special focus on the three most common childhood infections, namely chicken pox, measles and mumps. Infections of the gastrointestinal tract are discussed in Chapters 2 and 5 and respiratory tract infections are covered in Chapter 6.

Supporting Immune Function

A persistent controversy in herbal paediatrics is the use of immune modifiers to facilitate the maturation or function of an infant's immune system. Echinacea is the herb most often used for this purpose and can be the most controversial. Compared to adults, respiratory tract infections (RTIs) in infants are significantly more common and account for considerable morbidity, doctor visits, hospital admissions and healthcare costs.[1,2,3] Although antibiotic use has decreased in recent years, it still represents the standard treatment for respiratory tract infections in children.[4,5] There are concerns expressed by both doctors and parents over antibiotic resistance and the observation that antibiotics often do not alter the course of a respiratory illness.[5,6] With these prevailing issues in mind, many parents turn to herbal medicines and in particular Echinacea because it is one of the best known herbs. For example, a recent survey of complementary and alternative medicines in paediatric patients found a high use of Echinacea products.[7]

Some of the myths surrounding the use of Echinacea will be reviewed in the appropriate chapters in this text. Despite the controversy, adverse effects are not expected for Echinacea in paediatric use, although no specific trial information is available.[8] Echinacea is most certainly safe in pregnancy, as demonstrated by a large scale prospective study of the gestational use of Echinacea during organogenesis, which found no association with an increased risk of malformation.[9] Furthermore, a systematic review that drew on this study as well as expert opinion concluded that Echinacea is non-teratogenic, but advised cautious use during breast feeding until quality human studies can fully determine its safety.[10]

The authors have been using Echinacea for over 20 years in clinical practice and have observed few adverse reaction in paediatric patients. Based on such positive clinical experience it is proposed that Echinacea is the key paediatric herb for immune support.

Fever

Fever is the most common symptom of illness in childhood.[11] Most mildly feverish RTIs in children are minor and self limiting.[12] However, fever may also herald more serious disease, such as pneumonia or meningitis.[13] In addition, there is considerable parental concern about febrile seizures,[14] so it is understandable that many parents seek medical advice at the first sign of an elevated temperature.

For the purpose of this discussion, the following temperature readings for children younger than 11 years can be taken to signify fever: rectal temperatures above 38°C (100.4°F); oral temperatures above 37.5°C (99.5°F); axillary temperatures above 37°C (98.6°F) and tympanic temperatures above 37.9°C (100.2°F).[15] For children aged 11 years or older a temperature above 37.6°C (99.7°F) indicates fever.

Fever is an adaptive immune response to a pyrogenic stimulus, such as tissue trauma or infectious organisms.[16] The body produces a wide range of pyrogenic cytokines in response to infection, such as interleukins (IL-1, IL-6), interferon and tumour necrosis factor alpha (TNFα). The circumventricular organ system (CVOS) is neuronal tissue lying outside the blood-brain barrier that plays a key role in initiating increased synthesis of prostaglandins. When pyrogenic cytokines are detected by the CVOS, prostaglandin synthesis (especially cyclo-oxygenase-dependent prostaglandin E_2) is induced, activating the febrile response. Once the appropriate signal is received by the hypothalamus, it behaves in a similar manner to a thermostat and the temperature set point is elevated. As a consequence, autonomic, endocrine and behavioural processes are activated. For example, elevating the set point activates neurons in the vasomotor centre of the brain to initiate vasoconstriction which results in blood shifting from the periphery to the central compartment. Shivering increases heat production via muscular activity. The accompanying feeling of malaise reduces general activity and the reduction in sweating, together with seeking warmth, further contribute to heat production and conservation. Eventually the blood contacting the hypothalamus meets the new set point. The temperature remains raised until the hypothalamic set-point is reset downwards as a consequence of a reduction in pyrogen presence and/or antipyretic therapy, with subsequent associated heat loss.[16,17]

From an evolutionary perspective, the febrile response is a recently-evolved process preceded by what is termed the heat shock response. This heat shock response is an ancient and highly-conserved process essential for surviving environmental stresses, including extremes in temperature.[18] Heat stress, such as a high fever, has the ability to denature proteins vital for the maintenance of homeostasis. As a consequence specialised stress proteins are needed to ensure both the intracellular conservation and maintenance of protein homeostasis.[19] These stress proteins, also termed heat shock proteins (Hsp), are induced by fever. They augment the febrile response within the human febrile temperature range (38-41°C, 100.4-105.8°F).[18] In this manner fever, by inducing Hsp expression in host cells, increases their resistance to the chemical stresses generated in an infected environment.[20] Evidence is beginning to suggest that infected cells can release Hsp into the extracellular environment. Once there, they perform important immunoregulatory activities. This is thought to have two components: firstly the stimulation of an innate immune response (by an interaction with antigen-presenting cells) that results in the maturation of dendritic cells and secondly the chaperoning of antigens for cross-presentation on dendritic cell Major Histocompatibility Class I molecules, thereby inducing an adaptive T lymphocyte response.[18,21]

Is Fever Beneficial?

The life-threatening nature of a high fever is universally appreciated. However, it is not yet clear whether febrile elevations in body temperature per se can be lethal. It is known that the pathological events accompanying a high fever can precipitate a medical emergency and perhaps death.[22] This important distinction has long been recognised by natural therapists: fever is not the disorder, it is rather an adaptive response. As such, and where possible, it is something to be supported and not unduly suppressed.[23] This view has recently gained some support from the conventional medical community.

Substantial evidence has emerged supporting the hypothesis that a physiological antipyretic system exists, that employs both neuronal and humoral pathways.[22,24] It has long been recognised that fever seems to have an empirical upper limit, rarely exceeding 41°C (105.8°F). It has now been determined that endogenous antipyretic agents such as arginine vasopressin are secreted by thermoregulatory neurons in the preoptic region and anterior pituitary that attenuate fever and control the upper temperature limit.[22,24,25] The effect that conventional antipyretic therapy has on this endogenous antipyretic system is yet to be understood.

Perhaps more significantly in support of the concept of regulating fever, evidence exists that antipyretic therapies such as paracetamol (acetaminophen) are associated with post-infective complications.[26]

The Herbal Approach to Fever

Traditional herbalists used a strategy in managing fever that was directed at manipulating the skin. The skin can be an efficient regulator of core temperature, acting in effect like a radiator. This is due to the large and diffuse venous plexus that exists just below the skin surface.[27] Enormous amounts of heat can be transferred from the body core via the blood to the skin to effect radiant heat loss. Similarly, heat can be conserved by decreasing blood flow to the skin. Both processes are controlled by the autonomic nervous system.[17,27]

The traditional basis for manipulating the skin during the treatment of infection and fever management was inspired by Native American healing practices and promoted by Samuel Thomson.[23] An elegant description of Thomsonian philosophy has been provided by Wood.[28] Thomson drew a metaphorical picture of the body in health and disease. He likened it to a fountain, with the stomach at the centre, nourished by an inner fire that radiated to the periphery. Thus heat, life and nourishment depended on a radiant energy from the core to the periphery, with disease being interpreted as a disturbance to this natural flow.[28] As the blood is intimately involved with the radiant energy flow, great emphasis was placed on equalising the circulation when signs of disharmony appeared on the skin, such as excessive heat or cold. Thomson made use of the steaming practices of the Native Americans in an effort to open up the periphery, thus unblocking the channels to re-establish the fountain.[23] Herbal medicines with diaphoretic activity were most often prescribed in this context to further assist in opening the periphery to both blood and perspiration. In cases where it was perceived that the core temperature was inadequate to support a therapeutic fever, or the inner fire was lacking, heating remedies were also used. A strategy that usually preceded all these measures was the use of emetics in order to clear encumbrances on the digestive system.

In a more conservative modern world, the traditional sequence of emetics, steaming, diaphoretics and heating digestive/metabolic stimulants for treating acute infection needs to be radically modified. The emetic and steaming practices have all but disappeared. As a compensatory measure, modern phytotherapy is now more likely to employ diaphoretics in combination with diffusive stimulants and antimicrobial and immune-enhancing remedies. In many respects this represents an advance in practice, but it might have a greater impact on fighting infection were it to be combined with aspects of the traditional measures described by Thomson.

Practical Fever Management

The initial chill phase of a fever is characterised by a shutting down of the circulation to the surface, which produces shivering. It indicates that the core temperature is rising. This is an uncomfortable phase that ideally passes into a more comfortable stage as the core body temperature reaches the target set by the hypothalamus. Acceptable temperatures at this stage are between 37.8-38.9°C (100.0-102.0°F). At this temperature range, phagocytic activity increases and exogenous pyrogen production reduces. As a result, the upward stimulus on the hypothalamus set-point is reduced and it then begins to fall. The periphery starts to open up and the sweat glands begin operating. The patient feels hot, indicating the temperature is on the way down. The fever is said to have broken and recovery can commence.[23]

The clinician needs to be alert for these signs as they provide important pointers. For example, if the patient has a temperature of 40°C (104°F), its significance depends on whether the patient feels hot or cold. If the patient feels hot, the temperature is probably falling. However if the symptoms (or signs) indicate cold, the temperature is still rising and needs to be steadied. This can be achieved with tepid bathing and peripheral vasodilators/diaphoretics such as YEP (yarrow, elder flower and peppermint) tea or lime flowers. For a stronger reduction in temperature, the cooling bitters are additionally indicated, such as dandelion root, gentian or the stronger wormwood.[23]

Raising a Fever

If it is apparent that a therapeutic fever is not occurring and there is no serious underlying infection or pathology, it may be necessary to use warming remedies to support a febrile response. This is a useful strategy where low-grade chronic infections need some assistance to resolve. In the case of persistent catarrh, it is often advantageous to induce a therapeutic fever. The agents that can help to achieve this include diaphoretics together with warming remedies such as cinnamon, Angelica and the stronger ginger, garlic and cayenne.[23]

General Approach to Treating and Preventing Infections

By now, the themes involved in the herbal treatment of infection should be becoming apparent. It is now worthwhile to define the considerations for the herbal management of infections. These are as follows:

- Fundamentally, immune-enhancing herbs are the most important part of treating any infection, acute or chronic. The important herbs here are Echinacea, Andrographis and Astragalus. Astragalus should not be used during an acute infection

- As already noted diaphoretic herbs will help to focus the immune system during acute infections and ginger and other warming herbs can help their activity. Ginger is especially preferred as it is described as a diffusive stimulant, and the skin is a diffuse organ

- If the infection is located in a particular organ herbs to support that organ or its defensive functions are indicated: milk thistle (St Mary's thistle) for liver infections and expectorants for lung infections are two examples. It is not necessary to give diuretic herbs for urinary tract infections. Copious fluid intake will achieve the same result of flushing the bladder

- If the infection is located in a particular organ accessible to herbs and is bacterial, fungal or protozoal, those herbs which act against these microbes in these organs can be used. Note that the activity of antiseptic herbs will generally be mild, except on the skin and in the gut. Examples include buchu for urinary tract infections, golden seal for gastrointestinal infections and topical tea tree oil for skin infections

- If the infection is viral, systemic antiviral herbs can be prescribed. These include St John's wort (enveloped viruses only) and Thuja for the wart virus. Lemon balm and licorice have topical antiviral activity

Possibly the best herb for preventing an infection is Echinacea, but it must be the roots of *Echinacea angustifolia* and/or *Echinacea purpurea*. The idea that Echinacea can only be taken short-term is a myth which has no basis in fact. There is no evidence that Echinacea "wears out" the immune response when it is taken for long periods. In fact, it is probably the case that Echinacea works best as a preventative. The adult preventative dose is 5 mL per day of an Echinacea root combination or its equivalent in tablet form. This should be adjusted for children as outlined in Chapter 1. Ideally, this dose should be increased temporarily to 3 to 4 times in a day to ward off an infection. If the infection does take hold the Echinacea can be maintained at this higher level to shorten the duration of the infection and/or alternative immune herbs such as Andrographis can be introduced. If the infection is successfully prevented, the dose can be returned to the preventative dose. Patients are often amazed when they experience the ability of Echinacea to prevent infections. This herb, used properly, is a wonderful "practice builder".

Varicella (Chicken Pox)

Chicken pox is a common communicable disease of childhood caused by the varicella-zoster virus.[16,29,30] Varicella is highly infectious. After the primary infection the virus persists in the sensory nerve ganglia of the dorsal root and establishes a latent infection. The virus can reactivate years or decades later and spread unilaterally along a dermatome to cause herpes zoster (shingles), a painful localised vesicular rash.[30] The epidemiology of varicella differs between temperate and tropical climates. In most temperate climates more than 90% of people are infected before adolescence, whereas in tropical climates the disease is typically acquired later in life, with adults being more susceptible than children.[30] Varicella infection in temperate regions mostly affects children aged 1 to 9 years, although with the increased use of child care facilities, a shift to younger ages (≤ 5 years) has been observed.[31] However, there appears to be a reduced susceptibility in children with more siblings.[30]

Clinical Features

Chicken pox begins with a fever that is usually low grade and lasts for 2 to 3 days. Concurrent with the fever is the appearance of a self-limiting, pruritic, vesicular skin rash that can also affect mucosal sites. The rash begins as macules and progresses rapidly (24 to 48 hours) through papular and vesicular stages before beginning to crust. The vesicles appear in crops, so that on any part of the body the rash can be in different stages of development. Apart from fever, varicella commonly causes headache, malaise and loss of appetite. Bacteria or viruses can complicate varicella. Most commonly encountered are secondary bacterial infections caused by group A β-haemolytic streptococci or *Staphylococcus aureus*. An invasive infection can be life threatening. Central nervous system complications range from a benign cerebellar ataxia to the more serious meningoencephalitis, meningitis and vasculitis.[27,29,30]

Treatment Strategy

In almost all cases, varicella is a self-limiting disease[30] and treatments such as diaphoretic remedies, lotions for the pruritis and rehydration are all that is necessary. More comprehensive protocols would also include antimicrobial and immune-enhancing remedies.

Example Diaphoretic Formulations

There are several diaphoretic formulations worthy of mention. Weiss and Fintelmann advise that a diaphoretic tea prepared from meadowsweet 10 parts, lime flowers 70 parts, peppermint 15 parts and bitter orange peel 5 parts can be consumed hot and in large quantities.[32] For the sake of convenience, fluid extracts can be substituted, with the bitter orange peel replaced by chen pi. This mixture can be administered diluted with hot water and taken at the appropriate dosage. Lime flowers are particularly diaphoretic and due to the spasmolytic and mild sedative activities[33] will aid in reducing irritability.

Another time-honoured formulation is YEP, which in liquid form is as follows:

Yarrow	1:2	40 mL
Elder flowers	1:2	40 mL
Peppermint	1:2	20 mL
	Total	100 mL

Dose: Calculate the standard dose according to the most appropriate guideline in Chapter 1, using the adult dose of 5 mL. The dose is diluted with approximately 25 to 50 mL of warm to hot water and sipped by the child. Up to 5 doses can be taken in one day, while fever is present.

Yarrow, elder flowers and peppermint are traditional diaphoretics.[33] A dried herb infusion of the same herbs can also be used and both dosage forms are unlikely to pose compliance problems due to their relatively pleasant taste.

Topical Treatment for Rashes

Combine the following:

Licorice (high in glycyrrhizin)	1:1	2 mL
Rhubarb root or Cat's claw	1:2	2 mL
Echinacea angustifolia	1:2	2 mL
Natural cream base		50 g

Distilled water can be added to produce the consistency of a lotion. Apply to the rash twice a day.

The rationale for this formulation is as follows: glycyrrhizin, found in licorice root has been shown to be particularly active *in vitro* against several viruses, including the varicella-zoster virus.[23] Clinical experience also supports the use of licorice as a topical anti-inflammatory for pruritic skin conditions. Chickweed succus is traditionally used as a topical agent for pruritic skin conditions[34] and can be substituted for the licorice. Anthraquinones derived from *Rheum officinale* (rhubarb root) have displayed direct virucidal activity against a range of enveloped viruses, including the varicella-zoster virus.[35] The use of Echinacea is based on its traditional topical use and extrapolation from pharmacological studies (to improve wound healing and increase resistance to infection).[23] Cat's claw provides astringent and immune-supporting activities.[33]

A traditional topical approach is to bathe or sponge the affected areas with an infusion of burdock, golden seal and yellow dock root.[36] Physiomedicalists also used a salve prepared from balmony (*Chelone glabra*) to relieve the itch associated with chicken pox and measles and it was considered to be a most important remedy in this context.[37]

Supportive Herbal Treatment

It is often claimed that Echinacea is best used as a preventative, however its application should not be overlooked during acute paediatric infections. It has recently been clinically demonstrated that the oral use of a tablet containing 675 mg of *E. purpurea* root and

600 mg of *E. angustifolia* root (2 tablets per day) upregulated white blood cell count and the expression of heat shock protein 70 (Hsp 70) in blood samples subjected to heat shock.[38] There is clear evidence that Hsp 70 is involved in thermotolerance and cytoprotection of various organs exposed to heat stress.[39,40] Furthermore there is a strong traditional basis for prescribing *E. angustifolia* for fevers and common childhood conditions such as chicken pox and measles.[33] Based on this evidence and subjective clinical experience, either *E. angustifolia* root or a blend of both *E. angustifolia* and *E. purpurea* roots is recommended.

There is a clear role for the oral use of St John's wort in the treatment of chicken pox. The varicella-zoster virus is one of the eight herpes viruses and is surrounded by a lipid-containing envelope.[41] Both hypericin and pseudohypericin have demonstrated activity against several enveloped viruses including both herpes simplex viruses types 1 and 2.[23] It has been suggested that the mechanism for viral inactivation depends initially on the presence of a lipid-containing envelope.[23]

Example Herbal Formulations for Chicken Pox

1. Diaphoretic Formulation

See the formulation and doses for YEP outlined previously.

2. Topical Cream

See the licorice, rhubarb, Echinacea cream formulation outlined previously.

3. Antiviral Formulation

E. angustifolia root	1:2	50 mL
St John's wort high in hypericin	1:2	50 mL
	Total	100 mL

Dose: Calculate standard dose according to the most appropriate guideline in Chapter 1, using the adult dose of 5 mL. Three to four doses with water can be taken daily.

4. Combined Immune and Diaphoretic Formulation

An alternative to the above diaphoretic and antiviral formulations is the combined Immune/Diaphoretic Liquid formulation (adult dose 5 mL, see Appendix 1), containing *Echinacea angustifolia* root, elder flowers, lime flowers, yarrow, ginger and licorice. Calculate the standard dose for the child according to the most appropriate guideline in Chapter 1. The dose can be diluted in approximately 25 to 50 mL of warm to hot water and sipped. Up to 5 or 6 doses can be taken in one day while fever is present.

Case History

An unvaccinated 5-year-old male diagnosed with chicken pox was suffering a low grade fever with general malaise. Otherwise, the child's history was unremarkable, with a number of typical respiratory illnesses. He had been breast fed and was on a whole food diet.

The following formulation was prescribed:

Echinacea root blend	1:2	30 mL
Yarrow	1:2	35 mL
Elder flowers	1:2	35 mL
	Total	100 mL

Dose: 2 mL in juice 5 times a day.

Topical Lotion

Natural cream base (60%) diluted with distilled water (40%)		85 g
Calendula extracted with 25% alcohol	1:2	5 mL
St John's wort high in hypericin	1:2	5 mL
Licorice high in glycyrrhizin	1:1	5 mL
Lavender essential oil		5 drops

Application: The lotion was applied to the lesional crops as required and at least four times a day.

The child responded particularly well to the herbal treatment. The low-grade fever subsided within the first day of treatment, followed by an improvement in the malaise. The topical application was successful in alleviating the irritation from the lesions and seemed to hasten the scab formation and healing. The treatment as outlined above lasted 5 days. At this point the dose was reduced to 2 mL three times a day for another 5 days, after which Echinacea root blend as a simple at a dose of 2 mL twice daily was continued for another 4 weeks.

Rubeola (Measles)

Measles is an acute, highly communicable disease caused by the *Morbillivirus*.[16] A measles infection is acquired via the respiratory tract and occasionally through the conjunctivae. Virions enter the local lymphatic system and are transported to regional lymph nodes where they multiply before encountering the reticuloendothelial system. The reticuloendothelial infection is followed by a secondary viraemia, through which the skin and respiratory system become infected. The disease finally manifests after an incubation period of 10 to 12 days. A vasculitic rash develops as a consequence of an interaction between T cells and virus-infected cells.[42] Hence the major manifestations consist of a lymphoid proliferation (lymph glands, Peyer's patches, appendix, tonsils and adenoids) and a rash secondary to vasculitis.[29] Measles usually occurs in winter with epidemics following a 6-year cycle.[29,42]

The clinical progression of the disease follows several stages. The stage of invasion occupies the first three days and is marked by the three c's: coryza, cough, and conjunctivitis with photophobia. These symptoms are accompanied by fever of up to 39°C (102.2°F) and the patient feels miserable. During this stage a characteristic eruption, known as Koplik spots, appears at the gingivobuccal margin and spreads to the buccal mucous membrane. The fever can subside over the course of the first three days.[29,42] The second stage of eruption occurs over the following three days and the temperature can rise again, to about 40°C (104°F). The Koplik spots are by now fading and a maculopapular erythematous rash appears, first behind the ears and then on the face. Eventually this spreads to the whole body, including the palms and soles of the feet. During this stage it is not uncommon for the patient to experience abdominal pain, due to the lymphatic involvement.[29,42] The final stage of convalescence is heralded by a return to normal body temperature and the rash beginning to fade. However, the vasculitis leaves behind a ghost rash. Eventually there is a branny desquamation of the skin wherever the rash has been.[29,42]

Generally the prognosis of measles is good unless there are complications. The complication most often experienced is otitis media. However, pneumonia and encephalitis are less common but more serious complications.[29,42]

Treatment Strategy

The suggested treatment protocol for measles is similar to that described above for chicken pox. Diaphoretic therapy and Echinacea are particularly indicated. The Eclectics used black cohosh as a febrifuge and to "bring out" the rash of measles.[43] Due to the photophobia, sunlight avoidance is necessary. Irritability and abdominal discomfort can be treated with chamomile and/or lemon balm tea, or appropriate doses of these herbs as extracts. For the conjunctivitis, teas cooled to body temperature or suitably diluted extracts of eyebright and Calendula applied to the eye can help to reduce the inflammation. (Anything applied topically to the eyes needs to be relatively sterile and low in alcohol.) The topical treatment of conjunctivitis is further described in Chapter 6.

Vitamin A is a recommended therapy for measles in many developing countries and in developed countries under certain circumstances.[44] A controlled clinical trial conducted in the 1930s involving 600 children with acute measles used a whole food approach, with cod liver oil as the source of vitamin A. Mortality in the treated group was reduced to half that seen in the untreated group.[44] Preformed vitamin A as retinyl palmitate, can be found in animal dietary sources (liver, fish liver oils, eggs, and dairy products), whereas carotenoids (that can be converted to retinol) are obtained from dark-green leafy vegetables and deep-orange fruits and vegetables.[45] Cod liver oil provides about 85,000 IU of vitamin A per 100 g, 8,500 IU of vitamin D and 20 mg of vitamin E, as well as some elongated omega-3 fatty acids including eicosapentaenoic acid (EPA) and docosapentaenoic acid (DHA).[46]

Example Formulations for Measles

1. Diaphoretic Formulation

Diaphoretics are indicated during the febrile phases. See the formulation and doses for YEP outlined previously. Alternatively the Immune/Diaphoretic Liquid formulation (see Appendix 1) could be used as noted previously.

2. Immune/Skin Formulation

E. angustifolia root	1:2	50 mL
Baptisia or Cat's claw	1:2	40 mL
Pasque flower	1:2	10 mL
Total		100 mL

Dose: Calculate standard dose according to the most appropriate guideline in Chapter 1, using 5 mL as the adult dose. Up to 5 doses can be taken in one day. To be taken with water or juice.

Echinacea is included in the formulation for reasons previously described. Baptisia (wild indigo) is included based on traditional prescribing for septic conditions with lymphatic involvement.[43] Cat's claw is a suitable alternative. The inclusion of pasque flower (Pulsatilla) is based on its traditional indication for skin eruptions associated with infections.[34]

Rubella (German Measles)

German measles is caused by the erythrogenic *Rubivirus* and infection is acquired via inhalation. The virus spreads and replicates in the lymphoid tissue of the nasopharynx and upper respiratory tract and then invades all tissues, including unfortunately the placenta during pregnancy.[29,47] The virus is shed copiously via the respiratory, urinary and gastrointestinal tracts and the placenta. This shedding may continue for weeks or months after the disease.[29] Cold-like symptoms usually occur in the form of cough, congestion and coryza with lymphadenopathy. The post-auricular and occipital lymph nodes are typically enlarged and involvement of the joints is frequent.[29,48] Rubella is a disease that prefers winter and spring and has a peak incidence amongst school-age children, although younger patients are seen after exposure at home.[29] It usually has no long-lasting consequences, except in the event of infection occurring during early pregnancy. This may result in congenital rubella syndrome.[29,47]

During rubella infection signs vary from the typical to the almost imperceptible. There is usually a low-grade elevation in body temperature (38°C, 100.4°F) and, unlike measles, the maculopapular rash appears immediately, starting on the face and spreading to the whole body. The rash is generally completely resolved by day 3, giving rise to the common term of "3 day measles" for rubella.[29,47]

Herbal treatment of rubella should be based on the approaches provided above for measles, with diaphoretics required only during the mild febrile stage, if at all.

Parotitis (Mumps)

Mumps is caused by the *Rubulavirus* and is not just a disease of the parotid glands as commonly thought, but rather is a diffuse disease involving most of the exocrine glands.[29] Although the parotitis is considered to be the typical presentation, an estimated 40 to 50% of infected individuals have nonspecific symptoms, and another 20% are asymptomatic.[48] This can make diagnosis difficult. Viraemia can disseminate the virus to all exocrine glands including the salivary glands, pancreas, the choroid plexus and the mature ovaries and testes. The tissues affected display oedema and lymphocytic infiltration.[29]

Mumps is an endemic disease with a predilection for the late winter and spring months, with the incidence varying from year to year.[29] Exposure to the virus is through respiratory droplets that contain saliva, the primary shedding source. The incubation period is 12 to 24 days and infectivity begins 24 to 36 hours before clinical symptoms appear.[29]

The first symptom is frequently pain on chewing and swallowing, with a negligible elevation in temperature. As mentioned, the parotid glands are usually, but not always, involved. The enlargement of the parotid glands has a jelly-like feel and characteristically cups the pinna of the ear lobes. The submaxillary salivary glands are also affected, due to the involvement of the choroid plexus.[29] Mumps meningoencephalitis is a typical aspect of the disease, due again to the involvement of the choroid plexus, which produces a headache, the almost universal symptom of mumps. Nausea and vomiting are not unusual due to an acute pancreatitis that is self-limiting and not associated with long-term consequences.[29]

Since the gonads only become exocrine organs at puberty, their involvement is not expected in younger children. Approximately 25% of postpubertal and adult males are expected to have testicular involvement, with high fever, swelling, tenderness and pain. Approximately 5% of females have involvement of the ovaries.[29] Complications such as orchitis and oophoritis rarely, if ever, result in complete sterility. True encephalitis is a rare complication and may be fatal.[29]

Treatment Strategy

As chewing and swallowing are painful, food in the form of soups, broths, juices and smoothies is appropriate. If an elevated temperature is present, diaphoretic therapy is indicated. Either Echinacea or the herbal formulation recommended for measles is also appropriate, for reasons previously described. However pasque flower is particularly relevant if the testes or ovaries are involved. The herb was considered by both Physiomedical and Eclectic physicians as specifically indicated for orchitis and oophoritis as a result of mumps.[37,43] Due to the glandular involvement, poke root tincture is a worthy inclusion for older children and was considered a specific remedy for parotitis.[43] The safety of using poke root in paediatric conditions is controversial, but provided dosage guidelines are not exceeded any risk will be minimal.[8] Based on such traditional considerations the following formulation is recommended for mumps:

E. angustifolia	1:2	50 mL
Pasque flower	1:2	10 mL
Poke root	1:5	2 mL
Calendula	1:2	15 mL
Suitable flavouring mix		23 mL
Total		100 mL

Dose: Calculate the standard dose according to the most appropriate guideline in Chapter 1, using 5 mL as the adult dose. Up to 5 doses can be taken in one day. To be taken with water or juice.

An alternative to the above formulation is the combined Immune/Diaphoretic Liquid formulation (adult dose 5 mL, see Appendix 1) containing *Echinacea angustifolia* root, elder flowers, lime flowers, yarrow, ginger and licorice. Calculate the standard dose for the child according to the most appropriate guideline in Chapter 1. The dose can be diluted in approximately 25 to 50 mL of warm to hot water and sipped. Up to 5 or 6 doses can be taken in one day while fever is present, reducing to 3 to 4 doses once the mild fever has passed.

Vaccination

The public acceptance of vaccination programmes has been eroded by concerns over the safety risk, specifically the connection between autism and measles-mumps-rubella (MMR) vaccines containing thimerosal, a mercury-containing vaccine preservative (see Chapter 7).

Controversial research was published in 1998 that raised the possibility of a link between the MMR vaccine and a newly described syndrome of bowel disease and autism.[49] The authors of the study made it clear that the research did not prove a causal link, but raised the possibility based on parental and medical histories. They suggested further investigations were needed to examine the link between the MMR vaccine and autism. At a subsequent press conference the principle investigator suggested there was a case for splitting the MMR vaccine into its component parts.[50] This precipitated a collapse in confidence in the MMR vaccine and ever since the debate has been heated, with several careers and reputations damaged in the process.

Human exposure to ethylmercury thiosalicylate under the trade name of thimerosal began in the 1930s when it was introduced as a preservative for medicinal preparations and later vaccines.[51] It was not until 2001 that this application formally came into question as a possible toxic hazard to infants.[52]

Currently it has been removed from most vaccines, however it is still used, especially in developing countries.[51] The toxic effects of ethylmercury became evident in the 1870s as a result of animal experiments indicating that the central nervous system was a target. Incoordination was a common finding which was confirmed a century later as a result of human poisonings.[51] Acute exposure to thimerosal is associated with neurotoxicity and nephrotoxicity, however there are limited data on low dose exposure.[51,52] The effect that freshly deposited thimerosal exerts upon infants' brains after repeated exposures to vaccines is not known at this time. These issues and autism will be fully discussed in Chapter 7.

Varicella Vaccination and Increased Risk of Shingles

New research strongly suggests that varicella vaccination in childhood is associated with an increased risk of herpes zoster (shingles) infection amongst adults.[53] As noted previously both chicken pox and shingles are caused by the same varicella-zoster virus. Following a chicken pox infection, the virus becomes dormant, but can reactivate later in adulthood as shingles.[54] It has long been known that adults who have had chicken pox in the past receive a natural immune boost against both chicken pox and shingles by contact with children infected with chicken pox.[55] This continued contact helps to prevent the reactivation of the virus in the form of shingles.[54] Varicella vaccination programmes have substantially reduced the incidence of chicken pox and by so doing have reduced adult exposure to the virus.[55] This lack of exposure has prevented the opportunity for a natural immune boost, leading to a rise in shingles amongst adults.[53,54,55] The connection is significant, since shingles is known to cause three times the deaths and five times the number of hospitalisations than chicken pox.[53]

Minimising the Side Effects of Vaccination

To reduce the side effects of vaccination regardless of the type, Echinacea is the treatment of choice. Echinacea root in tablet or liquid form should be prescribed at appropriate doses (based on an adult dose of 7.5 mL/day for the 1:2 liquid or 3 tablets per day of the Echinacea Formula defined in Appendix 1) from three weeks prior to three weeks after the vaccination. Tincture of Thuja (1:5) is also useful after vaccination at low doses (based on an adult dose of 2 mL per day).

References

1   Wright AL, Taussig LM, Ray CG et al. *Am J Epidemiol* 1989; **129**(6): 1232-1246
2   Kaneko M, Watanabe J, Kuwahara M et al. *J Infect* 2002; **44**(4): 240-243
3   Kusel MM, de Klerk NH, Holt PG et al. *Pediatr Infect Dis J* 2006; **25**(8): 680-686
4   Palmer DA, Bauchner H. *Pediatrics* 1997; **99**(6): E6
5   De Sutter A, Lemiengre M, van Maele G et al. *Ann Fam Med* 2006; **4**(6): 486-493
6   Mainous AG, Hueston WJ, Davis MP et al. *Am J Pub Health* 2003; **93**(11): 1910-1914
7   Madsen H, Andersen S, Nielsen RG et al. *Eur J Pediatr* 2003; **162**(5): 334-341
8   Mills S, Bone K. *The Essential Guide to Herbal Safety.* Churchill Livingstone, Edinburgh, 2005.
9   Gallo M, Sarkar M, Au W et al. *Arch Int Med* 2000; **160**(20): 3141-3143
10   Perri D, Dugoua JJ, Mills E et al. *Can J Clin Pharmacol* 2006; **13**(3): 262-267
11   Russell FM, Shann F, Curtis N et al. *Bull WHO* 2003; **81**(5): 367-372
12   Freid VM, Makuc DM, Rooks RN. *Vital Health Stat 13* 1998; **137**: 1-23
13   Saunders NR, Tennis O, Jacobson S et al. *Can Med Assoc J* 2003; **168**(1): 25-30
14   Shinnar S, O'Dell C. *Pediatr Ann* 2004; **33**(6): 394-401
15   Ng DKK, Lam JCY, Chow KW. *HKMJ* 2002; **8**(1): 39-43
16   Porth CM. *Pathophysiology* 7th Ed, Lippincott Williams & Wilkins, Philadelphia, 2005, pp. 205-209.
17   Biddle C. *AANA J* 2006; **74**(2): 145-150
18   Hasday JD, Singh IS. *Cell Stress Chaperones* 2000; **5**(5): 471-480
19   Rao DV, Boyle GM, Parsons PG et al. *Mech Ageing and Dev* 2003; **124**: 55-69
20   Perdrizet GA. *New Horiz* 1995; **3**(2): 312-320
21   Srivastava P. *Nat Rev Immunol* 2002; **2**(3): 185-194
22   Tatro JB. *Clin Infect Dis* 2000; **31**(S1): 190-201
23   Mills S, Bone K. *Principles and Practice of Phytotherapy: Modern Herbal Medicine.* Churchill Livingstone, Edinburgh, 2000.
24   Richmond CA. *J Neurosci Nurs* 2003; **35**(5): 281-286
25   Mackowiak PA, Boulant JA. *Clin Infect Dis* 1996; **22**(3): 525-536
26   Mackowiak PA. *Ann Int Med* 1994; **120**(12): 1037-1040
27   Guyton AC, Hall JE. *Medical Physiology* 10th Ed, Saunders, Philadelphia, 2000, pp. 822-833.
28   Wood M. *The Practice of Traditional Western Herbalism,* North Atlantic Books, Berkeley, 2004.
29   Pomerance HH. *Fetal Pediatr Pathol* 2005; **24**(3): 169-189
30   Heininger U, Seward JF. *Lancet* 2006; **368**(9544): 1365-1376

31 Wharton M. *Infect Dis Clin North Am* 1996; **10**(3): 571-581
32 Weiss RF, Fintelmann V. *Herbal Medicine* 2nd Ed. Theime, Stuttgart, 2000
33 Bone K. *A Clinical Guide to Blending Liquid Herbs.* Churchill Livingstone, Edinburgh, 2003.
34 British Herbal Medicine Association's Scientific Committee. *British Herbal Pharmacopoeia.* BHMA, Bournemouth, 1983.
35 Sydiskis RJ, Owen DG, Lohr JL et al. *Antimicrob Agents Chemother* 1991; **35**(12): 2463-2466
36 Christopher JR. *Childhood Diseases,* Christopher Publications, Springville, Utah, 1978.
37 Clymer SR. *Nature's Healing Agents* 5th Ed. Humanitarian Society, Quakertown, 1973.
38 Agnew LL, Guffogg SP, Matthias A et al. *J Clin Pharm Ther* 2005; **3**(4): 363-369
39 Ostberg JR, Kaplan KC, Repasky EA. *Int J Hyperthermia* 2002; **18**(6): 552-562
40 Haveman J, Sminia P, Wondergem J et al. *Int J Hyperthermia* 2005; **21**(5): 473-487
41 Heininger U, Seward JF. *Lancet* 2006; **368**(9544): 1365-1376
42 Duke T, Mgone CS. *Lancet* 2003; **361**(9359): 763-773
43 Felter HW. *The Eclectic Materia Medica, Pharmacology and Therapeutics.* Eclectic Medical Publications, Portland, 1922, reprinted 1983.
44 Semba RD. *J Nutr* 1999; **129**(4): 783-791
45 Villamor E, Fawzi WW. *Clin Microbiol Rev* 2005; **18**(3): 446-464
46 Enig MG. *Know Your Fats* 7th Ed. Bethesda Press, Silver Spring, 2006.
47 Banatvala JE, Brown DWG. *Lancet* 2004; **363**(9415): 1127-1137
48 Andersen E. *AAHN J* 2006; **54**(10): 425-426
49 Wakefield AJ, Murch Sh, Anthony A et al. *Lancet* 1998; **351**(9103): 637-641
50 Horton R. *Lancet* 2004; **363**(9411): 747-749
51 Clarkson TW, Magos L. *Clin Rev Toxicol* 2006; **36**(8): 609-662
52 Ball LK, Ball R, Pratt RD. *Pediatrics* 2001; **107**(5): 1147-1157
53 Goldman GS. *Int J Toxicol* 2005; 24(4): 205-213
54 Goldman GS. *Vaccine* 2005; **23**(25): 3349-3355
55 Edmunds WJ, Brisson M. *J Infect* 2002; **44**(4): 211-219

CHAPTER FOUR

The Basis of Allergy in Children

THIS CHAPTER WILL DISCUSS Type 1 hypersensitivity and consider the emerging theories that attempt to explain the overall increase in the prevalence of allergic disorders. The treatment of specific allergic disorders is described elsewhere in the relevant chapters.

Incidence of Allergies in Children

Allergic disorders have increased so dramatically in Western countries that the rise has been described as an epidemic.[1,2] Moreover, the incidence of allergic disease in countries such as Australia, the UK and US are among the highest in the world.[2] Between 1993 and 2002, the Australian arm of the International Study of Asthma and Allergies in Children found an increase in the 12-month prevalence of allergic rhinitis from 9.7% to 12.7%, and eczema from 11.1% to 17.2%, but noted a fall in asthma prevalence from 27.2% to 20.0%. Since an earlier Australian study reported an almost doubling of asthma prevalence between 1984 and 1994 amongst Australian children,[3] the results of the latest study are puzzling. However the fall in asthma prevalence is supported by data from other recent studies. In New South Wales, the proportion of children diagnosed with asthma fell from 38% in 1992 to 32% in 2002.[4] Similar changes have been reported for the prevalence of current wheeze amongst schoolchildren in Hong Kong (from 12.4% in 1994 to 8.7% in 2002)[5] and in the UK (from 17.45% in 1997 to 14.2% in 2001).[6] In the US the prevalence of asthma in children increased between 1980 and 1996, but there was no discernible increase between 2001 and 2004.[7] US rates of asthma deaths in children also reflect this trend. The factors behind this recent downward trend in the prevalence of asthma are unclear. However two key reasons have been suggested: the increasing use of treatments that suppress asthma symptoms and the diagnosis of asthma being applied more sparingly since 2001.[8]

However, despite the recent anomaly for asthma, there is indeed an overall increase in the incidence of allergic diseases in industrialised countries over the past 30 years. This has often been explained by a decline in infections during childhood, which has given rise to the novel but speculative "hygiene hypothesis". Before discussing this hypothesis, it is worthwhile to briefly review the immunology of the allergic response.

Type 1 Hypersensitivity

Type 1 reactions are rapid IgE-mediated hypersensitivity responses that are a result of antigen challenge. The typical allergens are pollen, house dust mite, animal dander, foods (milk, peanuts, shellfish), antibiotics (penicillin, tetracycline), vaccines (pertussis, typhoid), venoms (bee, wasp), cosmetics and plant chemicals (poison ivy).[9,10] Exposure to the allergen can be through inhalation, ingestion, skin contact or injection. Depending on the portal of entry, Type 1 reactions can be an annoying local reaction (allergic rhinitis), severely debilitating (asthma) or a systemic and life-threatening response (anaphylaxis).[9]

Two basic types of immune cells are central to a Type 1 hypersensitivity reaction: the helper T subtype 2 (Th2) cells and the mast cells or basophils. Two subsets of helper T cells (Th1 and Th2), develop from the same precursor, the CD4+ T lymphocyte. Th1 cells differentiate in response to microbes and mediate the differentiation of B cells into IgM- and IgG-producing plasma cells. Th2 differentiation occurs in response to allergens and helminthes. Cytokines (IL-4, IL-5 and IL-13) secreted by Th2 cells stimulate the differentiation of B cells into IgE-producing plasma cells, act as growth factors for mast cells and recruit and activate eosinophils.[9,10]

Mast cells are normally distributed throughout connective tissue, especially in areas beneath the skin and mucous membranes of the respiratory, gastrointestinal and genitourinary tract and adjacent to blood and lymph vessels. Basophils are distributed throughout the blood and are one of the five major types of white blood cells.[9]

Type 1 hypersensitivity reactions begin with mast cell or basophil sensitisation. During the sensitisation or priming phase, allergen-specific IgE antibodies attach to receptors on the surface of mast cells and basophils.[9] IgE antibodies have a strong propensity to attach to mast cells and basophils, where a single mast cell or basophil can bind as many as half a million molecules of IgE.[11] With subsequent exposure, the sensitising allergen binds to the cell-associated IgE and initiates a series of events that ultimately leads to the degranulation of the sensitised mast cell or basophil. This causes the release of preformed mediators of the allergic response. Other mediators are released as a result of the activation of specific enzymes.[9,12] The well-known products of activated mast cells or basophils include histamine, acetylcholine, adenosine, chemotactic mediators and enzymes such as protease that lead to the generation of kinins.[9,12]

These mediators are said to orchestrate the symptoms of the allergic response. The end result is dilatation of local blood vessels, attraction of eosinophils and neutrophils to the reactive site, damage to local tissue by protease, increased permeability of the capillaries with loss of fluid into the tissues and contraction of local smooth muscle cells.[11] A number of abnormal tissue responses can then occur, depending on the type and location of the tissue in which the allergic reaction occurs.

The Hygiene Hypothesis

The hygiene hypothesis was first proposed in 1989 to explain the epidemiological features of hay fever and asthma and the rise in the prevalence of allergic disease.[13] In brief, the hypothesis states that over the past century declining family size, improved household amenities and higher standards of personal cleanliness have reduced the opportunities for cross-infection in young families. This may have resulted in a more widespread clinical expression of atopic disease.[14]

During the 1990's a plausible immunological basis for the hypothesis arose from the discovery of Th1 and Th2 lymphocyte populations in laboratory animals. It was subsequently recognised that natural immunity to bacterial and viral infections induces a Th1 pattern of cytokine release that suppresses the Th2 immune responses involved in IgE-mediated allergy.[14,15,16] This gave rise to the Th1/Th2 hypothesis, which placed these two types of immune cells as key supervisors of the immune system.[17] By way of extension, the Th1/Th2 hypothesis predicts a negative association between Th1 and Th2 associated diseases because of mutual inhibition.[18]

However a clearer understanding of the Th1/Th2 hypothesis is beginning to emerge. The Th1/Th2 hypothesis relies heavily on the dichotomy of cytokine profiles.[17] Most of these differences in cytokine profiles between Th1 and Th2 responses were derived from early work on mice and cultured cells.[17] More recent research involving human subjects strongly suggests that much of the earlier work is overly simplistic or inaccurate.[17,19] It is clear that Th1 and Th2 cells are critically positioned in the functional web of the immune system. However, it has now been established that they are situated downstream of events that initiate the primary immune drive, that is, the recognition of nonself or other antigens as potentially dangerous.[16,17] The recent increase in the prevalence of Th1 mediated disorders such as type 1 diabetes and Crohn's disease confounds matters further.[15,16,17] Most notably there appears to be a close correlation in the incidence of allergic disorders (Th2 mediated) and type 1 diabetes (Th1 mediated) both within and outside Europe, including Australia.[18] This has promoted a re-evaluation of both the hygiene and Th1/Th2 hypotheses.

Immunoregulatory Disorders

An emerging and unifying hypothesis that can explain the simultaneous increase in autoimmunity (Th1 mediated) and allergies (Th2 mediated) is the concept that modern living conditions can lead to a defective maturation of regulatory T cells (T_{reg}) and regulatory antigen-presenting cells (APC_{reg}).[15,16] It appears that the trigger to generate a productive systemic immune response, with the potential for inflammation and tissue damage, or alternatively a tolerogenic response, is largely determined by a specific microbial impact on antigen-presenting cells (APCs).[15,16] Naive TH cells are activated by APCs (chiefly dendritic cells) and act upstream to provide the appropriate stimulatory signals for differentiation into Th1 or Th2 cells. Conditioned APCs also induce T_{reg} that can suppress both Th1 and Th2 responses.15,16

Although not substantive, preliminary human data appears to support the concept of a defective T_{reg} activity in immunoregulatory disorders in western societies. For example, it has been demonstrated that in childhood cows milk allergy, the induction of immune tolerance is associated with the development of T_{reg} cells[20] and neonates with a hereditary allergy risk have deficient T_{reg} activity.[21] Further support is provided by experimental data that demonstrates that the induction of T_{reg} activity by various "friendly" micro-organisms can prevent or alleviate inflammatory disease.[15]

So what is the nature of this specific microbial impact that causes T_{reg} activity to regulate Th1 or Th2 cells?

The 'Old Friends' Hypothesis

The 'Old Friends' hypothesis suggests that the failure to develop adequate immunoregulatory pathways is a consequence of a diminished exposure to two categories of organisms. The first category is the harmless organisms associated with mud, untreated water and fermenting vegetable matter, such as saprophytic mycobacteria and lactobacilli.[15,16,22] These organisms have coexisted with humans throughout our evolutionary history, but are now less abundant with the advent of chlorinated water and relatively clean modern supermarket produce.[22] The second category is helminth infections, still common in developing countries, but almost completely absent from developed ones.[15,16,22] Helminthes needed to be tolerated by the immune system because most are relatively harmless and were constantly present in food and water throughout mammalian history.[22]

So while the 'Old Friends' hypothesis is essentially a refinement of the hygiene hypothesis, it represents an important advance in our understanding. The above mentioned organisms, rather than provoking aggressive immune responses, cause a pattern of maturation of dendritic cells so that these drive T_{reg} cells, rather than Th1 or Th2 effectors cells.[15,16,22] This in turn leads to mechanisms that help to control inappropriate inflammation. It is specifically thought that exposure to the 'Old Friends' is detected by pattern recognition receptors on dendritic cells. Dendritic cells thereby mature into regulatory dendritic cells, causing constant background activation of specific T_{reg} cells, resulting in bystander suppression of both Th1 or Th2 effectors cells.15,16,22

The validity of this pathway is supported by clinical trials and experimental models in which micro-organisms that are currently missing in the environment of developed nations are being proposed to treat allergy,[23,24,25] autoimmunity[26] and intestinal inflammation.[27,28]

The Gut and T$_{reg}$

The induction of the regulatory pathways involved with T_{reg} cells occurs primarily in the gut-associated lymphatic tissue (GALT). The presence of commensal micro-organisms is essential for the induction of this immune tolerance.[15] The gut is where the key events take place and its dynamic ecosystem appears to be crucial for the development of adequate individual/environment homeostasis. Accordingly, the gut represents the major immunological organ with the capacity for immune anergy or disruption, and hence modulation, of allergic responses.[15]

Probiotics

There is evidence that some probiotics can induce T_{reg} cells Some strains of lactobacillus actively participate in the maturation of dendritic cells, altering the cytokine profile in a beneficial way for T_{reg} activity. Furthermore, it has been found that there are less lactobacilli in the intestines of children with allergies.[29] A clinical study suggests that high doses of lactobacilli may inhibit the development of atopic dermatitis in genetically high-risk children.[30] A more recent double blind, randomised, placebo-controlled trial assessed the prevention of atopic dermatitis in genetically susceptible neonates. The mothers received probiotics from 36 weeks of gestation until birth and the neonates for the first 12 months of life. Results demonstrated significant protective effects against infantile eczema that continued through to 2 years of age.[31]

Clinical Implications

With regard to allergic disease, the evidence is reasonably clear that the fundamental disruption in the immune response is a gut-dependant phenomenon. This is consistent with the age-old herbal philosophy, as discussed in subsequent chapters. Hence any treatment should begin with a good diet, adequate fibre to encourage the growth of healthy organisms and if necessary probiotic therapy. Although not demonstrated from a scientific stance, it is also reasonable to assume that herbal remedies that enhance digestive function will have a positive impact in the holistic management of allergies. An obvious example is the association of both poor hydrochloric acid production and gastro-oesophageal reflux with asthma, where the prescription of bitter tonics to increase gastric acid production and antacids and demulcents to control reflux are a recommended strategy.[32] Herbal remedies such as *Albizia lebbeck* and *Scutellaria baicalensis,* that act downstream of T cells to stabilise mast cells to prevent the release of histamine,[32] provide a further strategy in the symptomatic relief of type 1 hypersensitivities. These and other strategies will be further discussed in subsequent chapters.

References

1   Isolauri E, Huurre A, Salminen S, Impivaara O. *Clin Exp Allergy* 2004; **34**(7): 1007-1010
2   Kemp AS, Mullins RJ, Weiner JM. *MJA* 2006; **185**(4): 226-227
3   Peat K, van den Berg RH, Green WF et al. *BMJ* 1994; **308**(6944): 1591-1596
4   Toelle BG, Ng K, Belousova E et al. *BMJ* 2004; **328**(7436): 386-387
5   Wong GW, Leung TF, Ko FW et al. *Clin Exp Allergy* 2004; **34**(10): 1550-1555
6   Anderson HR, Ruggles R, Strachan DP et al. *BMJ* 2004; **328**(7447): 1052-1053
7   Moorman JE, Rudd RA, Johnson CA et al. *MMWR Surveill Summ* 2007; **56**(8): 1-54
8   Toelle BG, Marks GB. *Thorax* 2005; **60**(2): 87-88
9   Porth CM. *Pathophysiology* 7th Ed. Lippincott Williams & Wilkins, Philadelphia, 2005, pp. 412-415.
10 Tortora GJ, Grabowski SR. *Principles of Anatomy and Physiology* 10th Ed, John Wiley & Sons, New York, 2003, pp. 798-799.
11 Guyton AC, Hall JE. *Medical Physiology* 10th Ed, Saunders, Philadelphia, 2000, pp. 411-412.
12 Gould HJ, Sutton BJ, Beavil AJ et al. *Ann Rev Immunol* 2003; **21**: 579-628
13 Strachan DP. *BMJ* 1989; **299**(6710): 1259-1260
14 Strachan DP. *Thorax* 2000; **55**(Suppl 1): S2-S10
15 Guarner F, Bourdet-Sicard R, Brandtzaeg P et al. *Nat Clin Pract Gastroenterol Hepatol* 2006; **3**(5): 275-284
16 Rook GAW, Brunet LR. *Gut* 2005; **54**(3): 317-320
17 Kidd P. *Alt Med Rev* 2003; **8**(3): 223-246
18 Stene LC, Nafstad P. *Lancet* 2001; **357**(9256): 607-608
19 Dent LA. *J Reprod Immunol* 2002; **57**(1-2): 255-272
20 Karlsson MR, Rugtveit J, Brandtzaeg P. *J Exp Med* 2004; **199**(12): 1679-1688
21 Haddeland U, Karstensen AB, Farkas L et al. *Pediatr Allergy Immunol* 2005; **16**(2): 104-112
22 Rook GA. *Trans R Soc Trop Med Hyg* 2007; **6** [Epub ahead of print]
23 Zuany-amorin C, Sawicka E, Manlius C et al. *Nat Med* 2002; **8**(6): 625-629
24 Wilson MS, Taylor MD, Balic A et al. *J Exp Med* 2005; **202**(9): 1199-1212
25 Ricklin Gutzwiller ME, Reist M, Peel JE et al. *Vet Dermatol* 2007; **18**(2): 87-93
26 Zaccone P, Fehervari Z, Jones FM et al. *Eur J Immunol* 2003; **33**(5): 1439-1449

27   Summers RW, Elliot DE, Urban Jr JF et al. *Gastroenterology* 2005; **128**(4): 825-832
28   Summers RW, Elliot DE, Urban Jr JF et al. *Gut* 2005; **54**(1): 87-90
29   Bjorksten B, Naaber P, Sepp E et al. *Clin Exp Allergy* 1999; **29**(3): 342-346
30   Kalliomaki M, Salminen S, Arvilommi H et al. *Lancet* 2001; **357**(9262): 1076-1079
31   Abrahamsson TR, Jakobsson T, Bottcher MF et al. *J Allergy Clin Immunol* 2007; **119**(5): 1174-1180
32   Bone K. *A Clinical Guide to Blending Liquid Herbs.* Churchill Livingstone, Edinburgh, 2003.

CHAPTER FIVE

Common Digestive Disorders in Children

HERBALISTS HAVE ALWAYS PLACED great emphasis on achieving and maintaining the optimal functioning of the digestive system.[1] The traditional position that the digestive system plays a fundamental role in health and disease is being increasingly validated by modern science. The gastrointestinal tract (GIT) performs many diverse functions, including of course the digestion of food and the absorption of nutrients. But the GIT is also the largest immune organ in the body and produces more antibodies than any other bodily system, as well as hosting 80% of all antibody producing cells.[2,3] In addition the GIT is host to an estimated 10^{14} microbes, representing some 400 to 500 species (of which 30 to 40 species comprise 99% of the population).[2,4] The relevance and impact of these resident microbes on the host's physiology and pathology is well documented. The presence of a normal bacterial flora is an essential requirement for normal gut physiology and mucosal immune cell education. The major host functions of the gut microflora include the production of nutrients, protection against invading organisms, trophic effects on the intestinal epithelium and the maturation and homeostasis of the immune response.[2,4,5]

In recent years the potential importance of increased intestinal permeability or a "leaky gut" has come into prominence. However this concept has it origins in the 19th century when the theory of auto-intoxication from gut bacteria was proposed.[6] With the notable exception of the skin, the epithelium of the GIT is exposed to a distinctly inhospitable milieu compared to other organ systems. The elements involved include the gastric acid and small bowel digestive enzymes, the bile and the gut flora and their degradation products.[6] An additional element in this inhospitable mix is the myriad of antigens presented by food.[7] These aggressors in the gut lumen have restricted access to the rest of the body due to the integrity of the tight junctions between the epithelial cells that line the gut wall.[7,8] Disruption of these tight junctions leads to increased intestinal permeability.[7,8] There is considerable evidence that implicates a leaky gut in several paediatric disorders including type 1 diabetes,[9,10] asthma[11,12] and eczema.[13,14] A fully functioning intestinal barrier is dependent on the normal balance of intestinal microbes[15] and hence the bowel flora is critically important in the prevention and treatment of increased intestinal permeability.

Factors Altering Gut Health

Dietary habits and environmental conditions exert a predominant influence over the gut microbial balance following weaning and into adolescence.[16] Oral antibiotic use can cause negative changes in gut ecology and the use of nonsteroidal anti-inflammatory drugs (NSAIDs) is associated with increased intestinal permeability.[17,18] In infancy the restricted use of antibiotics and antipyretics together with the consumption of vegetables fermented with lactobacilli is associated with fewer atopic disorders and higher numbers of lactic acid producing bacteria.[16]

Disease can also have a dramatic effect on the function of the GIT and can influence the composition of the intestinal microflora. An obvious example is infectious diarrhoea, where the presence of the organism causes the disease and temporarily changes the composition of the microflora.[2] In other examples a change in the composition of the bowel flora may act as a causative factor in a disease. For example infants with allergy have been observed to have a reduced faecal colonisation of *Bifidobacterium* and *Lactobacillus*.[19] The composition of the bifidobacteria flora has been observed to be different between atopic and healthy infants. Atopic infants are mainly colonised by *B. adolescentis* while healthy infants exhibit a more typical flora comprising mainly *B. bifidum*, *B. breve* and *B. infantis*.[20]

Paediatric Gastrointestinal Complaints Overview

Gastric upsets are relatively common in children and most are functional rather than organic in nature. An accurate diagnosis can be difficult, as most children under the age of 5 or 6 are unable to describe their symptoms accurately.[21] Therefore the clinician must be alert to symptoms that could suggest a higher probability of organic disease. These symptoms include weight loss, growth retardation, gastrointestinal blood loss, frequent vomiting, chronic severe diarrhoea, persistent fever and constant upper right or lower abdominal pain.[22]

The symptoms most frequently encountered with functional disorders include pain, which tends to move around the epigastric region, gastric spasm, a sensation of fullness, loss of appetite, nausea, occasional vomiting and constipation.[23]

Given the above mentioned symptoms, the following herbal actions and corresponding key herbs are most appropriate in the management of functional digestive disorders in children:

- Spasmolytic herbs to relieve gastric spasm such as chamomile, lemon balm and peppermint[24]
- Antacid herbs to reduce gastric irritation such as meadowsweet[24]
- Demulcent herbs to soothe the gut mucous membranes including slippery elm and marshmallow root[24]
- Carminative herbs to relieve the sensation of fullness such as chamomile, lemon balm and peppermint[24]
- Appetite stimulants to boost appetite such as fennel and fenugreek[24]
- Antinausea herbs for the symptomatic relief of nausea, including chamomile, peppermint and meadowsweet[1]

- Antiemetic herbs to relieve vomiting such as ginger (mild doses), globe artichoke and peppermint[24]
- Sedative herbs to generally calm and soothe the nervous system, most notably chamomile, lemon balm, passionflower and peppermint[24]

As can be seen from the above recommendations there is considerable overlap and a number of key herbs stand out, most notably chamomile, peppermint, lemon balm and meadowsweet.

Poor Appetite and Weak Digestion

Unusual eating habits and unpredictable appetites are typical childhood patterns and as a result parents often worry whether their child is eating enough.[25] The association between a prolonged lack of appetite and growth deficiency with impaired cognitive development is relevant in this context.[26] Loss of appetite can also be associated with the development of a respiratory tract infection or other illness, emotional stress such as results from school bullying, iron deficiency, intestinal parasites and snacking between meals on junk foods. On the other hand, uncomplicated loss of appetite can simply reveal a weakness of digestive function.[27] In such cases the aromatic digestive herbs and bitters are ideal remedies.

Treatment Strategy

The herbal treatment of a simple case of poor appetite with digestive weakness need not be overly complex. Clinical experience of one author (RS) has demonstrated that chen pi (*Citrus reticulata*) is an ideal remedy in such cases and covers a range of the commonly experienced symptoms. Chen pi is an important herb in Traditional Chinese Medicine (TCM) used to regulate Qi and strengthen the stomach and pancreatic digestive processes.[28] It is particularly useful for digestive weakness and stagnation presenting as abdominal distension, fullness, bloating and poor appetite.[28] Hence for these symptoms just chen pi 1:2 liquid extract can be used.

Calculate the chen pi dose according to the most appropriate guideline in Chapter 1. The liquid can be added to a small cup of peppermint tea to increase compliance, as well as taking advantage of the synergistic combination, and should be taken before meals.

Herbs which improve upper digestive function can be divided into five major groups:

- Simple bitters such as gentian and wormwood which improve most aspects of upper digestive function. For a child these can be used in quite low doses, even one or two drops
- Aromatic digestives such as Angelica, chen pi, cinnamon and Coleus which improve gastric acid secretions. Coleus also improves exocrine pancreatic function but it has a strong taste that could make compliance difficult
- Pungent herbs such as ginger and cayenne which are potent stimulators of gastric acid but are probably too strong for all but older children

- Choleretic herbs such as barberry, milk thistle and dandelion root which improve bile production by the liver. Dandelion root is ideally suited to children
- Cholagogue herbs such as peppermint which improve gallbladder function. Again peppermint is ideally suited to children

An example formulation for poor appetite and weak digestion in a child is as follows:

Wormwood	1:5	2 mL
Dandelion root	1:2	50 mL
Peppermint	1:2	25 mL
Cinnamon	1:2	25 mL
	Total	102 mL

Dose: Calculate the standard dose (based on an adult dose of 3 mL before meals) according to the most appropriate guideline in Chapter 1. To be taken with water or juice.

Alternatively, Upper Digestive Formula tablets (see Appendix 1) can be prescribed. Calculate the child's dose (based on an adult dose of 1 tablet sucked before each meal) according to the most appropriate guideline in Chapter 1. For younger children the tablets (or part thereof) can be crushed and mixed with honey or a suitable sweetener to improve compliance.

Case History

A mother presented with her 4-year-old female preschooler concerned about the child's poor appetite. She did not seem interested in food, picked at food whilst at the table and existed on a small range of preferred foods. The child seemed otherwise well. Although perhaps a little underweight, she could not have been described as a sickly child. There were no digestive symptoms or increased susceptibility to infection. It thus appeared to be a simple case of poor appetite, associated with an asymptomatic weakness in digestion. It seemed appropriate then to attempt to strengthen her digestion.

Chen pi 1:2 liquid extract was prescribed as a simple at 0.5 mL in a little juice before meals and at least twice a day. At first the child rejected the herbal treatment, but with parental persistence after about 5 days the child began to accept the liquid. Over weeks and months the child's digestive strength improved, as evidenced by an increase in appetite and a willingness to try new foods and consume good meals (as much as can be expected from a 4-year-old). The herbal treatment lasted 6 months at the recommended doses and was then gradually decreased over a 4-week period. The child came to like her "Chen poo", as the family termed the medicine, and continued to use it occasionally.

Functional Abdominal Pain (FAP)

Chronic abdominal pain is a common complaint among children and adolescents. In fact abdominal pain is so common that few children go through school without experiencing it at some stage.[29] However, as few as 50% of those experiencing recurrent abdominal pain ever present for treatment, presumably because the parents regard the symptom as trivial and transient in nature.[29] This is reflected in reports that only 2 to 4% of all paediatric office visits are for the evaluation of abdominal pain.[30] Children may experience abdominal pain when they are worried, excited or hungry. However, they may also complain when they have pain from an organic disorder.[31] A functional gastrointestinal disorder is typically diagnosed when no specific structural, infectious, inflammatory or biochemical cause can be found in a child with chronic abdominal pain.[32]

As the research into FAP has progressed, it is now evident that several types or subgroups of abdominal pain exist. These subgroups include functional dyspepsia, irritable bowel syndrome (IBS), abdominal migraine, functional abdominal pain and functional abdominal pain syndrome and are discussed below.[33]

With functional dyspepsia the child must experience all of the following symptoms at least once a week for at least 2 months:[33]

- Persistent or recurrent pain or discomfort centred in the upper abdomen above the umbilicus
- Pain not relieved by defecation or associated with a change in stool frequency or form

There should be no evidence of an inflammatory, anatomic, metabolic or neoplastic process.

In the case of IBS, the child must, at least once a week for at least 2 months, experience abdominal discomfort or pain that is associated with two or more of the following at least 25% of the time:

- Improvement with defecation
- Onset associated with a change in the frequency of the stool
- Onset associated with a change in the form of the stool

Again there should be no evidence of an inflammatory, anatomic, metabolic or neoplastic process.

Cases of abdominal migraine are more complex and the child must experience all of the following symptoms, at least twice in the preceding 12 months:[33]

- Paroxysmal episodes of intense, acute periumbilical pain that lasts for one hour or more
- Intervening periods of usual health lasting weeks to months
- The pain interferes with normal activities
- The pain is associated with two or more of the following: anorexia, nausea, vomiting, headache, photophobia and pallor

Again there should be no evidence of an inflammatory, anatomic, metabolic or neoplastic process.

In the case of functional abdominal pain, symptoms of episodic or continuous abdominal pain must be experienced at least once a week for at least 2 months.[33] There should be insufficient criteria for the other functional gastrointestinal disorders and no evidence of an inflammatory, anatomic, metabolic or neoplastic process.

Finally, for a diagnosis of functional abdominal pain syndrome symptoms should occur at least once a week for at least 2 months and abdominal pain must comprise 25% of pain complaints, in addition to one or more of the following symptoms:[33]

- Some loss of daily functioning
- Additional somatic symptoms such as headache, limb pain or difficulty sleeping

Pathophysiology of FAP

Most current research is in general agreement that FAP is a multifactorial disorder linked to an altered gut-brain interaction.[34,35,36] Children are naturally highly susceptible to influences around them and can experience pain as a response to these influences. For example stress from school and home increase the incidence of FAP.[31] The gut-brain connection suggests that a child with FAP has a dysregulation in the communication between the central and enteric nervous systems, which alters the perception of visceral sensations, resulting in the experience of abdominal pain.[37,38] The enteric nervous system is described as a local minibrain that contains a library of programs necessary for normal intestinal behavioural patterns.[38] Stimuli that would not normally cause pain can produce exaggerated symptoms in a child with an altered gut-brain connection.[32] These include physiological stimuli (such as altered bowel motility or intestinal gas), psychological stimuli (such as school problems, family problems, anxiety or excitement) or other stressful stimuli (such as low grade inflammation). This hypersensitivity to pain was demonstrated in a comparison with healthy children and those with chronic disease, where children with FAP reported both a lower pain threshold in response to painful stimuli on the surface of the body[39] and a hypersensitivity to intraluminal distension.[40]

Another focus of attention is the psychological environment within the family. This model proposes that recurrent abdominal pain is a biological response governed by an interaction between the child's temperament and the family and school environments.[29] It has been postulated that the child's symptoms might be influenced by the parents' conceptual model of illness.[41] An investigation involving the families of children with severe recurrent abdominal pain found that the child was more likely to have recovered if the parents attributed the symptoms to psychological factors. The researchers therefore concluded that an acceptance by parents of a biopsychosocial model of illness is an important factor in the resolution of symptoms.[41]

Another area of research that is particularly relevant to functional dyspepsia related to FAP is an abnormal transit time for the small intestine. A study involving 57 children with symptoms of functional dyspepsia found that 40% had slow small bowel transit. Children with fast small bowel transit times were less likely to report abdominal pain.[42] Slow gastric emptying is also implicated. It was found that 60% of the 30 children with functional dyspepsia had slow gastric emptying and this group was more likely to experience severe postprandial pain.[43]

Treatment Strategy

Simple functional dyspepsia can be successfully treated using just chen pi or cinnamon. Because herbs exert multiple effects, there is no reason why radically differing formulas need to be applied to the other types of FAP. For the more complex IBS type of FAP, the herbal approach requires the use of additional spasmolytics in order to calm the enteric nervous system, thus relieving pain. It is interesting to note in this context that one of the few therapeutic agents to be evaluated for paediatric FAP is peppermint essential oil. In a randomised, double blind, controlled trial, 42 children with IBS were given either enteric-coated peppermint oil capsules or placebo. Patients weighing more than 45 kg received 2 peppermint oil capsules (187 mg each) 3 times a day. The smaller children who weighed between 30 and 40 kg received one capsule 3 times daily. After 2 weeks, 75% of those receiving peppermint oil had reduced severity of pain associated with the IBS which was significantly better than placebo ($p < 0.002$).[44]

An example formulation for FAP is as follows:

Chen pi or Cinnamon	1:2	25 mL
Chamomile	1:2	20 mL
Lemon balm or Vervain	1:2	20 mL
St Mary's (milk) thistle	1:1	20 mL
Meadowsweet or Cramp bark	1:2	20 mL
Peppermint essential oil		1 drop
Total		105 mL

Dose: Calculate the standard dose (based on an adult dose of 5 mL) according to the most appropriate guideline in Chapter 1. To be taken with water or juice before meals.

An alternative formulation is as follows:

Chen pi or Cinnamon	1:2	25 mL
Chamomile	1:2	20 mL
Peppermint or Globe artichoke	1:2	20 mL
St Mary's (milk) thistle	1:1	20 mL
Meadowsweet or Cramp bark	1:2	20 mL
Total		105 mL

Dose: Calculate the standard dose (based on an adult dose of 5 mL) according to the most appropriate guideline in Chapter 1. To be taken with water or juice before meals.

In the case of FAP syndrome, mild anxiolytic and nervine tonic herbs such as passionflower, lemon balm, vervain and skullcap should be considered in addition to the above examples.

An alternative to the above liquid formulations is Smooth Muscle Relaxant tablets (adult dose 4 per day), perhaps in combination with Nervous System Tonic tablets for the nervy child (adult dose 4 per day) and Liver/Biliary Tonic tablets (adult dose 4 per day) or Upper Digestive Formula tablets (adult dose 1 before each meal) to improve digestion, as indicated.

Calculate the child's tablet dose according to the most appropriate guideline in Chapter 1. For younger children the tablets can be crushed and mixed with honey or a suitable sweetener to improve compliance. See Appendix 1 for the suggested formulations for these tablets.

Treatment Rationale

Peppermint essential oil and extracts are traditionally indicated for dyspepsia and spastic conditions of the gastrointestinal tract, and this is supported by various clinical evaluations for dyspeptic type conditions.[24] Cramp bark is ideal for abdominal spasm.[24]

Chen pi as noted is particularly useful for digestive weakness and stagnation presenting as abdominal distension, fullness, bloating and poor appetite.[28] Cinnamon also has similar properties.[24]

Chamomile is often considered to be the archetypal paediatric digestive remedy. It seems ideally suited to conditions where both the central and enteric nervous systems are involved. This concept is supported by well-documented traditional use for flatulent and nervous dyspepsia. The herb was an important ingredient in a formulation that successfully treated infantile colic.[24]

St Mary's (milk) thistle is also traditionally indicated for dyspeptic complaints[24] and clinical experience has demonstrated its usefulness where nausea is a feature. It has choleretic activity, as does globe artichoke.[24]

Meadowsweet rounds out the formulation because of its settling effects on gastrointestinal function, which is supported by traditional use for atonic dyspepsia and irritable bowel syndrome.[24]

Case History

A 6-year-old female child presented with her mother. The mother reported that since the beginning of the school year the child often complained of stomach pain before school and did not wish to go to school. The child was now in year 2 of school but was in a composite class with year 3 pupils. The mother reported the child was emotionally sensitive and had linked this new school stress with her child's symptoms. The mother had also talked to the teacher about the problem.

The following formulation was prescribed:

Chamomile	1:2	20 mL
Lemon balm	1:2	20 mL
Withania	1:2	60 mL
Total		100 mL

Dose: 2 mL in juice before breakfast, 2 mL after school and 3 mL before bed.

The combined actions of the herbs provided an almost immediate positive effect. There were two milder episodes of stomach pain after herbal treatment was initiated, then these ceased. The child was soon much more content to attend school and the problem never returned. In all the child took the formulation for 3.5 weeks and there were no compliance issues.

Food Allergy and Intolerance

Food allergies (FA) constitute a part of the increased prevalence of allergic disorders as discussed in Chapter 4. FA have become a major worldwide health concern over the past two decades and are associated with a significantly negative impact on the quality of life.[45] FA are much more common in the paediatric age group, however the real prevalence remains unclear.[46] Adults often misjudge their own FA because of confusion between true allergy as opposed to food intolerance.[47] Similarly, parents often overestimate FA in their children. Up to 25% of parents believe that their children are afflicted by FA, however studies indicate the real prevalence is likely to be much lower, somewhere between 6 and 8%.[48]

Food allergies are defined as abnormal immune responses to food proteins that result in adverse clinical reactions.[46,49,50] FA need to be distinguished from other adverse reactions to food that are not mediated by the immune system. These non-immune type reactions can result from a variety of mechanisms or defects. They include digestive enzyme deficiencies such as lactose intolerance, pharmacological reactions to food components, for example vasoactive amines, food poisoning including food-borne bacterial gastroenteritis, toxic reactions such as to staphylococcus enterotoxin and finally psychological aversion to certain foods.[46,49,50] The typical allergens of infancy and early childhood are eggs, cows milk, peanuts, wheat and soya, whereas allergens responsible for severe reactions in older children and adults are mainly peanuts and seafoods.[49] Allergic reactions to fruits and vegetables are relatively common, but are usually not severe.[51]

Pathophysiology

The precise pathogenesis of most food hypersensitivity reactions is not completely understood. Several factors play important roles, including genetics, the host's intestinal flora, the frequency of exposure to the various dietary allergens and the allergenicity of the various food proteins.[46] Immaturity of the intestinal mucosal barrier has been suggested as one mechanism that may explain the higher incidence of FA in infants and children.[46] As discussed in Chapter 4, oral tolerance appears to be dependent on the correct microbial stimulation of dendritic and T regulatory cells. It has been postulated that the increased prevalence of formula feeding and subsequent loss of the critical immunological factors present in breast milk have contributed to the rising incidence of immune based disorders, including allergy.[52] Further to this, it appears that the newborn cytokine profile is polarised away from cell-mediated immunity towards humoral immunity, which diverts the immunologic T cell memory to the Th2 phenotype, potentially leading to enhanced IgE production and atopic sensitisation.[53] Low grade intestinal inflammation and increased intestinal permeability induce changes in antigen handling that may lead to sensitisation.[53] The implication of this is that the allergic response is at least partially caused by a failure of gut associated lymphatic tissue (GALT) to maintain oral tolerance to antigens. In all, the data strongly suggest that the balance of microflora, mucosal integrity and GALT are important elements in the pathogenesis of food allergy.

Elimination/Challenge Diet

In general, the first approach in working with food allergies is to evaluate the patient with an elimination/challenge diet. The removal of a food that is recognised as problematic for 21 to 28 days should improve symptoms. However, since it is necessary to remove all offending foods, a modified elimination diet may not be effective.[54] After the removal of the potentially offending foods for 3 to 4 weeks, an offending food is carefully added back into the diet once every few days, with 2 to 4 days between the various foods, allowing for delayed hypersensitivity responses. The process is usually limited to the most common allergens such as cows milk, wheat, eggs, corn, soy and nuts and adapted to include any other suspicious food.

Obviously, any foods already known to cause a severe allergic response must be avoided completely and should not be part of any challenge.

Treatment Strategy

The primary difference in treating true FA and food intolerance is the use of specific antiallergic herbs for the former, otherwise the treatment goals are similar. The following actions and herbs summarise the overall strategy:[1]

- To improve upper digestive function (thereby improving the breakdown of food components which in theory reduces their allergenicity) the aromatic digestives such as cinnamon, Angelica and chen pi seem especially suited. A low quantity of a bitter herb such as gentian or wormwood may also be appropriate
- Antiallergic herbs such as Albizia and Baical skullcap to dampen the allergic response
- Immune modulating herbs particularly Echinacea to normalise the immune response
- Herbs with healing properties for the gut such as chamomile, Calendula and meadowsweet
- Herbs such as St Mary's (milk) thistle and Schisandra to assist hepatic screening and detoxification

Example Herbal Formulations

For food allergies the following formulation can be used:

Angelica or Cinnamon	1:2	10 mL
Baical skullcap or Albizia	1:2	30 mL
Echinacea root blend	1:2	20 mL
Chamomile	1:2	20 mL
Schisandra	1:2	25 mL
	Total	105 mL

Dose: Calculate the standard dose (based on an adult dose of 5 mL) according to the most appropriate guideline in Chapter 1. To be taken with water or juice before meals.

For food intolerance the following example formulation is more appropriate:

Angelica or Globe artichoke	1:2	10 mL
Chen pi or Cinnamon	1:2	25 mL
Echinacea root blend	1:2	20 mL
Chamomile	1:2	20 mL
Schisandra	1:2	25 mL
	Total	100 mL

Dose: Calculate the standard dose (based on an adult dose of 5 mL) according to the most appropriate guideline in Chapter 1. To be taken with water or juice before meals.

Choleretic herbs such as globe artichoke and dandelion root should also be considered, as noted above in the alternatives.

An alternative to the above liquid formulations is Upper Digestive Formula tablets (adult dose 4 per day) in combination with Allergy Support tablets (adult dose 4 per day) in the case of food allergies. For food intolerance the Upper Digestive Formula tablets can be combined with Liver Detox Assist tablets (adult dose 4 per day).

Calculate the child's tablet dose according to the most appropriate guideline in Chapter 1. For younger children the tablets can be crushed and mixed with honey or a suitable sweetener to improve compliance. See Appendix 1 for the suggested formulations for these tablets.

Common Intestinal Parasites

Intestinal parasites are relatively common amongst children, particularly those of preschool age. The most prevalent parasites are pinworms or threadworms (*Enterobius vermicularis*) and the protozoan *Giardia lamblia*.

Pinworms

Pinworm infestation is relatively common in children and is the most common helminthic infection in the US.[55] Infestation usually results from the transfer of ova from the perianal area to hands, clothing, bedding, furniture, rugs and toys, from which the ova are picked by the new host, transmitted to the mouth and then swallowed.[55,56] Reinfestation can easily occur through finger transfer of ova from the perianal area to the mouth, with thumb sucking a significant risk factor.[55,56] Pinworms reach maturity in the lower gastrointestinal tract within 2 to 6 weeks. The female worm migrates to the perianal region usually at night to deposit the ova. The sticky substance in which the ova are deposited and the movements of the female worm cause the major symptom of pinworm infestation, perianal pruritis.[55,56] Perianal pruritis and nocturnal restlessness are often the only signs indicating a pinworm infestation. Children with small worm loads are often asymptomatic, other than experiencing an ill-defined abdominal discomfort. Suspicion can be confirmed by the "cellophane tape test". This test consists of touching tape to the perianal area several times and examining it under a low power microscope for the presence of ova. The test should be performed on three consecutive mornings.[55,56] Clothing and bedding should be washed frequently and the environment thoroughly cleaned and vacuumed.

Example Formulation for Pinworms

Echinacea root blend	1:2	30 mL
Wormwood	1:5	15 mL
Black walnut hulls	1:10	20 mL
Cranesbill or Yellow dock	1:2	20 mL
Thyme or Cat's claw	1:2	25 mL
	Total	110 mL

Dose: Calculate the standard dose (based on an adult dose of 5 mL) according to the most appropriate guideline in Chapter 1. The dose is to be taken on an empty stomach 4 to 6 times a day, for 10 days. After a break of 10 days repeat for another 10 days. The second treatment is to kill any larvae that may have hatched after treatment.

Rationale

Echinacea is prescribed to assist with the immune response to worm infestation.[59] Wormwood is considered the archetypal herbal anthelmintic and both experimental and clinical evidence support this use.[24] The use of black walnut hulls is supported by its traditional use to expel worms[57] and an *in vitro* study has demonstrated larvicidal activity for plumbagin, a naphthoquinone found in the hulls.[58] Cranesbill is included in the formulation due to the presence of tannins. It has been established that tannins, although not larvicidal in themselves, synergise with larvicidal compounds (in this case black walnut hulls and wormwood) to cause bursting of larvae.[59] Thyme is included in the formula as a synergistic antimicrobial and anthelmintic remedy. Cat's claw provides astringency and immune support and yellow dock has a mild laxative action to assist with expulsion.[24]

Due to taste and the higher frequency of dose with a liquid formula, compliance issues may arise. In such cases and where the child is of the age to swallow tablets, this may be the most appropriate dosage form.

An example tablet formulation (Wormwood Combination, see also Appendix 1) is as follows:[60]

Wormwood	100 mg
Stemona	1 g
Black walnut hulls	100 mg
Essential oil of cloves	20 mg

Dose: Calculate the standard dose (based on an adult dose of 2 tablets) according to the most appropriate guideline in Chapter 1. This dose is to be taken on an empty stomach 2 to 3 times a day, for 10 days. The tablets can be crushed and mixed with honey or a suitable sweetener to improve compliance. After a break of 10 days repeat for another 10 days. The second treatment is to kill any larvae that may have hatched after treatment. These can be combined with immune support tablets (such as Short Term Immune Support, see Appendix 1) in similar doses.

Case History

Pinworms had been detected in 7 and 8–year-old sisters by their parents. Both were prescribed the liquid formulation as detailed below. There were some initial difficulties in the children's acceptance of the medicine, however persistence paid off. The parents were committed to herbal treatment and wished to avoid pharmaceutical anthelmintics.

Echinacea root blend	1:2	30 mL
Wormwood	1:5	15 mL
Black walnut hulls	1:10	20 mL
Cranesbill	1:2	20 mL
Thyme	1:2	25 mL
	Total	110 mL

Dose: Both children took 5 mL with water on an empty stomach 4 times a day for 10 days. After a break of 10 days this was repeated for another 10 days. At the completion of this treatment period no pinworms could be detected.

Giardia

Giardiasis is caused by the protozoan parasite *Giardia lamblia* and is considered to be the most common protozoal infection in humans, occurring frequently in both developing and industrialised nations.[61] The incidence is believed to range from 2 to 7% of the population in industrialised nations.[62] Giardia can exist in two forms, the cyst and the trophozoite. The cyst is the dormant form that is responsible for the transmission of giardiasis. Cysts are excreted from an infected host via the faeces and are exceptionally hardy, being able to tolerate extremes of temperature and pH.[62] Because giardiasis is spread by the faecal-oral route, the prevalence is higher in populations where sanitation is poor.[55] In industrialised nations the disease is commonly water borne, due to the organisms' resistance to normal chlorine levels in the water supply and its ability to survive in cold streams and rivers.[55] Infection with giardia is common among children and staff attending day care centres and kindergartens.[63]

Infection of the host is initiated when the cyst is ingested through contaminated water or, less commonly, food or direct faecal-oral contact. In response to the acidic environment of the stomach, the cysts transform into trophozoites in the proximal small intestine, where they replicate and cause the symptoms of giardiasis.[64] After exposure to biliary fluid, some of the trophozoites form cysts in the jejunum that are passed into the faeces, allowing the completion of the transmission cycle.[64]

The clinical presentation of giardiasis can vary greatly. Usually, after an incubation period of 1 to 2 weeks, symptoms of gastrointestinal distress begin to develop. These include intermittent nausea, low-grade malaise and anorexia, flatulence, cramping and malodorous watery diarrhoea. The gradual onset of a mild diarrhoea can differentiate giardiasis from other gastrointestinal infestations. Malabsorption of fats and carbohydrates can lead to significant weight loss in severe cases. Acute giardiasis usually lasts from 1 to 3 weeks.[55]

Herbal Formulation for Giardiasis

Echinacea root blend	1:2	25 mL
Pau d'arco	1:2	20 mL
Propolis	1:5	20 mL
Golden seal	1:3	20 mL
Peppermint or Chamomile	1:2	20 mL
	Total	105 mL

Dose: Calculate the standard dose (based on an adult dose of 5 mL) according to the most appropriate guideline in Chapter 1. The dose is to be taken on an empty stomach with water or juice 4 to 6 times a day, for 10 days. After a break of 10 days repeat for another 10 days. Extra Echinacea or pau d'arco can be added if propolis is not available.

Additional treatment: High Allicin Releasing Garlic tablets (see Appendix 1), 1 twice a day, are suitable for older children who can swallow tablets.

An alternative to the above liquid formulation is Cat's Claw Immune Formula tablets (adult dose 6 per day) in conjunction with Golden Seal tablets (adult dose 6 per day). Calculate the child's tablet dose according to the most appropriate guideline in Chapter 1. For younger children the tablets can be crushed and mixed with honey or a suitable sweetener to improve compliance. See Appendix 1 for the suggested formulations for these tablets.

Rationale

The Echinacea is included to assist with the immune response to giardiasis. Pau d'arco is anti-protozoal.[65] Propolis has clinical validation for its use in giardiasis, as demonstrated by an open comparison study involving 138 adults and children. The subjects received a 5-day regimen of either tinidazole or propolis. The children were given a 10% propolis solution, whereas the adults received either 20% or 30% propolis solutions. The cure rates, as evaluated by duodenal aspiration, were 52% in the propolis-treated children, 40% in the adults taking the 20% propolis solution and 60% in those taking the 30% propolis solution. In comparison the tinidazole (dose unspecified) produced a 40% cure rate. No side effects were noted for the propolis treatment.[66] Golden seal is included because of the traditional indications of infectious diarrhoea.[24] Its use in giardiasis is also supported by several *in vitro* studies. It has been demonstrated that berberine found in golden seal had an inhibitory activity against giardia trophozoites[67] and that berberine sulphate was shown to induce morphological damage to these.[68] Further support for the use of golden seal is provided by a placebo-controlled clinical study. Forty children received either placebo, berberine hydrochloride (5 mg/kg/day) or metronidazole (Flagyl) for 6 days. Berberine administration resulted in a marked decline in gastrointestinal symptoms, which was superior to metronidazole, and a 68% reduction in giardia positive stools. Metronidazole treatment resulted in 100% of the subjects being parasite free, however the authors speculated that an increase in dose or a longer duration of treatment would have increased berberine's therapeutic efficacy.[69] The formulation is completed with peppermint extract. Peppermint is indicated for many of the symptoms experienced as a result of giardiasis such as nausea, cramping and flatulence.[24] More recently an *in vitro* study demonstrated that an extract of peppermint induced morphological changes on the membrane surface of the parasite as well as inhibiting the adhesion of giardia trophozoites.[70] Peppermint is also a welcome addition into the formulation as a flavouring agent.

The traditional use of garlic as an antiparasitic agent has also received scientific validation.[60] A clinical investigation in 26 children infected with giardia using either 5 mL of crude extract of fresh garlic in 100 mL of water twice daily or 0.06mg capsules twice daily demonstrated symptom resolution within 36 hours.[71]

Case History

During the latter half of 1998, Sydney experienced a giardia outbreak due to a contamination of the water supply and children were the most affected. During that time many children were successfully treated with a similar protocol to the following:

Echinacea root blend	1:2	25 mL
Black walnut hulls	1:10	20 mL
Propolis	1:5	20 mL
Cranesbill	1:2	20 mL
Peppermint	1:2	20 mL
	Total	105 mL

The dose varied according to the child. However the common element was the frequency of doses. The formulation was taken with water or juice on an empty stomach 4 to 6 times a day, for 10 days. After a break of 10 days it was repeated for another 10 days. During that time not a single treatment was unsuccessful in removing symptoms.

Constipation

Constipation has been clinically defined as a delay or difficulty in defecation, which is present for two or more weeks and sufficient to cause significant stress to the patient.[72] As children age, normal physiological changes occur in the colon that decrease the daily stool number from a mean of 2.2 in infants younger that one year to a mean of 1.4 in one-to-three-year-old children.[73] Constipation in childhood is common, with reported prevalence ranging from 0.3 to 28%. It is more frequent when dietary fibre is lacking.[74] Amongst school age children, more boys than girls (3:1 ratio) suffer from constipation and this is usually of the functional type (see below).[74] Up to one third of children aged from 3 to 12 years will report constipation during any given year.[75]

Pathophysiology

Faecal continence is maintained by involuntary and voluntary muscle contraction. The internal anal sphincter has an involuntary resting tone that decreases when stool enters the rectum. The external anal sphincter is under voluntary control. The urge to defecate is triggered when the stool comes in contact with the mucosa of the lower rectum.[72,76] If a child does not wish to defecate, he or she can tighten the external anal sphincter and squeeze the gluteal muscles. This action can force the faeces higher in the rectal vault and reduce the urge to defecate. If a child frequently avoids defecating by using this technique, the rectum eventually stretches to accommodate the retained faecal mass and the propulsive power of the rectum is reduced.[72] The longer the faeces remain in the rectum the harder they become making defecation difficult and painful. The cycle of avoiding bowel movements because of the fear of painful defecation may progress to stool retention and infrequent bowel motions, a condition that is termed functional constipation.[72] As noted earlier, the majority of children (about 95%) over one year of age presenting with constipation have functional constipation.[72,74] However, when the warning signs are present, other causes of constipation must be considered. These include hypercalcaemia, hypothyroidism, gluten enteropathy, cystic fibrosis and lead toxicity.[72,76] Various medications such as opiates, phenobarbital and tricyclic antidepressants prescribed for children with developmental or behavioural disorders (such as mental retardation, autism, oppositional defiant disorder or depression) can also cause constipation.[72] Apart from a lack of fibre in the diet, cows milk intolerance is also associated with chronic constipation in children.[77]

Treatment Strategy

Bulk laxatives are first and foremost to be considered in the treatment of functional constipation in children. Remedies such as linseeds (flaxseed), slippery elm and psyllium aid in moistening and adding bulk to the stool, thereby facilitating defecation. Anthraquinone-type laxatives do have a role to play in the treatment of functional constipation in childhood and should not be dismissed outright. An appropriate dose of anthraquinone laxatives, usually in combination with carminatives, as a short term treatment will aid in softening the stool and facilitate the clearance of impacted faeces.[78] However, the age considerations noted in Chapter 1 should be observed for the stronger laxatives such as senna and cascara.

Example Treatments

Pour one cup of boiling water onto two teaspoons of chopped linseeds (flaxseed) and strain after 10 minutes. The child should drink one or two cups of this tea in the evening and in the morning if necessary.[79]

Alternatively slippery elm capsules (1 capsule 2 or 3 times a day) can be taken with meals and a glass of water. If the child cannot take capsules, then the dose can be emptied into water or juice.

For stubborn cases the following formulation may prove appropriate:

Dandelion root	1:2	20 mL
Butternut	1:2	25 mL
Yellow dock	1:2	20 mL
Chamomile	1:2	25 mL
Licorice	1:1	15 mL
	Total	105 mL

Extra yellow dock or dandelion root can be added if butternut is not available.

Dose: Calculate the standard dose (based on an adult dose of 5 mL) according to the most appropriate guideline in Chapter 1. To be taken with water or juice before meals 2 to 3 times a day.

An alternative to the above liquid formulation is Herbal Bowel Support tablets (adult dose for stubborn cases 2 to 6 tablets, depending on response, in the evening before bed). For milder cases Liver/Biliary Tonic tablets (adult dose 4 per day) can be tried. Calculate the child's tablet dose according to the most appropriate guideline in Chapter 1. For younger children the tablets can be crushed and mixed with honey or a suitable sweetener to improve compliance. See Appendix 1 for the suggested formulations for these tablets.

Rationale

The inclusion of dandelion is based on the traditional indication for constipation.[24] The mild laxative properties of dandelion root coupled with its gentle choleretic action will aid in the treatment of functional constipation. (Bile is a natural laxative). Butternut is a mild laxative useful for treating constipation in children where the bowel is sluggish.[60,78] Yellow dock is a mild laxative that contains low levels of anthraquinone glycosides and is indicated for sluggish bowel conditions.[24] Chamomile is included to provide spasmolytic activity to counteract the potential griping caused by anthraquinone type laxatives. It is also a relaxing nervine useful for tense children with contracted bowels.[78] Licorice rounds out the formulation as a mild laxative that provides some demulcent activity to soothe a tense bowel.[24]

An Additional Treatment

Probiotic supplementation is a useful additional strategy worthy of consideration. Two recent clinical trials have demonstrated a benefit for probiotics in chronic functional constipation in childhood. In a double blind, placebo-controlled comparative trial in 45 children under 10 years of age with chronic constipation, the probiotic (*Lactobacillus casei rhamnosus*) was found to be effective.[80] There was no significant statistical difference between the probiotic and magnesium oxide (the comparison treatment), however the probiotic group experienced less abdominal pain.[80] The second trial in 20 children (mean age 8 years) with chronic constipation demonstrated an efficacy for a mixed strain probiotic containing both *Bifidobacteria* and *Lactobacillus spp*. There was also a significant decrease in abdominal pain.[81]

Case History

An 8-year-old male presented with chronic constipation of several years' standing. After taking a diet history it was little wonder the child was constipated, with an abundance of processed foods in the diet which was also low in plant fibre. The mother was counselled over the plant fibre issue and an agreement was reached where no baked processed flour products would come into the home. More seasonal fruit and vegetables were to be consumed and the child was not to be offered other alternatives. Cheese was also removed, but a concession was made for milk. The following herbal formulation was prescribed:

Dandelion root	1:2	25 mL
Butternut	1:2	25 mL
Rhubarb root	1:2	25 mL
Chamomile	1:2	25 mL
	Total	100 mL

Dose: 2 mL with juice after the evening meal and 4 mL before bed.

Within several days the stool had softened to the point that it was not as difficult for the child to defecate. After 10 days the dose was reduced to the single 4 mL dose before bed. The dietary changes proved difficult, however over time and with assistance, a transition to a better diet with increased plant fibre was accomplished. The child took the formulation for approximately six weeks, without complaint. Once there were good signs that the bowel had relaxed and some tone was restored, the medicine was withdrawn without any adverse effects or return to constipation.

Diarrhoea

The guidelines outlined in the appropriate section in Chapter 2 can be followed.

References

1   Mills S, Bone K. *Principles and Practice of Phytotherapy: Modern Herbal Medicine.* Churchill Livingstone, Edinburgh, 2000
2   Ouweland A, Isolauri E, Salminen S. *Eur J Nutr* 2002; **41**(5): 32-37
3   Mayer L. *Pediatrics* 2003; **111**(6): 1595-1600
4   Guarner F. *Digestion* 2006; **73**(Suppl 1): 5-12
5   Cummings JH, Antoine JM, Azpiroz F et al. *Eur J Nutr* 2004; **43**(Suppl 2): 118-173
6   Bjarnason I, Takeuchi K, Bjarnason A et al. *Scand J Gastroenterol* 2004; **39**(9): 807-815
7   Liu Z, Li N, Neu J. *Acta Pediatrica* 2005; **94**(4): 386-393
8   Berkes J, Viswanathan VK, Savkovic SD et al. *Gut* 2003; **52**(3): 439-451
9   Bosi E, Molteni L, Radaelli MG et al. *Diabetologia* 2006; **49**(12): 2824-2827
10 Sapone A, de Magistris L, Pietzak M et al. *Diabetes* 2006; **55**(5): 1443-1449
11 Benard A, Desreumeaux P, Huglo D et al. *J Allergy Clin Immunol* 1996; **97**(6): 1173-1178
12 Hijazi Z, Molla AM, Al-Habashi H et al. *Arch Dis Child* 2004; **89**(3): 227-229
13 Caffarelli C, Cavagni G, Menzies IS et al. *Clin Exp Allergy* 1993; **23**(1): 28-31
14 Rosenfeldt V, Benfeldt E, Valerius NH et al. *J Pediatr* 2004; **145**(5): 615-616
15 Nazli A, Wang A, Steen O et al. *Infect Immunol* 2006; **74**(1): 192-201
16 Alm JS, Swartz J, Bjorksten B et al. *Pediatr Allergy Immunol* 2002; **13**(6): 402-411
17 Brismar B, Edlund C, Nord CE. *Eur J Clin Microbiol Infect Dis* 1993; **12**(9): 714-719
18 Treinen-Moslen M, Kanz MF. *Pharmacol Ther* 2006; **112**(3): 649-667
19 Bjorksten B, Naaber P, Sepp E, Mikelsaar M. *Clin Exp Allergy* 1999; **29**(3): 342-346
20 He F, Ouwehand AC, Isolauri E et al. *FEMS Immunol Med Microbiol* 2001; **30**(1): 43-47
21 Rasquin-Weber A, Hyman PE, Cucchiara S et al. *Gut* 1999; **45**(Suppl II): 1160-1168
22 Hyman PE, Danda CE. *Pediatr Annals* 2004; **33**(2): 97-104
23 Schilcher H. *Phytotherapy in Paediatrics.* Medpharm Scientific Publishers, Stuttgart, 1997.
24 Bone K. *A Clinical Guide to Blending Liquid Herbs.* Churchill Livingstone, Edinburgh, 2003.
25 Pitman T, Bennett H. *Today's Parent* 1998; 15(1): 74-75
26 Chatoor I, Surles J, Ganiban J et al. *Pediatrics* 2004; **113**(5): 440-447
27 Scott J, Barlow T. *Herbs in the Treatment of Children.* Churchill Livingston, Edinburgh, 2003.
28 Bensky D, Gamble A. *Chinese Herbal Medicine Materia Medica.* Eastland Press, Seattle, 1986.
29 Plunkett A, Beattie RM. *J Roy Soc Med* 2005; **98**(3): 101-106
30 Starfield B, Hoekelman R, McCormack M. *Pediatrics* 1984; **74**(6): 991-997
31 Scholl J, Allen PJ. *Pediatr Nurs* 2007; **33**(3): 247-259
32 Subcommittee on Chronic Abdominal Pain. *Pediatrics* 2005; **115**(3): 370-381
33 Rasquin A, Di Lorenzo C, Forbes D et al. *Gastroenterology* 2006; **130**(5): 1527-1537
34 Clouse R, Mayer E, Aziz Q et al. *Gastroenterology* 2006; **130**(5): 1492-1497
35 Drossman D. *Gastroenterology* 2006; **130**(5): 1377-1390
36 Saps M, Li B. *Pediatr Annals* 2006; **35**(4): 246-256
37 Jones M, Dilley J, Drossman D et al. *Neurogastroenterol Motil* 2006; **18**(2): 91-103
38 Wood JD. *World J Gastrointesterol* 2007; **13**(9): 1313-1332
39 Duarte M, Goulart E, Penna F. *Gastroenterol Nutr* 2000; **31**(3): 280-285
40 Di Lorenzo C, Youssef N, Sigurdsson L et al. *J Pediatr* 2001; **139**(6): 838-843
41 Crushell E, Rowland M, Doherty M et al. *Pediatrics* 2003; **112**(6): 1368-1372
42 Chitkara DK, Delgado-Aros S, Bredenoord AJ et al. *J Pediatr* 2003; **143**(5): 609-613

43 Friesen CA, Lin Z, Hyman PE et al. *J Pediatr Gastroenterol Nutr* 2006; **42**(3): 265-269
44 Kline RM, Kline JJ, Di Palma J et al. *J Pediatr* 2001; **138**(1): 125-128
45 Marklund B, Ahlstedt S, Nordstrom G. *Health Qual Life Outcomes* 2006; **4**: 48
46 Ferreira CT, Seidman E. *J Pediatr (Rio J)* 2007; **83**(1): 7-20
47 Young E, Stoneham MD, Petruckevitch A et al. *Lancet* 1994; **343**(8906): 1127-1130
48 Sampson HA. *Allergy* 2005; **60**(Suppl 79): 19-24
49 Sicherer SH. *Lancet* 2002; **360**(9334): 701-710
50 Allen KJ, Hill DJ, Heine RG. *MJA* 2006; **185**(7): 394-400
51 Ortolani C, Ispano M, Pastorello EA et al. *J Allergy Clin Immunol* 1999; **83**(3): 683-690
52 Kelly D, Coutts AGP. *Proc Nutr Soc* 2000; **59**(2): 177-185
53 Isolauri E, Sutas Y, Kankaanpaa P et al. *Am J Clin Nutr* 2001; **72**(Suppl 2): 444S-450S
54 Hanaway P. *Alt Ther Health Med* 2006; **12**(5): 52-60
55 Kucik CJ, Martin GL, Sortor BV. *Am Fam Physician* 2004; **69**(5): 1161-1168
56 Awasthi S, Bundy DAP, Savioli L. *BMJ* 2003; **327**(7412): 431-433
57 Felter HW, Lloyd JU. *King's American Dispensatory*. 18th Ed, 3rd revision, Volume 1. First published 1905, reprinted Eclectic Medical Publications, Portland, 1983.
58 Fetterer RH, Fleming MW. *Comp Biochem Physiol C* 1991; **100**(3): 539-342
59 Bone K, Morgan M. *Mod Phytother* 2003; **7**(2): 13-19
60 Bone K. *The Ultimate Herbal Compendium*. Phytotherapy Press, Warwick, Qld, 2007
61 Eckmann L, Gillin FD. *Am J Physiol Gastrointest Liver Physiol* 2001; **280**(1): G1-G6
62 Hawrelak J. *Alt Med Rev* 2003; **8**(2): 129-142
63 Ang LH. *Commun Dis Public Health* 2000; **3**(3): 212-213
64 Adam RD. *Clin Microbiol Rev* 2001; **14**(3): 447-475
65 Mills S, Bone K. *Principles and Practice of Phytotherapy: Modern Herbal Medicine*. Churchill Livingstone, Edinburgh, 2000, pp. 499, 500.
66 Miyares C, Hollands I, Castaneda C et al. *Acta Gastroenterol Latinoam* 1988; **18**(3): 195-201
67 Kaneda Y, Tanaka T, Saw T. *Tokai J Exp Clin Med* 1991; **15**(6): 417-423
68 Kaneda Y, Torii M, Tanaka T et al. *Ann Trop Med Parasitol* 1991; **85**(4): 417-425
69 Choudhry VP, Sabir M, Bhide VN. *Indian Pediatr* 1972; **9**(3): 143-146
70 Vidal F, Vidal JC, Gadelha AP et al. *Exp Parasitol* 2006; **115**(1): 25-31
71 Soffar SA, Mokhtar GM. *J Egypt Soc Parasitol* 1991; **21**(2): 497-502
72 Biggs WS, Dery WH. *Am Fam Physician* 2006; **73**(3): 469-477
73 Baker SS, Liptak GS, Colletti RB et al. *J Pediatr Gastroenterol Nutr* 1999; **29**(5): 612-626
74 Catto-Smith AG. *MJA* 2005; **182**(5): 242-246
75 Rubin G. *Clin Evid* 2004; **11**: 385-390
76 Croffie JM. *Ind J Pediatr* 2006; **73**(8): 697-701
77 Iacono G, Cavataio F, Montalto G et al. *NEJM* 1998; **339**(16): 1100-1104
78 McIntyre A. *Herbal Treatment of Children* Elsevier, Edinburgh, 2005.
79 Weiss RF, Fintelmann V. *Herbal Medicine* 2nd Ed, Thieme, Stuttgart, 2000.
80 Bu LN, Chang MH, Ni YH et al. *Pediatr Int* 2007; **49**(4): 485-490
81 Bekkali N, Bongers ME, Van den Berg MM et al. *Nutr J* 2007; **6**(1): 17 [Epub ahead of print]

CHAPTER 6

Common Respiratory Disorders in Children

Introduction

INFANTS AND CHILDREN ARE particularly prone to respiratory problems. The respiratory tract is not fully developed at birth, only reaching functional maturity at approximately 6 years of age.[1] For example, the number of alveoli increases from 24 million at birth to 257 million by age 4.[1] There are good physiological and anatomical reasons why infants are less able to cope with stress placed on the respiratory system. The processes of early growth and development demand a high basal metabolic rate, which translates into an increased requirement for oxygen.[2] On a body weight basis oxygen consumption is 2 to 3 times higher for a child than an adult. So the normal resting state in infants is one characterised by high respiratory and cardiovascular activities.[2]

Infants are obligatory nose breathers until 3 to 4 months of age, due to the configuration of the upper airways and a relatively large tongue that occupies most of the oropharynx.[2,3] This configuration of the upper airways changes with growth. The larynx and hydatid bone move down the posterior portion of the tongue, facilitating buccal respiration and the development of speech.[3] The eustachian tube is short and straight and closely communicates with the ear, placing the infant at a greater risk of middle ear infections.[3] The outcomes of the early growth and development of respiratory tissue are important for the future health of the child. Exposure at this time to noxious influences such as air pollution may have lasting deleterious effects on respiratory health.[1] Such an impact should not be underestimated, as it is now thought that 40% or more of the environmental burden of disease falls on children under 5 years of age.[4]

At the same time as the respiratory system is developing, the child's immune system, also immature at birth, is beginning to develop. This also accounts for the high incidence of respiratory tract infections in infants.[1]

Herbs for the Respiratory System

The materia medica for respiratory tract disorders has been reviewed elsewhere. Since this information is also relevant to paediatrics, readers are directed to that text for more detailed information.[5] Most acute and chronic respiratory paediatric diseases are associated with retained airway secretions. They are in turn due to increased production of a viscous mucus, impaired mucociliary transport and/or a weak cough.[6] Hence herbs that modulate mucus production and consistency and increase mucociliary transport such as eyebright, aniseed, cinnamon, fennel and thyme will feature prominently in treatments. As many respiratory tract infections are associated with a bacterial influence, respiratory antimicrobials such as thyme (again) and elecampane in conjunction with immune modulators such as Echinacea and Andrographis are also relevant. Diaphoretics will also be indicated during the acute phase of respiratory infections.

The major actions for the respiratory system and the corresponding herbs are listed below. Some herbs may fall into several categories. This is either a result of the fact that they contain several active components and/or the fact that a group of active components can act in several different ways. For example, mullein contains saponins which are expectorant, mucilage which is demulcent and iridoids which are anticatarrhal. So although mullein will be mainly viewed as an anticatarrhal herb in this therapeutics section, its other actions also reinforce its value as a therapy.

Expectorants

- Expectorants facilitate the removal of secretions from the lungs
- Major expectorant herbs include fennel, anise, elecampane, white horehound, senega and Grindelia. *Pelargonium sidoides* is particularly useful for children

Respiratory Demulcents

- These herbs contain mucilage and have a soothing and anti-inflammatory action mainly on the lower respiratory mucosa (lungs, trachea and pharynx)
- The major respiratory demulcent herbs are marshmallow root or leaves and slippery elm, but also include Irish moss

Respiratory Spasmolytics

- Respiratory spasmolytics relax the bronchioles of the lungs
- These include elecampane, thyme, Grindelia, Euphorbia, Coleus and licorice

Anticatarrhals

Anticatarrhal herbs have the following beneficial properties:

- They reduce excessive discharge from mucous membranes. This discharge may vary from clear and thin to thick and yellowish depending on the condition
- They decrease airways hypersensitivity
- They can also decrease nasal congestion and mucosal oedema
- Anticatarrhal herbs for the upper respiratory tract include eyebright, ribwort, elder, peppermint, ground ivy and golden seal. Golden seal is particularly indicated where there is copious yellow to green discharge of a chronic nature. Golden rod may also fit into this category
- Anticatarrhal herbs for the lower respiratory tract include mullein and ribwort

- Sage has a general drying effect on bodily secretions including the mucous membranes and may be indicated where secretions are particularly copious and watery

Respiratory Antiseptics

- Respiratory antiseptics provide a weak antimicrobial action which can assist to resolve or control a bacterial or fungal infection in conjunction with other treatments and the body's innate defences
- The main respiratory antiseptic herbs include thyme, elecampane, *Pelargonium sidoides* and garlic. Inhalations based on tea tree and Eucalyptus oils also come under this category

Antitussives

- Antitussives allay cough, either through soothing (demulcents) or removing (expectorants) the irritation, or depressing the cough reflex
- Antitussive herbs therefore include anticatarrhals, expectorants and demulcents together with wild cherry, sundew, licorice and hops
- In treating cough, the source of the irritation should always be located. If the cough is coming from a sore throat and there is no lung involvement, it is pointless to give expectorants. A demulcent gargle or lozenge is indicated, together with appropriate treatment of the source of the sore throat

Antiallergic Herbs

The principal antiallergic herbs for respiratory tract allergies are Albizia and Baical skullcap. Nettles is another herb with antiallergic properties which can sometimes be useful, especially for allergic rhinitis

Mucolytics

- Mucolytic herbs decrease the viscosity of mucus by decreasing the effectiveness of its structural elements (mainly mucopolysaccharides). They mainly include sulphur-containing herbs such as onions, garlic and horseradish
- The mucolytic action probably explains the popularity of garlic and horseradish tablets for the treatment of rhinitis and sinusitis. However, this approach on its own is only superficial and symptomatic

Mucous Membranes Trophorestoratives

- The main herb in this category is golden seal. Its use is believed to restore the healthy function of mucous membranes

Pelargonium sidoides: An Important Children's Respiratory Herb

A relatively "new" and clinically proven herb for children's respiratory disorders is *Pelargonium sidoides*. Of course this herb is only new to the English-speaking world. The tincture has been used for decades in Europe and it is a traditional African herb.

The use of the root of this plant was originally introduced into Europe in the early 20th century by Charles Henry Stevens as a cure for tuberculosis. Stevens had been successfully treated for this disorder in Africa by a traditional Zulu medicine man. For a long time it was known under the mysterious names of "Stevens Cure" and "umckaloabo" before its true botanical identity was revealed in only 1974.[7]

In the 1920s, the Swiss doctor Seehehaye treated around 800 tuberculosis patients over a period of 9 years. Successful outcomes were reported, culminating in the publication of 64 case histories.[7] In the 1950s and onwards in Germany, the herb became popular for the treatment of respiratory conditions and appeared to be particularly suitable for children. More recently its value for adults (as originally promoted by Stevens) has been established in clinical trials.[7]

There is considerable clinical evidence for the value of this herb in acute bronchitis. A recent systematic review of 6 randomised, double blind, controlled trials found that the methodology of the trials was generally good.[8] Meta-analysis of the 4 placebo-controlled trials suggested that *Pelargonium sidoides* had significantly reduced bronchitis symptoms scores by day 7 in patients with acute bronchitis.[8]

Recently an open, post-marketing surveillance study in children aged less than 12 years was undertaken in Germany.[9] Children up to 2-years-old with acute bronchitis were treated with *Pelargonium sidoides* tincture at 5 drops three times a day (TDS). The dose was higher for older children, with those over age 6 receiving 20 drops TDS. The children were evaluated initially and after 7 and 14 days of herbal treatment. Results for 742 children indicated a significant decrease (p<0.001) in bronchitis-specific symptoms over the time course of the treatment. Treatment with the herb was deemed effective by the supervising doctors in 88.3% of cases. Adverse events were minor and transitory in nature.

The benefits of *Pelargonium sidoides* in children extend to infections of the upper respiratory tract. There are several clinical trials of *Pelargonium sidoides* in acute tonsillopharyngitis in children.[10] For example one trial from the Ukraine examined the efficacy of the tincture in 143 children aged 6 to 10 years with acute non-group A β-haemolytic streptococcus (non-GABHS) tonsillopharyngitis.[11] A randomised, double blind, placebo-controlled design was used and treatment outcomes were assessed according to a tonsillopharyngitis severity score (TSS). The decrease in TSS from baseline to day 4 of treatment was 7.1±2.1 points in the Pelargonium group compared to only 2.5±3.6 for placebo. This finding was statistically significant (p<0.0001). Adverse events were mild and not considered to be related to the treatment.

Randomised, double blind, placebo-controlled trials in adults have also proven the efficacy of *Pelargonium sidoides* in the management of acute bacterial maxillary sinusitis and the common cold.[12,13] These applications would also apply to children, since the herb has been shown to be safe in children of all ages in the trials described above.

The Common Cold and Influenza

The common cold is the conventional term for a mild upper respiratory tract illness characterised by nasal stuffiness and discharge, sneezing, sore throat and cough.[14] Although the illness is usually self-limiting, it can predispose to bacterial complications.[14] Influenza is typically regarded as a disease entity separate from the common cold. However, the clinical presentation can be similar to the common cold, where the only difference is often the severity of symptoms and the myalgia, a typical influenza symptom.[14]

Epidemiology

The occurrence of the common cold shows a clear seasonality. In temperate regions the frequency of respiratory tract infections (RTIs) increases rapidly in autumn (fall), remains high throughout winter and decreases in spring. In tropical regions, most colds arise during the rainy season.[14]

On average infants have 6 to 8 RTIs per year, whilst adults have 2 to 3 per year.[15,16] During the first years of life it appears that boys have more RTIs than girls, a trend that is reversed later in life.[17] Day care facility attendance is a major risk factor for RTIs in children and the frequency of infection increases with the number of children in the group.[18,19] It has been suggested that those children who suffer more frequent RTIs are more likely to also have intestinal dysbiosis and respiratory allergic disorders.[20]

Although the terms "common cold" and "influenza" respectively imply that there is a single cause for each illness, RTIs are caused by numerous viruses belonging to several different families. Rhinoviruses comprise over 100 different serotypes and are the most common cause of RTIs in all age groups, followed by parainfluenza virus, respiratory syncytial virus, adenovirus and enteroviruses.[14]

Pathogenesis

The pathogenesis of the common cold involves a complex interplay between the host's inflammatory response and the replicating virus. The primary site of replication for the parainfluenza virus is in the tracheobronchial epithelium,[21] whereas rhinovirus replication occurs primarily in the nasopharynx.[22]

Viral infection of the nasal mucosa results in vasodilation and increased vascular permeability, which in turn causes nasal obstruction and rhinorrhoea, the primary clinical symptoms of the common cold.[14] Tracheal neurons form an airways intrinsic nervous system that help to control mucous gland secretion. Under the influence of the various viruses that impact the respiratory system, these neurons secrete vasoactive intestinal peptide (VIP). VIP acts as a powerful secretagogue, inducing an increase in mucus production.[23]

Viral infection of the upper respiratory tract in children often causes dysfunction of the eustachian tube, an important factor in the pathogenesis of acute otitis media.[24]

PATHOGENS ASSOCIATED WITH THE COMMON COLD[25]

Association	Pathogen	Relative frequency of infections caused by the agent
Agents primarily associated with the common cold	Rhinovirus	Frequent
	Coronavirus	Occasional
Agents primarily involved with other clinical syndromes that also cause common cold symptoms	Respiratory syncytial virus	Occasional
	Human metapneumovirus	Occasional
	Influenza virus	Uncommon
	Parainfluenza virus	Uncommon
	Adenovirus	Uncommon
	Enterovirus	Uncommon
	Bocavirus	Uncommon

Clinical Manifestation and Complications

Rhinovirus infections typically start with a sore or "scratchy" throat, which is soon accompanied by nasal stuffiness and discharge and sneezing.[14] The soreness of the throat usually decreases over 2 or 3 days, while the initial watery secretions turn thicker and more purulent.[26] Surprisingly, it has been found that the purulence of the nasal discharge is not associated with changes in the nasopharyngeal bacterial flora and is therefore not considered indicative of a secondary bacterial infection.[27,28] Fever is a frequent finding in children, along with headache and malaise.[14] Cough is associated with approximately 30% of colds and usually begins after the onset of the nasal symptoms.[21]

Although the common cold is usually a self-limiting illness of short duration, it is sometimes accompanied by a secondary bacterial complication. Acute otitis media is the most common complication and affects approximately 20% of children with viral upper respiratory tract infections.[29,30] Sinusitis is another bacterial complication of the common cold.[14] A self-limiting sinus inflammation is part of the pathophysiology of the common cold, however 5 to 13% of children will experience an acute bacterial sinusitis complication, a frequency much greater than in adults (0.5 to 2%).[21] Differentiation of the common cold from bacterial sinusitis is difficult. A diagnosis of bacterial sinusitis should be considered if rhinorrhoea or daytime cough persists without improvement for at least 10 to 14 days, or if signs of more severe sinus involvement are present, such as fever, sinus or facial pain or facial swelling.[21] The exacerbation of asthma is a potentially serious complication of colds: the majority of asthma exacerbations occur as a result of the common cold.[21,31,32]

Although not a complication, another unfortunate consequence of the common cold is the inappropriate use of antibiotics for these illnesses and the associated contribution to the problem of antibiotic resistance.[21] Systematic reviews have shown that antibiotics have no role in the treatment of the common cold.[31,32] Despite this information, it is estimated that 30% of visits to primary care clinics for the common cold result in the inappropriate prescription of antibiotics.[21]

Herbal Treatment

The herbal treatments of the common cold and influenza follow a similar pattern. However, in the case of more severe forms of influenza, treatment should be more vigorous in terms of amount and frequency of dose.[5] The use of St John's wort as an antiviral agent should be considered in these circumstances.

Diaphoretics are the cornerstone of the treatment of acute RTIs characterised by fever. Guidelines for the use of diaphoretics were provided in Chapter 3 and are relevant here. These agents include peppermint, yarrow, lime flowers and elder. They work best when administered as a hot tea and in conjunction with ginger as a diffusive stimulant. Pleurisy root is indicated if there are pulmonary or bronchial complications. Chamomile is also a good diaphoretic for children.

Other essential aspects of treatment are as follows:

- Immune-enhancing herbs such as Echinacea and Andrographis to support the body's fight against the virus. Note that Astragalus and tonics such as Korean ginseng are contraindicated in the acute stage of infection
- Anticatarrhal herbs for upper respiratory catarrh, especially eyebright, elder flowers and golden seal. Traditionally, golden seal was said to be contraindicated in the acute stage of infection. So its use may be best in the later stages of any secondary bacterial infection. Also garlic, because of its mucolytic and possible antiviral properties, can be a useful treatment if the child is old enough
- St John's wort as an antiviral treatment for influenza

Since these are acute disorders, dosages should be high and often.

Diaphoretic Formulation

Yarrow	1:2	40 mL
Elder flowers	1:2	40 mL
Peppermint	1:2	20 mL
	Total	100 mL

Dose: Calculate the standard dose according to the most appropriate guideline in Chapter 1, using the adult dose of 5 mL. The dose is diluted with approximately 25 to 50 mL of warm to hot water and sipped by the child. Up to 5 or 6 doses can be taken in one day.

Example Liquid Formulation for RTIs Affecting the Upper Respiratory System

The following formulation contains diaphoretics, therefore a separate diaphoretic treatment like the one described above is not necessary.

Echinacea root blend	1:2	35 mL
Golden rod 1:2 or Pelargonium	1:5	20 mL
Elder flowers or Eyebright	1:2	20 mL
Lime flowers or Chamomile	1:2	20 mL
Peppermint or Cinnamon	1:2	10 mL
	Total	105 mL

Dose: Calculate the standard dose according to the most appropriate guideline in Chapter 1, using the adult dose of 5 mL. Up to 5 or 6 doses can be taken in one day, in warm to hot water as previously described.

An alternative to the above diaphoretic and immune formulation is the combined Immune/ Diaphoretic Liquid formulation (adult dose 5 mL, see Appendix 1) containing *Echinacea angustifolia* root, elder flowers, lime flowers, yarrow, ginger and licorice. Calculate the standard dose for the child according to the most appropriate guideline in Chapter 1. The dose can be diluted in approximately 25 to 50 mL of warm to hot water and sipped. Up to 5 or 6 doses can be taken in one day while fever is present.

Alternative Tablet Formulations

For the older child or the younger one who will not take liquids, herbal tablets or capsules may provide a useful alternative.

Providing only immune support during an infection can be highly effective and a good suggested combination is one based on Andrographis, Echinacea and holy basil. See the Short Term Immune Support formulation in Appendix 1. Calculate the child's dose (based on an acute adult dose of 4 to 6 tablets per day) according to the most appropriate guideline in Chapter 1. These can be supplemented with extra Echinacea Formula tablets (see Appendix 1) based on an adult dose of 2 to 3 per day. For younger children the tablets (or part thereof) can be crushed and mixed with honey or a suitable sweetener to improve compliance.

Example Liquid Formulation for RTIs Affecting the Lower Respiratory System Characterised by Unproductive Cough and Fever

Echinacea root blend	1:2	35 mL
Thyme	1:2	15 mL
Grindelia	1:2	15 mL
Marshmallow root	1:5	20 mL
Pleurisy root or Chamomile	1:2	23 mL
Ginger	1:2	2 mL
	Total	110 mL

Dose: Calculate the standard dose according to the most appropriate guideline in Chapter 1, using the adult dose of 5 mL. Up to 5 or 6 doses can be taken in one day in warm to hot water as previously described.

An alternative to the above liquid formulation for RTIs affecting the lower respiratory system is the Short Term Lower Respiratory Support Liquid (standard adult dose 5 mL, see Appendix 1) containing *Echinacea angustifolia* root, licorice, pleurisy root, thyme, ginger and white horehound. Calculate the standard dose for the child according to the most appropriate guideline in Chapter 1. This dose can be diluted in approximately 25 to 50 mL of warm to hot water and sipped. Up to 5 or 6 doses can be taken in one day while fever is present.

Alternatively the Short Term Immune Support tablets can be prescribed, possibly with Echinacea Formula tablets, as noted above.

Decongestant Topical Preparation

Natural cream base	45 g
Eucalyptus essential oil	1 mL
Tea tree essential oil	1 mL
Essential oil solubiliser	4 mL

Directions: Blend the essential oils with the essential oil solubiliser and then simply blend into the natural cream base, using suitable sterile equipment. The cream base should be an aqueous cream. Therefore in order to blend lipid-soluble essential oils into such a base in the quantities described, the use of an essential oil solubiliser is advised, as noted above.

The decongestant cream is used in a similar manner to any proprietary vapour rub. However, it provides an alternative topical preparation that is not based on paraffins. An alternate base of laponite gel (clay gel) can also be used. Laponite gel readily takes up essential oils without the use of a solubiliser. The cream or gel applied to the chest and thoracic regions especially at night before bed provides anticatarrhal and anti-infective vapours that complement the oral herbal medicines, hastening the road to recovery.

Clinical experience of the authors has demonstrated the value of topical essential oils used in the manner described above.

Rationale for the Formulations

The use of Echinacea is based on its immune supporting activity and the traditional indication for preventing and treating URTIs.[33] Although the weight of scientific evidence for the use of Echinacea in the treatment and prevention of URTIs in adults is positive, it is less so for children.[34] Nonetheless, clinical experience suggests a key role for Echinacea root in children. Golden rod, eyebright and elder flowers provide an anticatarrhal action that relieves the mucus buildup that characterises upper RTIs. As well, elder flowers provide diaphoretic activity to aid in the management of fever.[33] Further diaphoretic activity is contributed by the lime flowers or chamomile and peppermint, or pleurisy root supported by ginger, with the added benefit that lime flowers or chamomile will provide a mild sedative activity in those cases where nervous system agitation arises as a result of the RTI. Grindelia in the formulation for the lower respiratory tract provides expectorant and bronchospasmolytic activities. Thyme provides these activities as well but also provides expectorant and antimicrobial activities. The marshmallow root is a demulcent to soothe the cough. Cinnamon is traditionally indicated for the common cold and influenza and there is clinical evidence noted previously to support the use of Pelargonium.

Case History

A 7-year-old female presented with a history of repeated lower respiratory tract infections. The child had constantly congested mucous membranes, particularly in the lower respiratory tract and a persistent cough but with no evidence of wheeze. Other relevant issues were a history of antibiotic use and the child appeared thin and devitalised. At the time of presentation the child was free of infection.

The following formulation was prescribed:

Echinacea root blend	1:2	40 mL
Thyme	1:2	20 mL
Grindelia	1:2	20 mL
Marshmallow root glycetract	1:5	20 mL
	Total	100 mL

Dose: 3 mL with water three times a day, with instructions to increase the dose to 5 times a day should the child contract an RTI.

A decongestant gel was also dispensed that included eucalyptus oil, lemon scented tea tree oil and the essential oil of *Melaleuca ericifolia*. The gel was applied to the chest and back before bed.

Dietary instruction included the elimination of dairy products and processed wheat products, and a probiotic was prescribed.

This protocol did not alter over the course of treatment. The catarrhal congestion of the mucous membranes and the cough were fully resolved after 4 weeks of treatment. The child suffered only one RTI during the following winter.

Bacterial Sinusitis

The developmental immaturity of the sinuses places infants at greater risk of sinus inflection, as evidenced by the statistics quoted previously. Both the ethmoid and maxillary sinuses are present at birth, but only the ethmoid sinuses are pneumatised (have air-filled cavities).[21,35] The maxillary sinuses are not pneumatised until 4 years of age. The sphenoidal sinuses are present by 5 years of age, whereas the frontal sinuses only begin development at age 7 to 8 years and are not completely developed until adolescence.[21,35]

As previously noted, acute bacterial sinusitis (ABS) usually follows a viral upper RTI. The bacterial pathogens typically associated with ABS are *Streptococcus pneumoniae*, *Haemophilus influenzae* and *Moraxella catarrhalis*.[21,35] Forceful nose blowing has been shown to generate enough force to propel nasal secretions into the sinus cavities.[21] Bacteria from the nasopharynx that enter the sinuses are normally readily cleared. However, inflammation and oedema during viral rhinosinusitis may block sinus drainage and impair mucociliary clearance.[21] These are favourable conditions for the growth of bacteria.

Herbal Treatment

Diaphoretic herbs are essential if fever is present. Otherwise the use of immune supporting, anticatarrhal and mucolytic herbs is recommended.

Example Liquid Formulation

Echinacea root blend	1:2	40 mL
Eyebright	1:2	30 mL
Golden seal 1:3 or Pelargonium	1:5	20 mL
Ribwort or additional Eyebright	1:2	20 mL
	Total	110 mL

Dose: Calculate the standard dose according to the most appropriate guideline in Chapter 1, using the adult dose of 5 mL. Up to 5 doses can be taken with water in one day.

There may be compliance issues due to the presence of golden seal. If this is the case, use the concept of blending the herbal mixture with jelly as discussed in Chapter 1. Alternatively, *Pelargonium sidoides* is a useful substitute as noted.

Rationale for the Herbal Treatment

Echinacea is for immune support. Eyebright is considered to be the most important anticatarrhal remedy for nasal catarrh and sinusitis.[36] This herb can be supported in this activity by ribwort. Golden seal is prescribed along traditional lines and is considered a specific remedy for inflammations of the mucous membranes, particularly when accompanied by catarrh.[33] It would be most relevant if the sinusitis is subacute or chronic. Elder flowers could be used instead, especially for acute sinusitis accompanied by fever, as can *Pelargonium sidoides*.

Example Tablet Formulations

An alternative to the above liquid formulation is Upper Respiratory Tract Support tablets containing *Echinacea purpurea* root, eyebright, golden rod, golden seal and cayenne (see Appendix 1). Calculate the child's dose (based on an acute adult dose of 6 tablets per day) according to the most appropriate guideline in Chapter 1. These can be supplemented with extra Short Term Immune Support tablets (see Appendix 1) based on an adult dose of 4 per day. For younger children the tablets (or part thereof) can be crushed and mixed with honey or a suitable sweetener to improve compliance.

Essential Oil Inhalation

A key to treating acute bacterial sinusitis is the use of essential oil inhalation. Clinical experience has demonstrated that the most effective apparatus is an aerosol diffuser. Undiluted essential oils such as tea tree oil or eucalyptus oil are placed in an aerosol diffuser and positioned in the bedroom overnight. The vapours from the diffuser can also be inhaled through the nose for several minutes three times during the day.

Tonsillopharyngitis

Approximately one third of upper RTIs in children feature a sore throat as the primary symptom.[21] The agents most frequently associated with tonsillopharyngitis are the viruses that typically cause respiratory tract infections.[37] It can occasionally be caused by Epstein-Barr virus, herpes simplex virus or cytomegalovirus.[21] However, a most important source of concern is bacterial infection with group A β-haemolytic *Streptococcus* (GABHS) such as *Streptococcus pyogenes*, which can progress to acute rheumatic fever.[37] Effective treatment of GABHS tonsillopharyngitis with penicillin has been seen to reduce the risk of rheumatic fever by approximately 90%.[38] Studies demonstrate that GABHS remains present in the throat after antibiotic treatment in approximately 10% of cases.[38] The association of GABHS tonsillopharyngitis with rheumatic fever is thought to be via molecular mimicry. The accepted theory is that, after an apparent recovery, the host initiates an inappropriate autoimmune response against a number of streptococcal degradation products that exhibit a molecular mimicry with host tissue. The tissues are thereby damaged by an immunological cross reaction. The three tissues commonly involved are the heart, the joints and the central nervous system.[38]

GABHS tonsillopharyngitis is uncommon in children under 3 years of age, as is rheumatic fever.[37] Children between the ages of 5 to 15 years are more commonly impacted.[37]

Scarlet fever, the upper RTI with characteristic skin rash, is also associated with a group A streptococcus.[21,37] It is now uncommon and less virulent than in the past.[21]

Clinical Manifestations

The onset of streptococcal tonsillopharyngitis is often rapid and is characterised by a sore throat and an absence of cough and fever. Headache and gastrointestinal symptoms such as abdominal pain and vomiting are frequent. The pharynx is red and the tonsils are enlarged and covered with yellow blood-tinged exudates. There may be petechiae or 'doughnut' lesions on the soft palate and posterior pharynx and uvula may be red, stippled and swollen. The anterior cervical lymph nodes are enlarged and tender.[21,37] Some patients may have the additional stigmata of scarlet fever, which include a red, fine papular rash that feels like sand paper and resembles sunburn with goose bumps, and a strawberry tongue.[21]

The onset of viral tonsillopharyngitis is usually more gradual and symptoms typically include rhinorrhoea, cough and occasionally diarrhoea. A viral aetiology is suggested by the presence of conjunctivitis, coryza, hoarseness and cough.[21]

Herbal Treatment

The main aspects of treatment are:

- Immune-enhancing herbs. If a chronic condition, Astragalus may be considered otherwise Echinacea and Andrographis are key. Echinacea is best taken as a liquid to obtain a local effect on the throat. *Pelargonium sidoides* should also be considered in this context

- Diaphoretic herbs if fever is present, such as YEP

- Anticatarrhal herbs such as eyebright and golden seal. The golden seal can also work locally as an antiseptic (either by taking it in liquid form or chewing the occasional tablet)

- Lymphatic and depurative herbs are particularly indicated in tonsillitis and these include Echinacea, poke root, clivers, burdock and Baptisia

- A local treatment such as a throat spray or lozenge using herbs such as:
  - Sage – astringent and antiseptic to the mucous membranes
  - Clove oil – local anaesthetic to provide a soothing effect
  - Echinacea – immune-enhancing, anti-inflammatory
  - Marshmallow root – demulcent and soothing to the inflamed throat
  - Myrrh – vulnerary and antiseptic, induces local leucocytosis
  - Propolis – vulnerary and antiseptic

Example Liquid Formulation

Echinacea root blend	1:2	40 mL
Sage 1:2 or Pelargonium	1:5	20 mL
Baptisia or Eyebright	1:2	20 mL
Propolis 1:5 or Calendula	1:2	20 mL
Poke root	1:5	5 mL
	Total	105 mL

Dose: Calculate the standard dose according to the most appropriate guideline in Chapter 1, using the adult dose of 5 mL. Up to 5 doses with water can be taken in one day.

There may be compliance issues due to the soreness of the throat. If this is the case, the recommendation of blending the herbal mixture with jelly, as discussed in Chapter 1, may be useful.

Example Tablet Formulations

Providing only immune support during an infection can be highly effective and a good suggested combination is one based on Andrographis, Echinacea and holy basil. See the Short Term Immune Support formulation in Appendix 1. Calculate the child's dose (based on an acute adult dose of 4 to 6 tablets per day) according to the most appropriate guideline in Chapter 1. These can be supplemented with extra Echinacea Formula tablets (see Appendix 1) based on an adult dose of 2 to 3 per day. For younger children the tablets (or part thereof) can be crushed and mixed with honey or a suitable sweetener to improve compliance.

Rationale for Herbal Treatment

Echinacea is prescribed for its immunomodulatory and lymphatic activities.[33] Sage has astringent and antimicrobial properties and is indicated for inflammation and infection of the throat.[33] Baptisia is similar to Echinacea in that they both have influence on the immune and lymphatic systems and are indicated for acute and chronic respiratory infections.[39] Propolis has antiviral and antibacterial activity and is indicated for infections such as tonsillitis.[39] Further support for the use of propolis is provided by two *in vitro* studies that demonstrate that ethanolic extracts of propolis are active against both *S. pyogenes* and *H. influenzae* as well as inhibiting bacterial adhesion to human oral cells.[40,41] Poke root is considered a specific for inflammation of the upper respiratory tract[36] with a particular influence on glandular structure including the tonsils.[33] It should only be included in formulations for older children.

Topical Throat Spray or Gargle

As noted above, diluted herbal extracts are recommended as a gargle for the older child. Alternatively, throat sprays are useful in cases where the child is unable to gargle. An example gargle is given below.

Echinacea root blend	1:2	40 mL
Sage	1:2	30 mL
Propolis 1:5 or Calendula	1:2	30 mL
	Total	100 mL

Directions: Dilute 2 mL in 10 to 20 mL of water and gargle 2 to 4 times a day, depending on severity. Note that gargling with Echinacea can produce temporary difficulty in swallowing and is only suitable for older children. Alternatives to the Echinacea and propolis are Calendula or myrrh.

Otherwise a proprietary herbal throat spray (with potential ingredients as noted previously) can be used.

Case History

A 6-year-old male presented with chronic tonsillitis. He had suffered numerous episodes over the previous 18 months. The child appeared otherwise well with a good appetite. He consumed a healthy diet, but seemed particularly prone to tonsillitis, especially during the colder months. The following formulation was prescribed:

Echinacea root blend	1:2	40 mL
Sage	1:2	30 mL
Baptisia	1:2	30 mL
Poke root	1:5	5 mL
	Total	105 mL

Dose: 2 mL with water three times a day.

Only two acute episodes occurred over the following 18 months and these were treated with *Belladonna* 6X and *Mercurius solubilis* 5C homoeopathic remedies. Hence the herbal treatment markedly reduced the frequency of acute episodes.

Conjunctivitis

Conjunctivitis is a catch-all description of an inflammation and/or infection of the conjunctiva caused either by an infectious agent or as a result of an allergic reaction.[42] The conjunctiva are the most immunologically active tissues of the external eye.[21] They can react to a wide range of bacterial and viral agents, allergens, irritants, toxins and systemic disturbances. As there are potentially two different issues involved in the pathogenesis of conjunctivitis, namely infectious or allergic, these will be discussed separately. Ophthalmia neonatorum is a form of conjunctivitis that occurs in infants younger than 4 weeks of age and is the most common ocular disease of newborns.[21] The folk medicine treatment for this type of conjunctivitis is breast milk, where a drop of milk is place in the affected eye at each breast feed. Interestingly, there is a level of scientific support for such a practice. Two *in vitro* studies have demonstrated that colostrum from human milk has a significant inhibitory effect on the organisms associated with ophthalmia neonatorum.[43,44]

Acute Purulent Conjunctivitis (APC)

APC is one of the most common diseases in childhood, occurring in approximately one in eight children each year.[45] It is characterised by a generalised conjunctival hyperaemia, oedema, mucopurulent exudates, glued eyelids (lids stuck together after sleeping) and varying degrees of ocular pain and discomfort.[21,37] The most frequent causes of APC are *Haemophilus influenzae,* pneumococci, staphylococci and streptococci. Epidemics of APC among children usually occur as a result of *Haemophilus influenzae* or pneumococci.[21] Apart from the localised symptoms, children suffering from APC are otherwise usually well.[45] In order to prevent contagion, patients should be encouraged to wash hands frequently, not touch their eyes and avoid direct contact with others.[37]

Viral Conjunctivitis

Viral conjunctivitis is generally characterised by a watery discharge. Follicular changes resulting from small aggregates of lymphocytes are often found in the conjunctiva of the eyelids.[21] The most common causative agent is the adenovirus. Conjunctivitis is also commonly associated with systemic viral infection, particularly measles.[21]

Allergic Conjunctivitis

Allergic conjunctivitis condition is common, affecting approximately 30% of atopic children. Often mistaken for infectious conjunctivitis, it is caused by the direct exposure of the mucosal surfaces of the eyes to environmental allergens.[21,37] Children usually complain of ocular itching rather than pain and there is conjunctival swelling and a watery discharge.[21,37] Allergic conjunctivitis occurs in several forms. Seasonal allergic conjunctivitis is typically associated with allergic rhinitis and is most often triggered by plant pollens.[21,42] Perennial allergic conjunctivitis, present all year round, is caused by animal dander or dust mite. The symptoms are usually less severe than seasonal allergic conjunctivitis.[21]

Herbal Treatment of Conjunctivitis

An example approach for infectious conjunctivitis using only Echinacea is given below. It can also be combined with eyebright or golden seal in an oral preparation.

Echinacea root blend   1:2   100mL

Or

Echinacea purpurea glycetract   1:3   100mL

Dose: Calculate the standard dose according to the most appropriate guideline in Chapter 1, using the adult dose of 3 mL for the Echinacea root blend or 4 mL for the *Echinacea purpurea* glycetract. Up to 5 doses can be taken in one day with water.

Providing only immune support during an infection can be highly effective and a good suggested tablet combination is one based on Andrographis, Echinacea and holy basil. See the Short Term Immune Support formulation in Appendix 1. Calculate the child's dose (based on an acute adult dose of 4 to 6 tablets per day) according to the most appropriate guideline in Chapter 1. These can be supplemented with extra Echinacea Formula tablets (see Appendix 1) based on an adult dose of 2 to 3 per day. For younger children the tablets (or part thereof) can be crushed and mixed with honey or a suitable sweetener to improve compliance.

For allergic conjunctivitis the following liquid formulation can be considered:

Echinacea root blend	1:2	25 mL
Eyebright	1:2	30 mL
Baical or Chinese Skullcap	1:2	25 mL
Albizia	1:2	20 mL
Total		100 mL

Dose: Calculate the standard dose according to the most appropriate guideline in Chapter 1, using an adult dose of 5 mL. Up to 4 doses can be taken in one day with water.

An alternative to the above liquid formulation is Upper Respiratory Tract Support tablets containing *Echinacea purpurea* root, eyebright, golden rod, golden seal and cayenne (see Appendix 1). Calculate the child's dose (based on an adult dose of 4 tablets per day) according to the most appropriate guideline in Chapter 1. For younger children the tablets (or part thereof) can be crushed and mixed with honey or a suitable sweetener to improve compliance.

A topical eyewash can also be considered for all types of conjunctivitis. An example is given below:

Eyebright	1:2	30 mL
Golden seal	1:3	20 mL
Calendula	1:2	20 mL
Chamomile	1:2	30 mL
Total		100 mL

Directions: Place 5 mL in 80 mL of sterile water. The solution is used to bathe the conjunctiva three times a day. Prepare fresh each day.

Treatment Rationale

Echinacea is prescribed for its immunomodulatory and lymphatic activities.[33] Topical eyebright is considered a specific for conjunctivitis and possesses anti-inflammatory and astringent activities.[33,36] The use of eyebright is also supported by a prospective, open label, multicentre cohort study. The trial was carried out in the clinics of 12 experienced anthroposophical general practitioners and ophthalmologists in Germany and Switzerland. Patients with inflammatory or catarrhal conjunctivitis were treated with one drop of Euphrasia single-dose eye drops 1 to 5 times a day. The efficacy variables were redness, swelling, secretion, burning of the conjunctiva and a foreign body sensation. Tolerability variables assessed included conjunctival reddening, burning of the conjunctiva, foreign body sensation and veiled vision. All symptoms were given for the right or left eye separately, with the degree of severity measured in relation to baseline after approximately 7 and 14 days. If all symptoms had disappeared after the first follow-up, no second follow-up was done. Sixty-five patients fulfilled the inclusion criteria. A complete recovery was seen in 53 patients (81.5%) and a clear improvement in 11 patients (17.0%). A slight worsening was observed in only one patient in the second week of treatment (1.5%). No serious adverse events were observed during the entire trial. The efficacy and tolerability were evaluated by the patients and doctors as "good" to "very good" in more than 85% of cases.[46]

Topical golden seal, Calendula and chamomile are prescribed according to the traditional indications for conjunctivitis.[36] Golden seal is a mucous membrane tonic with antimicrobial and anti-inflammatory activities well supported by the antimicrobial and anti-inflammatory activities of Calendula.[33] Chamomile is included for its anti-inflammatory activity.[33] Note that alcoholic extracts should not be applied directly to the eye.

Case History

A 4-year-old male child attending preschool presented with acute purulent conjunctivitis. The eyelids had been glued for the past two mornings. They had been bathed in warm salty water. The following formulation was prescribed:

Echinacea purpurea glycetract	1:3	40 mL
Eyebright	1:2	30 mL
Flavouring mixture		30 mL
	Total	100 mL

Dose: 2 mL in water four times a day until symptoms resolved.

A topical eyewash was also recommended.

Eyebright	1:2	30 mL
Golden seal	1:3	20 mL
Calendula	1:2	20 mL
	Total	70 mL

Directions: Place 5 mL in 80 mL of warm, sterile, salty water and bathe the affected area three times a day. Prepare fresh each day.

By the completion of the first day of treatment there was a marked reduction in inflammation and oedema. The second day of treatment saw a resolution of the infection. However, the oral formulation was continued for a few more days.

Otitis Media

Otitis media (OM) is one of the most common childhood infections and is the leading cause of doctor visits by children.[47] It is also the most common reason for prescribing antibiotics to children and is often the primary basis for operations such as myringotomy, with the insertion of tympanostomy tubes (grommets), and adenoidectomy.[21] An important characteristic of OM is its propensity to become chronic. The earlier in life a child experiences the first episode of OM, the more likely the child will experience recurrence, severity and persistence of middle ear effusion.[21]

OM has two primary manifestations: acute infection, termed suppurative or acute otitis media (AOM), and inflammation accompanied by effusion, termed nonsuppurative or secretory otitis media, or otitis media with effusion (OME).[48] AOM and OME are interrelated, in that acute infection is usually followed by residual inflammation and effusion. This in turn predisposes the child to further infection.[21] AOM is associated with upper respiratory symptoms in 95% of cases, pain in 75% of cases, fever in 25% of cases and otorrhoea in less than 5%.[49] OME is associated with upper respiratory symptoms in 75% of cases, but pain, fever and otorrhoea are not characteristic.[49] The tympanic membrane is often discoloured, bulging and thickened in AOM. It is relatively normal in OME, although fluid may be seen behind the membrane.[49] The fluid is most often purulent in AOM and serous in OME.[49]

OM can be responsible for serious infectious complications, middle and inner ear damage, hearing impairment and indirect impairment of speech, language and cognitive and psychosocial development. However, most cases of OM are not severe and are self-limiting.[21]

Epidemiology

Most children will have at least one episode of AOM, with a peak incidence between the ages of 6 and 11 months.[48] Recurrent AOM (≥ 3 episodes) is common, affecting 10 to 20% of children in their first year. Nearly 40% of older children will have 6 or more episodes of AOM.[21,48] The most likely reasons for the higher rates of AOM in infants and younger children include less mature immunological defences and a less favourable structural and functional eustachian tube development.[21]

Microbiology

AOM is usually caused by bacterial pathogens. Three predominate: *Streptococcus pneumoniae* is found in approximately 40% of cases, *Haemophilus influenzae* in approximately 25 to 30% and *Moraxella catarrhalis* in approximately 10 to 15%.[21,48] Evidence of a viral cause can be found either alone or more commonly in association with pathogenic bacteria. Rhinovirus and respiratory syncytial virus are found most often.[21] Viral co-infection can substantially worsen the symptoms of OM.[45] The way in which this comes about is not clear, however bacterial OM with viral co-infection exhibits a higher concentration of inflammatory mediators than bacterial OM alone.[45]

Eustachian Tube Dysfunction

Under normal circumstances the eustachian tube is passively closed and only opens by the contractions of the veli palatine muscle.[21] In the context of the middle ear, the eustachian tube has three main functions: protection, clearance and, most importantly, ventilation.[21] The middle ear mucosa depends on a continuous supply of air from the nasopharynx delivered by the eustachian tube. Interruption of the ventilation process by tubal obstruction initiates a complex inflammatory response leading to secretory metaplasia, compromise of the mucociliary transport system and effusion of liquid into the tympanic cavity. Impaired middle ear ventilation is thereby considered to be an important contributing factor to both OME and AOM.[21]

Infants and young children have eustachian tubes that are short, compliant, horizontal and poorly functional, making them prone to OM.[21,45] Maturation of the tube is a gradual process, evidenced by a progressive reduction in tubal compliance with increasing age. This explains the decline in the occurrence of OM as children grow older.[21,45]

The OM-prone child can suffer frequent colonisation with potential middle ear pathogens and fails to develop a broad-based immune response. As a result the child experiences repeated episodes of colonisation and infection.[49]

Risk Factors

Poverty has long been considered to be an important factor in both the development and the severity of OM. Various elements are thought to contribute to this relationship, including crowding, poor hygiene, suboptimal nutrition and limited access to medical care.[21] Exposure to other children, whether at home or in day care centres, poses a significant risk factor.[21,50] Most studies examining the relative protective effects of breast-feeding versus formula or cows milk feeding demonstrate a protective effect against OM for breast milk.[21] Breast-feeding duration is also important, as it appears that feeding for more than 6 months provides a greater protection than feeding between 4 months and 6 months.[51] Congenital abnormalities such as an unrepaired cleft palate, submucosal cleft palate and other craniofacial anomalies, and Down's syndrome are associated with a high incidence of OM.[21]

Gastro-oesophageal reflux appears to be linked to chronic OME. Numerous studies have found the presence of pepsin protein in the effusion collected from children with OME.[52,53,54] It also appears that this can occur without any significant gastrointestinal symptoms.[53] Even under normal conditions fluid from the rhinopharynx can penetrate the nasopharyngeal orifice of the eustachian tubes during swallowing.[55] Exposure to gastric juices causes inflammation, oedema and epithelial ulceration, which in turn may favour the development of OM by inhibiting tubal function.[56]

A positive association between allergic rhinitis and OM has been noted. For example, a case control study of 76 children admitted for the insertion of tympanostomy tubes found a high incidence of atopic symptoms compared to matched controls.[57] A meta-analysis found that the use of a pacifier increased the risk of OM by 24%.[58]

Clinical Manifestations

The signs and symptoms of AOM can be highly variable, especially in infants and young children. Ear pain may be present, as evidenced by irritability, a change in sleeping and/or eating patterns and occasionally tugging or holding the ear. Fever may also be a feature and (rarely) rupture of the tympanic membrane with purulent otorrhoea. Symptoms associated with an upper RTI can also occur. Occasionally there may be no symptoms at all. In contrast, OME is often not accompanied by overt complaints, but usually causes some hearing loss.[21]

Herbal Treatment

The treatment of AOM and its chronic manifestation follow a similar pattern. However, treatment for AOM will be more frequent, particularly if accompanied by pain and fever. OME should be considered either as part of an allergic pattern or as a sign of vicarious elimination.[5]

The following herbs should be considered during treatment:

- Antiallergic herbs such as Albizia and Baical skullcap (mainly for OME)
- Upper respiratory anticatarrhal herbs such as eyebright, golden rod, golden seal, ribwort, elder flowers and ground ivy (for both AOM and OME)
- Depurative and lymphatic herbs including poke root (for older children) and clivers (for both AOM and OME)
- Immune-enhancing herbs such as Echinacea and Andrographis (for both) and Astragalus (for OME only). *Pelargonium sidoides* should be considered for AOM
- Diaphoretic herbs for fever management in AOM: elder flowers and peppermint are ideally suited

Example Herbal Liquid Formulation for AOM

Echinacea root blend	1:2	30 mL
Elder flowers or Chamomile	1:2	25 mL
Ribwort or Eyebright	1:2	25 mL
Clivers	1:2	25 mL
	Total	105 mL

Dose: Calculate the standard dose according to the most appropriate guideline in Chapter 1, using the adult dose of 5 mL. Up to 5 doses can be taken in one day with warm water in the case of acute episodes.

Example Tablet Formulations

An alternative to the above liquid formulation is Upper Respiratory Tract Support tablets containing *Echinacea purpurea* root, eyebright, golden rod, golden seal and cayenne (see Appendix 1). Calculate the child's dose (based on an acute adult dose of 6 tablets per day) according to the most appropriate guideline in Chapter 1. These can be supplemented with extra Short Term Immune Support tablets (see Appendix 1) based on an adult dose of 4 per day. For younger children the tablets (or part thereof) can be crushed and mixed with honey or a suitable sweetener to improve compliance.

Topical Application

Infused oil of fresh mullein flowers

Infused oil of fresh St John's wort flowers or flowering tops

Infused oil of fresh peeled garlic cloves

Infused oil of dried or fresh Calendula flowers

The four infused oils are blended in equal parts

Dose: One to two drops are placed in the affected ear at least twice a day.

Rationale for the Formulations

Echinacea is prescribed to aid immune defence, which is particularly important for children with acute and chronic infections that relate to immune system immaturity. Echinacea is also beneficial as a preventative remedy for children prone to OM. Elder flowers, eyebright and ribwort possess anti-catarrhal properties and are indicated for OM.[39] Elder flowers is also diaphoretic as is chamomile. Furthermore, ribwort is a mucous membrane tonic and restorative similar to golden seal.[59] It avoids the paediatric compliance issues associated with golden seal. Clivers is an excellent lymphatic remedy for chronic respiratory tract catarrh.

The example topical application is based on both traditional prescribing practices and clinical evidence. Infused oils of the fresh flowers of mullein and fresh garlic cloves are traditional applications for ear pain and OM.[39,60] Two clinical studies have demonstrated the efficacy of herbal infused oils for OM. Children between the ages of 6 and 18 years (n=103) with ear pain (otalgia) and eardrum problems associated with AOM were randomly assigned to be treated with Otikon (infused oils of garlic, mullein, Calendula and St John's wort) or anaesthetic ear drops. Ear pain was assessed using two visual analogue scales and this took place over the course of three days. Both treatments significantly reduced ear pain. The pain scores in the two groups were comparable to each other both before and throughout the treatment phases. The researchers concluded that Otikon was as effective as the anaesthetic ear drops and appropriate for the management of AOM-associated ear pain.[61]

The second study of double blind design was conducted in an outpatient community clinic and enrolled 171 children aged between 5 and 18 years. The children, who had otalgia and other clinical findings associated with middle-ear infection, were randomly assigned to receive treatment with Naturopathic Herbal Extract Ear Drops (NHED) or anaesthetic ear drops, with or without amoxicillin. NHED contained garlic, mullein flowers, Calendula, St John's wort, lavender and vitamin E in olive oil. There were four treatment groups: NHED at 5 drops 3 times daily (group A), NHED with a topical anaesthetic at 5 drops 3 times daily (group B), oral amoxicillin 80 mg/kg/day (maximum

500 mg/dose) divided into 3 doses with either NHED (group C) or the topical anaesthetic (group D). The presence or absence of ear pain was assessed over 3 days using a visual analogue scale. At the beginning of the trial there were no significant between-group differences in patient age or gender, degree of fever, main symptoms, associated symptoms and severity or laterality of acute otitis media. After treatment, each group demonstrated a statistically significant improvement in ear pain. Patients given ear drops alone had a better response than patients who were given ear drops together with amoxicillin. Results were better in the NHED groups than in the respective control groups.[62]

Case History

An 8-year-old male presented with a 4-year history of chronic OM impacting the right ear. There was a history of antibiotic use and a tympanostomy tube insertion had been recommended. The parents were not supportive of this approach. The child was already taking a probiotic formulation.

Treatment consisted of:

Echinacea purpurea glycetract	1:3	40 mL
Elder flowers	1:2	30 mL
Golden rod	1:2	30 mL
Poke root	1:5	5 mL
	Total	105 mL

Dose: 4mL with water three times a day

The following topical application was also prescribed:

Infused oil of fresh mullein flowers	50 mL
Infused oil of fresh St John's wort flowering tops	25 mL
Infused oil of fresh garlic cloves	25 mL
Liquid CO_2 extract of Calendula	4 drops

Directions: Place 1 drop of the infused oil in the affected ear morning and night.

The above protocol resulted in a significant reduction in the frequency and duration of the acute episodes. The core herbal treatment went on for 10 months and the child is now free of OM and has avoided grommet insertion.

Allergic Rhinitis

Allergic rhinitis (AR) is an inflammatory disorder of the nasal mucosa characterised by nasal congestion, rhinorrhoea and itching and is often accompanied by sneezing and conjunctival irritation.[21,63]

The two prerequisites for the expression of AR are the sensitivity to an allergen and its presence in the environment. Currently AR is classified as seasonal or perennial, terms that may soon be replaced by intermittent and persistent.[21] Seasonal or intermittent

AR follows a well-defined course of cyclical exacerbations, while perennial or persistent AR causes year-round symptoms.[21] Approximately 20% of all cases are seasonal, 40% perennial and 40% mixed (that is, perennial with seasonal exacerbations).[21] However other data exist that suggest that these percentages do not reflect current trends and that up to 80% of patients with AR have the mixed type.[64]

In temperate climates airborne pollens responsible for seasonal AR appear in distinct phases as trees pollinate in the spring, grasses in early summer and weeds in late summer. Mould spores in temperate climates persist outdoors only in summer, whereas in warm climates they can be present throughout the year.[21,65] In contrast, perennial AR is most often associated with indoor allergens such as house dust mite, mould and allergens from domestic animals (dogs and especially cats).[21,65]

Epidemiology

The past four decades have seen a marked increase in the prevalence of AR in urban settings, with a relatively smaller increase in rural settings.[21] This is thought to be for the reasons discussed in Chapter 4. In prosperous societies, 20 to 40% of children suffer from AR.[66] Its prevalence peaks in late childhood, with a diagnosis generally established by 6 years of age. Symptoms resolve within 10 years of onset in only 10 to 20% of children.[67] Risk factors include a family history of atopy, introduction of foods or formula in early infancy, food allergy, exposure to tobacco smoke and heavy exposure to indoor allergens.[21] There is also a significant relationship between AR and allergic and non-allergic asthma (see later in this chapter).[68]

Pathogenesis

In susceptible children, the inflammatory cascade begins with allergen deposition on the nasal mucosa and consists of early phase and late phase responses.[69] For the early phase response, the bridging of IgE molecules by allergens initiates the degranulation of mast cells and release of both preformed and newly-generated inflammatory mediators.[21] These mediators cause sensory neural stimulation and plasma exudation from blood vessels, with the patient experiencing itching, sneezing, nasal discharge and congestion.[69] The late phase response appears 4 to 8 hours after allergen exposure and is associated with cellular infiltration and the release of proinflammatory cytokines and chemokines that serve to sustain the allergic response.[21,69]

Clinical Manifestations

Symptoms of AR in children are often mistaken for respiratory infections. While older children are able to blow their noses to clear the congestion, younger ones tend to sniff and snort. Nasal itching brings on grimacing, twitching and picking the nose that may result in epistaxis. Children with AR often perform the 'allergic salute', which is the upward rubbing of the nose with an open palm or extended index finger. This practice can result in a horizontal skin crease over the bridge of the nose, termed a nasal crease. Typical complaints include intermittent nasal congestion, itching, sneezing, clear rhinorrhoea and conjunctival irritation. Symptoms increase with longer and higher levels of allergen exposure. Patients may eventually experience headaches, wheezing, coughing and may lose their sense of smell and taste. Nasal congestion is often worse at night, causing mouth breathing and snoring, which interferes with sleep and leads to irritability.[21]

Interactions between AR and Asthma

Allergic asthma and AR are often considered clinical manifestations of the same condition, termed the chronic allergic respiratory syndrome.[70,71] The vast majority of patients with AR also have asthma and cross-sectional and longitudinal studies have established that AR is a major independent risk factor for asthma.[71,72,73] Clinical studies also provide evidence that AR and asthma are different expressions of the same disharmony. For example inflammatory infiltration, characterised by the presence of eosinophils and CD_4 T cells, was similar in the nasal mucosa of all patients with AR, irrespective of the presence of asthma or the allergic status of the patient.[74] An earlier study demonstrated that eosinophil infiltration was present in the nasal mucosa of asthmatic patients in the absence of AR.[70] In other words, eosinophil infiltration is a common feature in patients who have only AR and patients who have only asthma.

Overall, possible mechanisms by which AR may exert an influence over the lower airways include interference with the beneficial role of the nasal mucosa in conditioning the air entering the respiratory tree, irritant effects from nasal secretions impacting the lower airways and systemic propagation of nasal inflammation to the bronchial tree (or vice versa).[69,75]

Impact of AR on School Children

Allergies are among the most cited reasons for missed school days in the US, accounting for more than 2 million school days lost annually.[76] The symptomatic burden of AR can be compounded by the problem that many antihistamine and decongestant drugs used in the treatment of AR can cause either sedation or irritability, potentially impairing school performance and learning.[77] The symptoms of AR may impair cognitive function and compromise learning, with many children suffering 'presenteeism', where the child is physically present at school but cognitively absent.[67] Children with AR can be more irritable and tired, which leads to inattention and difficulty concentrating in class. Recently, interest has been raised in investigating a possible correlation between AR and attention deficit hyperactivity disorder (ADHD), given the similarities in classroom symptoms.[67] ADHD is fully discussed in the following chapter.

General Treatment Strategies

Allergen avoidance should be included in any treatment plan for AR. For example, sealing the mattress, pillows and covers in allergen-proof encasings and hot water laundering (> 54°C or 130°F) of bedding have been shown to reduce exposure to dust mite allergen.[63] Diet can create a state of hypersensitivity and catarrh of the mucous membranes which predisposes to rhinitis.[5] Moreover, the dietary components that contribute to this process do not necessarily give a positive reaction to the RAST or skin prick test.[5] These dietary components typically include dairy products, refined wheat products and salt.[5] Whole grains and whole grain products are less of a problem, except when baked with yeast. In a cross-sectional survey performed on 690 children aged from 7 to 18 years, it was found that a high level of adherence to the Mediterranean diet was protective against AR.[78]

Herbal Treatment of AR

The herbal treatment of AR consists mainly of immune-modulating herbs, along with antiallergic and anticatarrhal remedies. Treatment at a deeper level may involve the use of depuratives or lymphatics, or the promotion of digestion with bitters, choleretics and aromatic digestives.

Example Herbal Liquid Formulation for AR

Echinacea root blend	1:2	30 mL
Eyebright	1:2	20 mL
Nettle leaf	1:2	20 mL
Baical or Chinese skullcap	1:2	30 mL
	Total	100 mL

Dose: Calculate the standard dose according to the most appropriate guideline in Chapter 1, using the adult dose of 5 mL. Up to 5 doses can be taken with water in one day in the case of intense episodes, but the baseline dosage is 3 per day.

Example Tablet Formulations

An alternative to the above liquid formulation is Upper Respiratory Tract Support tablets containing *Echinacea purpurea* root, eyebright, golden rod, golden seal and cayenne (see Appendix 1). Calculate the child's dose (based on an acute adult dose of 4 tablets per day) according to the most appropriate guideline in Chapter 1. These can be supplemented with Allergy Support tablets (see Appendix 1) based on an adult dose of 4 per day. For younger children the tablets (or part thereof) can be crushed and mixed with honey or a suitable sweetener to improve compliance.

Rationale

Echinacea is prescribed because of its immune-modulating effects. Eyebright is useful in the treatment of AR due to its anti-inflammatory and anticatarrhal activity and is considered a priority for AR.[33] Nettle leaf and Baical skullcap both possess antiallergic activity.[33] Sixty-nine volunteers completed a randomised, double blind, placebo-controlled study investigating the effect of a freeze-dried preparation of nettle leaf on allergic rhinitis. Patients were advised to take nettle leaf (600 mg) or placebo at the onset of symptoms. Nettle was rated higher than placebo in the global assessments, but was only slightly higher in diary data after one week.[33]

Case History

A 13-year-old female presented with a 5-year history of AR. There was also a family history of AR. The child suffered headaches and sinus pain and was worse in cold and windy weather. She felt cold, had cold extremities and had a low appetite.

Treatment consisted of:

Echinacea angustifolia	1:2	25 mL
Astragalus	1:2	25 mL
Golden seal	1:3	25 mL
Bayberry	1:2	15 mL
Poke root	1:5	5 mL
Ginger	1:2	5 mL
	Total	100 mL

Dose: 5mL with water three times a day. (Given her age and the chronicity of her condition, the full adult dose was recommended).

The treatment protocol remained unchanged for a 5-month period. During that time the patient suffered only two acute episodes. The patient is now 18 years old and remains free of AR. She is currently taking Echinacea root blend tablets and a probiotic formulation.

Childhood Asthma

Asthma is a chronic inflammatory condition of the lower airways resulting in episodic airflow obstruction.[21,79] It is recognised to be the result of a complex interaction between several cells, mediators and neural pathways, leading to inflammation with airway hyper-responsiveness, wheeze, cough and breathlessness.[80] Allergic asthma can occur at any age, however the incidence is highest in childhood.[79]

There are two main types of respiratory disease characterised by wheeze and/or coughing. The first is a recurrent wheeze primarily triggered by common viral infections of the respiratory tract. The second, and most common type, is chronic asthma associated with allergy that persists into late childhood and often adulthood.[21] A third less common type typically emerges in females who develop obesity and early onset puberty (by 11 years of age).[21]

Aetiology

A number of factors have been proposed as causative in childhood asthma. The research stresses the relevance of a combination of environmental exposures with biological disturbances, along with genetic vulnerabilities. Respiratory exposures include inhaled allergens, respiratory viral infections and chemical and biological air pollution such as tobacco smoke, grain dust, wood smoke, ambient air pollution, dust mite, mould, cockroach droppings and cats.[21,81] In terms of the hygiene hypothesis, and particularly the old friends hypothesis (see Chapter 4), exposure to a wide range of potentially beneficial micro-organisms has decreased in the modern world as a result of increased urbanisation and indoor living.[82] This, coupled with antibiotic use, has possibly led to a deficiency in bystander suppression of both Th1 or Th2 effectors cells, leading to the observed rise in the incidence of childhood inflammatory disorders, particularly those of an allergic nature.[82,83,84] Epidemiological studies provide support for this theory, including those observations demonstrating that exposure to farm animals and raw milk early in life reduces the likelihood of developing asthma, AR and atopic sensitisation.[85,86] Paradoxically, early and extensive exposure to cats and their epidermal allergens may replicate the protective effects of farm animals by modifying Th2 responses.[87]

Diet and Asthma

Current diets in most westernised countries differ considerably from those of previous generations, for whom the prevalence of asthma and allergy was significantly lower.[82] The modern diet is dominated by food that has been processed, modified, stored and transported great distances. This is in contrast to a traditional diet characterised by food that was locally-grown and consumed shortly after harvesting. Therefore seasonal eating was the norm.[82] The nutritional hypothesis attributes the increase in respiratory allergies to changes in dietary intake and particularly focuses on the antioxidant and lipid intake of both the child and the mother. Antioxidants feature because the lungs are continually exposed to relatively high concentrations of oxygen in comparison to other organs and lung tissue is quite sensitive to pro-oxidant effects.[88] From birth, the human lung is subject to many hazardous oxidative events as a result of exposure to inhaled irritants, allergens and pollutants. It has been established that a higher maternal or child intake of the antioxidant vitamins A, C and E, as well as zinc and selenium, particularly when taken as components of food, was associated with a lower risk of wheezing illness or asthma in children.[89,90] Further to this, another study demonstrated that a low maternal dietary vitamin E intake is associated with asthma in 5-year-old children.[91] A study of school-age children found a significant decrease in asthma risk from the early introduction of daily fresh fruit and vegetables.[92]

The lipid aspect of the dietary hypothesis involves the concept of an increased intake of omega-6 fatty acids through margarine and vegetable oil derivatives, as well as a decreased intake of omega-3 and fish oil derivatives. This is thought to have the potential to alter the inflammatory pathways involved in allergy and asthma.[93] Observational studies have shown a protective effect for omega-3 fatty acid intake and an increased risk of asthma associated with a high intake of omega-6 fatty acids.[94,95] Furthermore, fish oil supplementation in pregnancy has been shown to reduce infant allergy in children with a high risk of atopy.[96] Trans fatty acid consumption in margarine, fried foods and fast food is also associated with an increased risk of allergy and asthma in children.[95,97,98]

Finally, there is a significant correlation between exclusive breast-feeding during the first several months following birth and a lower asthma rate during childhood.[99] This effect is probably due to the immunomodulatory effect of breast milk, together with the avoidance of the allergens found in breast milk substitutes.[99]

Obesity and Asthma

Most prospective studies suggest that childhood obesity increases the risk of subsequent asthma.[100] A recent meta-analysis of the effect of body weight on asthma in children demonstrated that a high body weight, either at birth or later in childhood, was associated with a future asthma risk.[101] Gastro-oesophageal reflux (GER) is a possible causal link between obesity and asthma. There is a significant association between GER and obesity, and GER is linked to asthma.[102,103] There is also a possible hormonal association since leptin, a proinflammatory cytokine produced by adipose tissue, is associated with asthma in children.[104] Serum leptin levels are strongly correlated with measures of body fat.

Gastrointestinal Microbiota and Asthma

An increasing accumulation of epidemiological and clinical data supports the hypothesis that disturbances in the gastrointestinal microbiota, resulting from antibiotic use and dietary influences, have lead to an increase in allergic airways disease.[105] Asthma is significantly more likely to develop in children at age 7 years who received antibiotics in their first year of life. This is independent of other well-known asthma risk factors and was observed even for antibiotic use in non-respiratory tract infections. The risk of asthma was highest in children who received more than four courses of antibiotics, especially among rural children or in the absence of maternal asthma.[106] A recent meta-analysis of several studies examining antibiotic use in the first year of life reported a twofold increase in the risk of childhood asthma following antibiotic use.[107] Adding further support to this link are several studies in children demonstrating a positive correlation between altered faecal microbiota and atopic disorders.[108,109]

Stress and Asthma

Clinical observation and evolving research support the hypothesis that psychosocial and emotional factors, particularly stress, may impact disease expression in asthma.[110] Stress may contribute to early life lower respiratory tract infection, which is predictive of repeated wheeze in infancy.[111] Parental stress is also a predictor of wheezing in infancy. For example, the evidence suggests that a child's asthma morbidity is greater when the mother has symptoms of depression.[112] Stressful life events have been shown to have an association with increased asthma attacks in children, in many instances weeks after the event.[113] Amongst inner-city children with asthma, parental psychosocial problems and distress are associated with increased asthma morbidity.[114]

Epidemiology

Whichever criteria are used, the prevalence of wheeze and physician-diagnosed asthma has increased in most populations in the world in the past 20 to 30 years (see Chapter 4). However, higher prevalence rates are especially reported in more westernised countries, with wheezing occurring in more than 30% of infants in the first year of life and physician-diagnosed asthma rates of over 20% in children.[80] If a child develops a wheeze in the first year of life, they have about a 50% chance of developing asthma. If the child suffers from recurrent wheeze, then the chance rises to 80%.[80] Approximately 80% of all asthmatics report the onset of symptoms before 6 years of age.[21]

Immunology

It is widely accepted that allergic inflammation is driven by the activation of Th2 cells producing the cytokines IL-4 and IL-13. These cytokines contribute to IgE production, mucus hypersecretion and airway hyper-responsiveness (AHR), together with IL-5 that promotes eosinophilic inflammation.[115,116] As discussed in Chapter 4, the newly described regulatory T cell (T_{reg}) hypothesis has emerged. This theory proposes that the active suppression of inappropriate Th2 responses to allergens by both $CD_4^+CD_{25}^+$ T cells and IL-10-producing T_{reg} is either defective or overcome in those who develop allergic disease.[116,117,118]

A recent immunoepidemiological survey of 172 children rated their blood T cell responses to allergens in terms of atopic sensitisation, AHR and clinical symptoms of asthma (wheeze). Atopy was closely associated with Th2 cytokine production, whereas both atopic and non-atopic children also exhibited IFN-γ, TNF-a and IL-10 responses. Skinprick test wheal size was related to IL-5 and IFN-γ responses and negatively correlated with IL-10 production. Asthma symptoms were associated with eosinophilia and IL-5 production, whereas AHR was associated with IFN-γ.[119] The implications of this study are that, while atopic sensitisation is clearly associated with Th2 responses, other factors including Th1 cytokines such as IFN-γ, may be important for the clinical expression of asthma. Eosinophilic inflammation might also amplify the Th2 response to allergens.[116]

An additional factor has recently been described involving complement and eosinophilic inflammation. The complement system is a primary effector system for both innate and adaptive immune responses and its activation results in an enhanced inflammatory response.[3] It had been demonstrated that complement pathways are activated in the lungs of individuals with asthma,[120] in the serum of children exposed to cigarette smoke,[121] in the plasma of aspirin-sensitive subjects[122] and in various experimental models of asthma.[120] It is thought that this activation of complement via exposure to allergens enhances eosinophilic inflammation and contributes to the clinical expression of asthma.[120]

Clinical Manifestations

Intermittent dry cough and/or expiratory wheeze are the most common chronic symptoms of asthma. Older children will report shortness of breath and chest tightness, while younger children are more likely to report intermittent, nonfocal chest pain.[21] Respiratory symptoms can be worse at night, especially during prolonged exacerbations triggered by RTIs or inhaled allergens. Daytime symptoms linked to play and physical activities are reported with great frequency by children.[21] Other symptoms can be subtle, including self-imposed limitations on physical activity, difficulty in keeping up with peers in physical activities and general fatigue.[21]

General Treatment Strategies

Aeroallergens play an important role in the pathogenesis of AR and asthma. The avoidance of these allergens is an important strategy in the treatment and prevention of both AR and asthma. Readers are directed to a free full text paper: Wu F, Takaro TK. 'Childhood Asthma and Environmental Interventions' *Environmental Health Perspectives,* 2007; **115**(6): 971-975 (accessible through the PubMed database) that covers environmental interventions aimed at reducing contact with aeroallergens in the home.

Herbal Treatment of Asthma

Herbal treatment of asthma involves the use of immune modulators, anti-inflammatory herbs, respiratory spasmolytics, antiallergics, antioxidants and expectorants, among others. Issues such as bowel flora dysbiosis, gastro-oesophageal reflux, repeated viral infections, poor digestion and allergic rhinitis or chronic sinusitis need to be considered and addressed as appropriate. The dietary considerations described for allergic rhinitis are also relevant.

Important Herbs in Asthma Management

The following is a list of important herbs to choose from in asthma management. The relevant actions of each herb are also provided.

HERB	ACTION
Adhatoda vasica	Expectorant Bronchodilator Respiratory stimulant
Albizia lebbek	Antiallergic
Allium cepa (onion)	Anti-inflammatory Antiallergic Anti-PAF Mucolytic
Althaea officinalis (marshmallow root)	Demulcent Reflex demulcent
Andrographis paniculata	Immune enhancing Resolving bacterial and viral infections
Boswellia serrata	Anti-inflammatory (inhibits leukotriene production and cytokines)
Bupleurum falcatum	Anti-inflammatory Antitussive Reflex expectorant Adaptogenic
Coleus forskohlii	Bronchodilator Digestive
Echinacea spp	Immune enhancing Resolving bacterial and viral infections Lymphatic
Euphrasia officinalis (eyebright)	Anticatarrhal
Ginkgo biloba	Anti-PAF

Glycyrrhiza glabra (licorice)	Anti-inflammatory Antitussive Mucoprotective Bronchodilator Adrenal tonic Mild reflex expectorant
Grindelia camporum	Expectorant Bronchial spasmolytic
Hydrastis canadensis (golden seal)	Mucous membrane trophorestorative Anticatarrhal Digestive
Hypericum perforatum (St John's wort)	Antiviral (enveloped viruses) Nervine tonic
Inula helenium (elecampane)	Respiratory antiseptic Bronchial spasmolytic Expectorant
Passiflora incarnata (passionflower)	Sedative Spasmolytic
Pelargonium sidoides	Antibacterial Immune modulating Expectorant
Plantago lanceolata (ribwort)	Anticatarrhal
Rehmannia glutinosa	Anti-inflammatory Adrenal tonic
Scutellaria baicalensis (Baical skullcap)	Antiallergic Antiviral Antioxidant
Valeriana officinalis (valerian)	Sedative Spasmolytic
Verbascum thapsus (mullein)	Anticatarrhal
Zingiber officinale (ginger)	Anti-inflammatory Diffusive stimulant (facilitates expectoration and diaphoresis) Digestive

Protocol Construction

Asthma is a deep-seated, protracted condition that requires herbal treatment in pharmacological doses. Hence a high dosage protocol is proposed. Based on the herbs outlined above, it is suggested that ideally two liquid formulations or tablet or capsule products, each of 4 to 6 herbs are developed for the individual patient.

One formulation can be a long-term treatment aimed at treating the underlying factors behind the asthmatic condition. The second formulation can be aimed at the symptoms and sustaining causes, including the inflammation.

The herbs in the two formulations should be chosen so that there is as much overlap of the required actions as possible. This reduces the number of herbs needed to give a broad range of required actions. For example:

- Ginger has expectorant, digestive-stimulant and anti-inflammatory activities
- Adhatoda is expectorant and bronchodilating

The treatment should be varied over time, depending on the patient's response. Also not every factor can necessarily be treated at the one time, so particular treatment goals may need to be changed from time to time. This is a dynamic interactive model.

However, two formulations may not always be practical, so the following example formulation is aimed at treating both long-term and short-term issues in asthma.

Example Herbal Liquid Formulation for Asthma

Echinacea root blend	1:2	30 mL
Eyebright	1:2	20 mL
Grindelia	1:2	15 mL
Ginkgo	2:1	20 mL
Baical or Chinese skullcap	1:2	20 mL
	Total	105 mL

Dose: Calculate the standard dose according to the most appropriate guideline in Chapter 1, using the adult dose of 5 mL. Up to 5 doses can be taken with water in one day in the case of intense episodes.

Rationale for the Liquid Formulation

The use of Echinacea in asthma remains controversial with many warnings in the popular press against its use in asthma. This misconception has come about because of *in vitro* research demonstrating that isolated polysaccharides stimulated TNF-γ, a proinflammatory cytokine involved in asthma.[5] These studies are unlikely to be relevant to the oral use of Echinacea products. Specifically, the polysaccharides used differ markedly from those found in Echinacea and are largely irrelevant to the therapeutic action of Echinacea root, since it is now widely accepted that polysaccharides are not present in ethanolic extracts of Echinacea.[5] In later research it has been shown that a mixture of alkylamides, the bioavailable phytochemicals in Echinacea largely responsible for its therapeutic action, actually decrease acute TNF-γ production.[123] The authors' clinical experience demonstrates that Echinacea is safe in asthma and is particularly beneficial in reducing the incidence of RTIs associated with asthma.

Grindelia is a respiratory expectorant and spasmolytic indicated for respiratory conditions characterised by spasm.[33] Ginkgo is prescribed because of its anti-PAF (platelet activating factor) activity.[33] The anti-PAF effects of the ginkgolides in *Ginkgo biloba* are well-documented. Oral treatment using standardised Ginkgo extract normalised pulmonary functions in extrinsic asthma in children. This was correlated with a significant improvement in spirometric parameters.[124] Baical skullcap contains the flavonoids baicalin and baicalein which have both demonstrated antiallergic and antiasthmatic activity.[33] Eyebright is included for the sinusitis/rhinitis often associated with childhood asthma.

Example Tablet Formulations

For the older child or the younger one who will not take liquids, herbal tablets or capsules may prove a useful alternative for asthma management.

Key herbal formulations (examples provided in Appendix 1) which should be considered in asthma are Chronic Lung Support (adult dose 4 per day), Boswellia Combination (adult dose 4 per day) and Echinacea Formulation (adult dose 2 per day). Other formulations to be consideration as appropriate to the case are Upper Respiratory Tract Support (adult dose 4 per day) if sinusitis or sinus allergy is present, Clear Lung Formula (adult dose 4 per day) if the lungs are highly congested with mucus and Upper Digestive Formula (adult dose 1 tablet sucked briefly before each meal) if there is evidence of functional hypochlorhydria. In general, no more than 3 different formulations should be prescribed at the one time. Calculate the standard dose for the child according to the most appropriate guideline in Chapter 1. For younger children the tablets (or part thereof) can be crushed and mixed with honey or a suitable sweetener to improve compliance.

Case History

Susie, aged 3½ on presentation, was diagnosed as asthmatic 18 months prior after an unresolved viral infection. It started as a persistent cough. Disodium cromoglycate was ineffective and she was currently taking six puffs of inhaled steroids a day and used a bronchodilator by nebuliser three times a day. She was alway tired due to a nocturnal cough which interfered with her sleeping. She often complained of a "sore tummy" which probably indicated gastro-oesophageal reflux. Her father had asthma. On examination she was underweight, looked devitalised, her nose was constantly blocked and she was mouth breathing. Chest examination showed the presence of wheezes. She had swollen neck lymph glands.

Two formulations were prescribed, the first for the underlying issues and the second for the night cough/gastro-oesophageal reflux:

Elecampane	1:2	20 mL
Ginkgo biloba standardised extract	2:1	25 mL
Eyebright	1:2	20 mL
Echinacea angustifolia	1:2	35 mL
	Total	100 mL

Dose: 2.5 mL with water twice a day

Licorice	1:1	20 mL
Meadowsweet	1:2	25 mL
Marshmallow root glycetract	1:5	55 mL
	Total	100 mL

Dose: 2 mL with a small quantity of water two to three times in the evening

Also her mother was advised to reduce her dairy product intake.

The day after initial presentation she had a bad time with increased bronchodilator medication required. This settled down to her normal medication. Her sleep at night was better and the night mixture was helping her cough. She was mouth breathing less.

At the next consultation 4 weeks later she had been well with no acute problems. Conventional medication had been reduced to inhaled steroids only. Her mother asked if she could use night mixture during the day as it seemed to help considerably. The prescription was repeated, but the second mixture was increased to 2 mL three to four times, including during the day.

After 4 more months there was considerable progress. Inhaled steroid dose was substantially reduced, with no need for other conventional medication. People commented how well she looked. Attacks of nocturnal coughing were infrequent and mild.

Croup

Croup is a generic term encompassing a heterogenous group of illnesses affecting the larynx, trachea and bronchi.[125] Laryngotracheitis, laryngotracheobronchitis, laryngotracheobronchopneumonitis and spasmodic croup are all included in the croup syndrome. In children with croup, upper airway obstruction causes a barking cough, a hoarse voice, inspiratory stridor and varying degrees of respiratory distress.[21,125]

Viral croup affects children six months to 12 years of age, with a peak incidence at two years of age. Boys are affected more often than girls, and although the disease can occur throughout the year, it predominates in the autumn and winter months.[21,125]

The anatomic makeup of the child's larynx helps explain how the symptoms of croup develop. The subglottic region of the larynx is held within a narrow ring of cartilage. In children with croup, viral infection causes this area to become inflamed and oedematous, which can lead to obstruction. Because children have a very narrow larynx, even a small decrease in the airway radius causes a large decrease in airflow, leading to the typical symptoms.[125]

Aetiology

The parainfluenza viruses are the most frequent cause of croup, accounting for approximately 75% of cases. Adenovirus, respiratory syncytial virus, rhinovirus, enteroviruses and influenza viruses A and B may also cause laryngotracheo-bronchitis.[21,125]

Clinical Manifestations

It can be difficult to differentiate between the common patterns of spasmodic croup and viral croup. Both occur most frequently in the evening or during the night. Spasmodic croup is more likely to appear suddenly without a clearly identifiable viral prodrome, but may be preceded by mild to moderate coryza and hoarseness.[21,125] The child awakens with a characteristic barking, metallic cough, noisy inspiration and respiratory distress, is afebrile and may be anxious and frightened. Usually the symptoms diminish within a few hours and the following day the child may appear well. Attacks can occur several nights in a row and may represent an allergic reaction to viral antigens, rather than an infection.[21] Viral croup on the other hand is usually preceded by 12 to 72 hours of low grade fever and coryza.[125] As the illness progresses, hoarseness and the characteristic barking cough will develop. Symptoms are worse at night, peak between 24 to 48 hours, and generally resolve within 5 to 7 days.[125]

General Treatment Strategy

Humidification is the time-honoured therapy for croup. The child is encouraged to inhale the steam generated from a kettle or hot water tap. Even a hot shower can serve this requirement well. This is thought to soothe the air passages and relieve the spasm.[60] However, the practice is not supported by clinical evidence. In fact, the evidence demonstrates that humidification is actually not effective for croup.[126] Despite this, practical experience by one of the authors (RS) has observed a good efficacy for humidification.

Example Herbal Formulations for Croup

The herbal treatment of croup should follow a similar pattern to that described for acute tonsillopharyngitis.

References

1   Schwartz J. *Pediatrics* 2004; **113**(Suppl 4): 1037-1043
2   Hammer J, Eber E. *Prog Respir Res* 2005; **33**: 2-7
3   Porth CM. *Pathophysiology* 7th Ed, Lippincott Williams & Wilkins, 2005.
4   Valent F, Little D, Bertollini R et al. *Lancet* 2004; **363**(9426): 2032-2039
5   Mills S, Bone K. *Principles and Practice of Phytotherapy: Modern Herbal Medicine*. Churchill Livingstone, Edinburgh, 2000.
6   Hess DR. *Respir Care* 2007; **52**(10): 1392-1396
7   Kolodziej H. *Planta Med* 2008; [Epub ahead of print]
8   Jimoh T, Guo R, Ernst E. *Planta Med* 2007; **73**(9) Abstract P050, p.839
9   Haidvogl M, Heger M. *Phytomed* 2007; **14**(Suppl 6): 60-64
10   Kolodziej H, Schulz V. *Dtsch Apoth Zeit* 2003; **143**(12): 55-64

11   Bereznoy VV, Riley DS, Wassmer G et al. *Altern Ther Health Med* 2003; **9**(5): 68-79
12   Bachert C, Schapowal A, Kieser M. *Focus Alternat Complement Ther* 2006; **11**(Symposium); Abstract 04
13   Lizogub VG, Riley DS, Heger M. *Explore* 2007; **3**(6): 573-584
14   Heikkinen T, Jarvinen A. *Lancet* 2004; **361**(9351): 51-58
15   Monto AS, Sullivan KM. *Epidemiol Infect* 1993; **110**(1): 145-160
16   Monto AS. *Epidemiol Rev* 1994; **16**(2): 351-371
17   Monto AS, Ullman BM. *JAMA* 1974; **227**(2): 164-169
18   Wald ER, Dashefsky B, Byers C et al. *J Pediatr* 1998; **112**(4): 540-546
19   Ball TM, Holberg CJ, Aldous MB et al. *Ach Pediatr Adolesc Med* 2002; **156**(2): 121-126
20   Markova T, Chuvirov D. *Adv Exp Med Biol* 2007; **601**: 301-306
21   Moscona A. *J Clin Invest* 2005; **115**(7): 1688-1698
22   Dreschers S, Franz P, Dumitru C et al. *Cell Physiol Biochem* 2007; **20**(1-4): 241-254
23   Wine JJ. *Auton Neurosci* 2007; **133**(1): 35-54
24   Heikkinen T. *Vaccine* 2000; **19**(1): 51-55
25   Kleigman RM, Behrman RE, Jenson HB, Stanton BF. *Nelson Textbook of Pediatrics* 18th Ed, Saunders Elsevier, Philadelphia, 2007.
26   Igarashi Y, Skoner DP, Doyle WJ et al. *J Allergy Clin Immunol* 1993; **92**(5): 722-731
27   Winther B, Brofeldt S, Gronborg H et al. *Acta Otolaryngol* 1984; **98**(3-4): 315-320
28   Winther B. *Dan Med Bull* 1994; **41**(2): 193-204
29   Heikkinen T, Ruuskanen O, Ziegler T et al. *J Pediatr* 1995; **126**(2): 313-316
30   Autret-Leca E, Giraudeau B, Ployet MJ et al. *Br J Clin Pharmacol* 2002; **54**(6): 652-656
31   Fahey T, Stacks N, Thomas T. *Arch Dis Child* 1998; **79**(3): 225-230
32   Arrol B, Kenealy T. *Cochrane Database Syst Rev* 2005; **20**(3): CD000247
33   Bone K. *A Clinical Guide to Blending Liquid Herbs.* Churchill Livingstone, Edinburgh, 2000.
34   Braun L, Cohen M. *Herbs and Natural Supplements* 2nd Ed. Churchill Livingstone, Edinburgh, 2007.
35   American Academy of Pediatrics. *Pediatrics* 2001; **108**(3): 798-808
36   British Herbal Medicine Association's Scientific Committee. *British Herbal Pharmacopoeia*, BHMA, Bournemouth, 1983.
37   Kasper DL, Braunwald E, Fauci AS et al. *Harrison's Principles of Internal Medicne* 16th Ed. McGraw-Hill, New York, 2005.
38   Olivier C. *JAC* 2000; **45**(1): 13-21
39   Bone K. *The Ultimate Herbal Compendium,* Phytotherapy Press, Warwick, Qld, 2007.
40   Bosio K, Avanzini C, D'Avolio A et al. *Lett Appl Microbiol* 2000; **31**(2): 174-177
41   Drago L, De Vecchi E, Nicola L, Gismondo MR. *J Appl Microbiol* 2007; **103**(5): 1914-1921
42   Broide DH. *Allergy Asthma Proc* 2007; **28**(4): 398-403
43   Ibhanesebhor SE, Otobo ES. *J Trop Pediatr* 1996; **42**(6): 327-329
44   Ramsey KH, Poulsen CE, Motiu PP. *J Reprod Immunol* 1998; **38**(2): 155-167
45   Norman EK. *Lancet* 2005; **366**(9479): 6-7
46   Stoss M, Michels C, Peter E et al. *J Altern Complement Med* 2000; **6**(6): 499-508
47   Freid VM, Mukuc DM, Rooks RN. *Vital Health Stat* 1998; **13**(137): 1-23
48   Rovers MM, Schilder AGM, Zielhuis GA, Rosenfeld RM. *Lancet* 2004; **363**(9407): 465-473
49   Faden H. *Eur J Pediatr* 2001; **160**(7): 407-413
50   Takala AK, Jero J, Kela E et al. *JAMA* 1995; **15**(273): 859-864
51   Chantry CJ, Howard CR, Auinger P. *Pediatrics* 2006; **117**(2): 425-432
52   Tasker A, Dettmar PW, Panetti M et al. *Laryngoscope* 2002; **112**(11): 1930-1934
53   Lieu JE, Muthappan PG, Uppaluri R. *Otolaryngol Head Neck Surg* 2005; **133**(3): 357-361
54   Crapko M, Kerchener JE, Syring M, Johnston N. *Laryngoscope* 2007; **117**(8): 1419-1423
55   Lubianca Neto JF, Hemb L, Silva DB. *J Pediatr (Rio J)* 2006; **82**(2): 87-96
56   Cherry J, Morguiles S. *Laryngoscope* 1968; **73**(11): 1937-1940
57   Kraemer MJ, Richardson MA, Weiss NS, et al. *JAMA* 1983; **249**(8): 1022-1025
58   Uhari M, Mantysaari K, Niemeia M. *Clin Infect Dis* 1996; **22**(6): 1079-1083
59   Burgess N. *Mod Phytother* 1995; **1**(2): 6-7
60   McIntyre A. *Herbal Treatment of Children.* Elsevier Butterworth Heinemann, Edinburgh, 2005.
61   Sarrell EM, Mandelberg A, Cohen HA. *Arch Pediatr Adolesc Med* 2001; **155**(7): 796-799
62   Sarrell EM, Cohen HA, Kahan E. *Pediatrics* 2003; **111**(5 Pt 1): e574-579
63   Plaut M, Valentine MD. *NEJM* 2005; **353**(18): 1934-1946
64   Ciprandi G, Cirillo I, Vizzaccaro A et al. *Allergy* 2005; **60**(7): 882-887
65 . Schoenwetter WF. *Allergy Asthma Proc* 2000; **21**(1): 1-6
66   Sly RM. *Clin Rev Allergy Immunol* 2002; **22**(1): 67-103
67   Blaiss MS. *Curr Med Res Opin* 2004; **20**(12): 1937-1952
68   Demoly P, Bousquet J. *Lancet* 2006; **368**(9537): 711-713

69   Jeffery PK, Haahtela T. *BMC Pulm Med* 2006; **6**(1): S5
70   Gaga M, Lambrou P, Papageorgiou N et al. *Clin Exp Allergy* 2000; **30**(5): 663-669
71   Togias A. *J Allergy Clin Immunol* 2003; **111**(6): 1171-1183
72   Dixon AE, Kaminsky DA, Holbrook JT et al. *Chest* 2006; **130**(2): 429-435
73   Thomas M. *BMC Pulm Med* 2006; **6**(1): S4
74   Lambrou P, Zervas E, Oikonomidou E et al. *Ann Allergy Asthma Immunol* 2007; **98**(6): 567-572
75   Togias A. *J Allergy Clin Immunol* 2004; **113**(1): S8-14
76   Schoenwetter WF, Dupclay L, Appajosyula S et al. *Curr Med Res Opin* 2004; **20**(3): 305-317
77   Kay GG. *J Allergy Clin Immunol* 2000; **105**(6): S622-627
78   Chatzi L, Apostolaki G, Bibakis I et al. *Thorax* 2007; **62**(8): 677-683
79   Tattersfield AE, Knox AJ, Britton JR, Hall IP. *Lancet* 2002; **360**(9342): 1313-1322
80   Landau LI. *MJA* 2002; **177**(6 Suppl): S38-S39
81   Etzel RA. *Pediatrics* 2003; **112**(1): 233-239
82   Devereux G. *Nat Rev Immunol* 2006; **6**(11): 869-874
83   Umetsu DT, McIntire JJ, Akbari O et al. *Nat Rev Immunol* 2002; **3**(8): 715-720
84   Droste JH, Wieringa MH, Weyler JJ et al. *Clin Exp Allergy* 2000; **30**(11): 1547-1553
85   Von Ehrenstein OS, Von Mutius E, Illi S et al. *Clin Exp Allergy* 2000; **30**(2): 187-193
86   Riedler J, Braun-Fahrlander C, Eder W et al. *Lancet* 2001; **358**(9306): 623-624
87   Plats-Mills T, Vaughan J, Squillace S et al. *Lancet* 2001; **357**(9258): 752-756
88   Schneider AP, Stein RT, Fritscher CC. *J Bras Pneumol* 2007; **33**(4): 454-462
89   Litonjua AA, Rifas-Shiman SL, Ly NP et al. *Am J Clin Nutr* 2006; **84**(4): 903-911
90   Arshad SH. .*J Allergy Clin Immunol* 2005; **116**(1): 3-14
91   Devereux G, Turner SW, Craig LC et al. *Am J Respir Crit Care Med* 2006; **174**(5): 499-507
92   Nja F, Nystad W, Lodrup Carlson KC et al. *Acta Paediatr* 2005; **94**(2): 147-154
93   Devereux G, Seaton A. *J Allergy Clin Immunol* 2005; **115**(6): 1109-1117
94   McKeever TM, Britton J. *Am J Respir Crit Care Med* 2004; **170**(7): 725-729
95   Bolte G, Frye C, Hoelscher B et al. *Am J Respir Crit Care Med* 2004; **163**(1): 277-279
96   Dunstan JA, Mori TA, Barden A et al. *J Allergy Clin Immunol* 2003; **112**(6): 1178-1184
97   Weiland SK, von Mutius E, Husing A, Asher MI. *Lancet* 1999; **353**(9169): 2040-2041
98   Wickens K, Barry D, Friezema A et al. *Allergy* 2005; **60**(12): 1537-1541
99   Gdalevich M, Mimouni D, Mimouni M. *J Pediatr* 2001; **139**(2): 261-266
100 Story RE. *Curr Opin Pediatr* 2007; **19**(6): 680-684
101 Flaherman V, Rutherford GW. *Arch Dis Child* 2006; **91**(4): 334-339
102 Chinn S. *J Asthma* 2003; **40**(1): 1-16
103 Stordal K, Johannesdottir GB, Bentson BS et al. *Acta Paediatr* 2006; **95**(10): 1197-1201
104 Sood A, Ford ES, Camargo CA. *Thorax* 2006; **61**(4): 300-305
105 Noverr MC, Huffnagle GB. *Clin Exp Allergy* 2005; **35**(12): 1511-1520
106 Kozyrskyj AL, Ernst P, Becker AB. *Chest* 2007; **131**(6): 1753-1759
107 Marra F, Lynd L, Coombe, M et al. *Chest* 2006;**129**(3):610-618
108 Bjorksten B, Naaber P, Sepp E, Mikelsaar M. *Clin Exp Allergy* 1999; **29**(3): 342-346
109 Sepp E, Julge K, Mikelsaar M, Bjorksten B. *Clin Exp Allergy* 2005; **35**(9): 1141-1146
110 McEwen BS. *Physiol Rev* 2007; **87**(3): 973-904
111 Wright RJ, Cohen S, Carey V et al. *Am J Respir Crit Care Med* 2002; **165**(3): 358-365
112 Klinnert MD. *Pediatr Pulmonol* 1997; **24**(4): 234-236
113 Sandberg S. *Thorax* 2004; **59**(12): 1046-1051
114 Weil CM. *Pediatrics* 1999; **104**(6): 1274-1280
115 Robinson DS. *Br Med Bull* 2000; **56**(4): 956-968
116 Ahern DJ, Robinson DS. *Curr Opin Allergy Clin Immunol* 2005; **5**(6): 531-538
117 Robinson DS, Larche M, Durham SR. *J Clin Invest* 2004; **114**(10): 1389-1397
118 Hawrylowicz CM, O'Garra A. *Nat Rev Immunol* 2005; **5**(4): 271-283
119 Heaton T, Rowe J, Turner S et al. *Lancet* 2005; **365**(9454): 142-149
120 Wills-Karp M. *Proc Am Thorac Soc* 2007; **4**(3): 247-251
121 Shima M, Adachi M. *Prev Med* 1996; **25**(5): 617-624
122 Lee SH, Rhim T, Choi YS et al. *Am J Respir Crit Care Med* 2006; **173**(4): 370-378
123 Stevenson LM, Matthias A, Banbury L et al. *Molecules* 2005; **10**(10): 1279-1285
124 Bowgain-Rouse M. 6th International Conference on Prostaglandins, Florence. 1986.
125 Knutson D, Aring A. *Am Fam Physician* 2004; **69**(3): 534-540
126 Lavine E, Scolnik D. *CJEM* 2001; **3**(3): 209-212

CHAPTER 7

Common Nervous System Disorders in Children

IN CONTRAST TO MANY other body systems, the nervous system grows proportionally more rapidly before birth.[1] The quickest period of growth is between 15 and 20 weeks gestation, at which time there is a significant increase in the number of neurons. A second growth spurt occurs between 30 weeks gestation and 1 year of age.[1,2] At birth, the average brain weighs approximately 325 g (11.5 oz). By 1 year of age this weight has tripled.[1] Head circumference, one of the best indicators of brain growth, increases 6 times as much during the first year of life as it does during the second year.[1]

At birth the nervous system is not completely integrated, but is obviously sufficiently developed to sustain extra-uterine life.[1] Most of the neurological reflexes are primitive. These reflexes comprise a group of behavioural motor responses or adaptive reactions that are part of normal early development and will disappear as the brain and nervous system mature.[3] Such automatic movements are directed by the brain stem, the primitive part of the brain. As they fulfil their function, they are inhibited and replaced by postural reflexes controlled by the cortex.[2] Such reflexes include the Moro or the startle reflex, the rooting or suckling reflex and the stepping reflex. They are used to evaluate the newborn or infant system.[1]

The maturation of the nervous system also includes an increase in the size of neurons, the size and number of glial cells and the number of interneuron connections.[1] As this maturation continues, the level of functioning develops from the simple to the complex: from primitive reflexes to purposeful movement controlled by the cortex.[1,3]

The first year of life is marked by psychosocial developmental milestones, facilitated by the satisfaction of basic needs.[1] There are many theoretical constructs concerning human development; one of the most commonly used is the Erikson theory. Erik Erikson, a student of Freud, proposed that personality development is a continual process throughout life that is determined by the interaction of the internal maturation process with external social demands, in other words, the expected interplay of nature and nurture.[4] He proposed eight stages of development, listed in the table below.

THE EIGHT STAGES IN ERIKSON'S THEORY[4]

Psychosocial stage	Age	Challenge
Basic trust vs mistrust	Birth to 1 year	To develop a sense that the world is a safe place
Autonomy vs shame and doubt	1 to 3 years	To realise that one is an independent person who can make decisions
Initiative vs guilt	3 to 6 years	To develop the ability to try new things and to handle failure
Industry vs inferiority	6 to adolescence	To learn basic skills and work with others
Identity vs identity confusion	Adolescence	To develop a lasting sense of self
Intimacy vs isolation	Young adulthood	To commit to another in a relationship
Generativity vs stagnation	Middle adulthood	To contribute to younger people, through child rearing or other productive work
Integrity vs despair	Late life	To view one's life as satisfactory and worth living

Contemporary Parenting/Childhood Issues

Parenting, including parenting fashions, clearly has the ability to impact on the emotional and social development of the child. Few would disagree that we live in changing times and the integration of mind, body and social issues that should underpin a holistic approach necessitates a brief discussion of some contemporary issues in parenting. Shifting economic structures have led to profound changes in the organisation of family life.[5] Urbanisation and economic demands have resulted in greater mobility, less time for family life and a breakdown of the extended family.[6] Many families are isolated from traditional sources of child-rearing information, where parenting was learnt by example.[6] At the same time there has been a loss of information about traditional folk/family medicine. This information void has been rapidly filled by various medical, psychological and psychiatric health professionals offering highly subjective views on child rearing, resulting in the area becoming "professionalised".[5] Further to this, parenting information is often gained via the modern media, with a proliferation of television programmes, such as *Supernanny*, and websites. Presumably this is in response to a demand from modern parents, who believe that parenting is tougher now than for previous generations.[7]

Recently, western culture's attitude to child rearing has changed radically, from discipline and authority to permissiveness and individual rights.[8] This new culture has, among other things, seen a commercialisation of childhood. Whole industries of consumer goods for children have developed.[9] As a result, children now have access to adult information and entertainment and the boundaries between what are considered adulthood and childhood have become blurred. This has lead to the opinion in some quarters that children are in effect miniature adults.[9] One notable result of these changing expectations of childhood is that behaviour previously considered normal, such as inattention and distractibility, are now viewed as problematic. These perceived problematic behaviours are now more likely to draw medical attention.[5,9] Contemporary language also reflects this change, as we are more likely to use medical labels to describe a child's feelings, such as "depression", than less pathological descriptions such as "unhappy".[9]

Cognition, Behaviour and the Environment

There is considerable concern over the long-term consequences of modern toxic threats from air, water, food and soil pollution.[10] The foetus, infant and child are particularly vulnerable to such threats. There are numerous practical reasons behind this vulnerability. For example, more food and water is consumed per unit of body weight and children breathe in relatively more air.[11] Their immature organ systems, especially the developing nervous system, are more sensitive to toxins and the blood/brain barrier is immature and porous, allowing greater access to these chemicals.[10] The skin surface absorbs relatively more toxic material and has lower levels of some chemical binding proteins, allowing more of the chemical to reach target organs.[10,11] This is compounded by the normal behaviour of infants and toddlers that sees them ingest soil and floor dust. Finally, rapid growth increases the long-term accumulation of chemicals.[10] Although this discussion will focus primarily on effects in children, it is thought that end organ vulnerability may be greatest in the foetus and that for some compounds the toxic effects seen in childhood are primarily the result of foetal exposure.[10]

Persistent Organic Pollutants (POPs)

POPs are chemicals that are extremely stable, can be transported over large distances, accumulate in high concentrations in fatty tissue and are magnified through the food chain.[10,12] Due to their semi-volatility, POPs evaporate from the warmer regions of the earth and condense in the polar regions, thus posing a major threat to the people and other life forms living in those areas.[10,12] Some POPs are pesticides and nine, including DDT, have been banned from use in western countries. However their persistence and accumulation in the food chain, especially from foods high in fat, have resulted in continued widespread human exposure in these regions.[10,12] Dioxins and polychlorinated biphenyls (PCBs) are example of POPs that continue to be of great concern. They exhibit similar biological activity to each other.[10] Although PCBs are now banned, we are left with their legacy.[10] Because of the biopersistence of POPs, children remain actively exposed to organochlorin pesticides, dioxins and PCBs. They are present in most foods (unless organic) especially meat, fish, eggs and breast milk.[10]

The adverse effects of dioxins result from their ability to bind to the aryl hydrocarbon receptor,[10] a ligand-activated transcription factor that regulates the genes involved in xenobiotic metabolism, cellular proliferation and differentiation.[13] It is also known as the dioxin receptor and is distributed in the central nervous system, the cardiovascular system and in reproductive tissue.[14] Children suffering increased exposure to dioxins and PCBs have exhibited impaired neurodevelopment at 7 months[15] and (in another cohort) at 42 months.[16] At 7 years of age, boys exposed to high levels of PCBs demonstrated less masculine play and girls less feminine play.[17]

Lead

The effect of environmental lead exposure on children's health is one of the most clearly understood issues. However, there is still a great deal of controversy over what is considered to be a safe level of exposure. Children appear to be especially sensitive to lead. In comparison to adults, more is absorbed via the gastrointestinal tract, a greater proportion of systemically circulating lead reaches the brain (especially for children under 5 years) and the developing nervous system is particularly vulnerable to lead exposure.[10] Although lead's toxicity cannot be explained in terms of a single mechanism, it appears that its ability to substitute calcium is a factor common to many of its toxic effects.[18] For example, lead's ability to cross the blood/brain barrier is primarily due to its ability to substitute for calcium ions.[19,20] With the banning of lead in petroleum, industrial emissions have become the major contributor to environmental contamination.[10] The effects of lead are thought to be related to blood concentrations and safe blood lead limits have progressively decreased from 60 μg/dL in the 1960s to the current WHO guideline of a maximum of 10 μg/dL.[10] This level is still controversial and a current question is whether any level of blood lead is safe (see below).

With respect to lead's neurotoxicity, the amount of lead in the brain is of most interest. Because this cannot be measured in humans, the surrogate exposure biomarker most often used is blood lead.[23] Only 5% of an individual's total burden of lead is in the blood and is tightly bound to erythrocytes. The most important toxic fraction is in the plasma, due to its access to soft tissues such as the brain.[23] Hence blood lead as an index of exposure is likely to significantly underestimate the potential neurotoxicity.[23] A relatively recent review concluded that detrimental effects can occur at levels below 10 μg/dL and a safe level of lead is yet to be established.[18]

A consistent message in the findings from the comparative and pooled data of 7 prospective studies on lead is that it reduces IQ.[18,21] More recent work has demonstrated that blood lead concentrations correlate to lower IQ, externalising behaviour (aggression and hyperactivity) and school problems. The study was conducted in 780 urban 5- to 7-year-olds.[22]

At the lower doses characteristic of community exposure, it is thought that lead disrupts the role of neurotransmitter systems in sculpting the brain.[23] Specifically, by increasing the normal basal release of neurotransmitters and inhibiting the release evoked by depolarisation, the presence of lead in the neuronal environment increases the level of background noise in excitatory synapses.[24]

Methyl Mercury

Like lead, mercury is a heavy metal that exists naturally in the environment. Exposure levels have risen because of discharges from the hydroelectric, mining, pulp and paper industries, the incineration of municipal and medical waste and the emissions from power plants, especially those burning coal.[25] The US Environmental Protection Agency (EPA) estimates that 50 to 75% of the total input of mercury into the atmosphere results from human activities.[25] Mercury exists in the environment in several different forms, namely metallic, organic and inorganic and interconversion between these forms can occur.[23] Microbes in soil and in river and lake sediments can convert elemental or inorganic mercury into organic methyl mercury (MeHg), the most toxic and bioavailable form of mercury.[12] MeHg accumulates most efficiently in the aquatic food chain, with predatory fish at the top of the chain containing the highest concentrations, such as shark, swordfish and tuna.[25] Consumption of marine life is the major route of human exposure to MeHg, and when ingested almost all of it is absorbed.[12]

The recognition of the devastating effects of high-dose MeHg exposure has led investigators to ask whether low-dose *in utero* exposure, more typical of the seafood consumer, is associated with neurological effects. There is strong evidence from animal studies that *in utero* exposure has significant neurotoxic activity.[12,23,25] The WHO has identified maternal hair levels of 10 to 20 µg/g as the range for which the risk of adverse neurodevelopmental outcomes, such as delayed walking or speech, begin to rise.[23] However, there is strong criticism of using hair mercury as a biomarker, since this compartment is, biologically speaking, considerably remote from the brain.[23] Several longitudinal, prospective studies evaluated the above conclusion of the WHO by studying birth cohorts in populations with a high seafood diet. Studies from New Zealand and the Faroe Islands demonstrated an inverse association between prenatal exposure to MeHg and a child's neurodevelopment.[23] A follow-up study in the Faroe Islands cohort concluded that the neurodevelopmental problems observed during the first intervention as the result of prenatal MeHg exposure were multifocal and permanent.[26] An Australian study clearly demonstrated the risk to small children from eating more than one serving of fish per fortnight. The study found that children under the age of six who regularly eat large predatory fish had mercury levels up to seven times the safe level.[27] The subjects of the study were Chinese infants living in Sydney who had all been weaned on fish congee up to eight times a week. They presented with developmental delays or neurological problems. One of the fathers was also diagnosed with mercury poisoning after complaining of rashes, abdominal pain and diarrhoea.[27] A recently published ecological study in Texas revealed alarming results. It found that for every 1000 lbs of environmentally-released mercury in a region, there was a 43% increase in the need for special education services and a 61% increase in the rate of autism.[28]

Potential New Threats

In 1995, Greenpeace conducted a study that demonstrated the presence of medium-chain-length chlorinated paraffins (MCCPs) in human breast milk.[10] MCCPs are used to make a wide range of products including PVC plastics, paints, sealants, glues, flame retardants, rubber and leather goods. They are released into the environment when the products are manufactured.[29] It is thought that MCCPs are absorbed by animals and humans via soil, water and food. Studies on fish and rodents have demonstrated harmful effects, although effects on humans are as yet unknown.[29]

Mixed Exposures

Most of the research into the detrimental effects of chemicals on biological systems is focussed on one substance at a time. However, in the real world we are exposed to mixtures, not single compounds. Much of the contemporary concern about chemical mixtures stems from the possibility that pollutants might have synergistic or additive effects.[30] A recent study, the first to measure multiple toxins in umbilical cord blood, revealed some potentially alarming results. The cord blood from 10 newborns was found to contain 287 chemicals, of which 180 are known to cause cancer in humans or animals, 217 are toxic to the brain and nervous system and 208 cause birth defects or abnormal development in animals.[31] Exposure does not necessarily have to be at a cytotoxic level, as low-dose exposure can still have a significant impact at both molecular and cellular levels.[32]

Detoxification for Children

Effective herbal therapy for heavy metal detoxification should involve those herbs that both prevent heavy metal absorption and those that are capable of mobilising them from soft tissue. On current knowledge, there are few herbal remedies that fit this requirement, most notably St Mary's thistle and garlic. No paediatric studies have been performed on those, so the reliance is on experimental and adult data.

Garlic is now well known to antagonise lead and to protect against cadmuim toxicity in animal models, comparable to drugs such as D-penicillamine used to treat heavy metal toxicity.[33] Garlic given to chicken either exposed to natural or experimental lead toxicity had a superior effect as a post-exposure treatment, which suggests that garlic is capable of mobilising lead from the tissues.[34] After 1 to 3 months of treatment with garlic, signs of chronic lead toxicity were reduced by 83% in workers with occupational lead poisoning.[34] Following on from research that demonstrated silymarin in St Mary's (milk) thistle could strongly bind iron, test tube experiments established that it could also strongly bind heavy metals.[35]

For those children who have been exposed to heavy metals or consume a high seafood diet and/or high meat diet, treatment is relevant. This will also be the case for children showing high levels of exposure to organochlorines and heavy metals in body tissues. In addition, high POP exposure can be suspected where there is evidence of endocrine disruption, poor neurodevelopment or a relevant diagnosis such as autism. In other words the requirement for POP treatment can either be presumptive or diagnostic.

Key herbs to help facilitate the removal of POPs are those that boost phase I/II detoxification by the liver. These include Schisandra, rosemary, green tea and turmeric.[36]

Stress

The human response to stress is well documented[1] and it is linked to deviations in immune function and several diseases in adults, including a heightened risk of cardiovascular disease[37] and an increased susceptibility to infectious diseases.[38] The impact of stress on the health of children is less documented. Several studies have reported increased levels of respiratory infection associated with school stress amongst children.[39,40] For children predisposed to atopy and asthma, high levels of parental stress predicted increases in proliferative responses to selected allergens[41] and were a predictor of wheezing in infancy.[42] Low socioeconomic status and stress were associated with elevations in the inflammatory cytokines IL-5 and IFN-γ in asthmatic adolescents.[43] More recently, chronic family stress was associated with an increase in the frequency of illnesses and enhanced natural killer cell (NKC) cytotoxicity in children.[44] This impact of chronic stress on NKC cytotoxicity in children is in contrast to that usually found in adults, where decreases in activity are consistently found.[45]

Herbal Treatment

An example liquid formulation is as follows:

Withania	1:1	25 mL
Skullcap	1:2	25 mL
Spiny jujube or Bacopa	1:2	25 mL
Chamomile	1:2	25 mL
	Total	100 mL

Dose: Calculate the standard dose according to the most appropriate guideline in Chapter 1, based on an adult dose of 5 mL. To be taken with water three times a day.

Rationale

Withania is an indicated remedy for the stressed, underweight child.[46] Its adaptogenic properties will aid in modifying the stress response, whilst not overly stimulating the child. Spiny jujube or Zizyphus provides gentle nervous system tonic and calming activity.[47] Another herb with similar properties is Bacopa. Skullcap has traditional indications for restlessness and wakefulness and possesses nervous system tonic properties.[46] Chamomile is the classical herbal remedy for restlessness and nervous irritability in children.[46,48]

Alternatives to the above liquid formulation are Nervous System Tonic tablets (adult dose 4 per day), Sleep/Anxiety Support tablets (adult dose 4 per day) or Stress Control tablets (adult dose 4 per day). See Appendix 1 for the suggested formulations. A judicious combination of 2 of these formulations may be appropriate. Calculate the child's tablet dose according to the most appropriate guideline in Chapter 1. For younger children the tablets can be crushed and mixed with honey or a suitable sweetener to improve compliance.

Common Sleep Problems

Infant sleep difficulties are among the most prevalent problems presenting to paediatricians and other child-care professionals.[49] The consolidation of sleep, referred to as sleeping through the night, is a maturation process that occurs over the first year of life.[50] However, surveys show that as many as 20 to 30% of all infants and toddlers do not achieve this goal and their sleep pattern continues to be fragmented and characterised by multiple and/or prolonged night wakings.[51] Other studies show that 25 to 50% of preschoolers display bedtime resistance and delayed sleep onset.[52,53] There is also increasing evidence that school-age children and adolescents suffer sleep disturbances that are associated with significant impediments to learning, cognition and memory.[54]

Recent data suggest that a significant percentage of children displaying symptoms of attention-deficit/hyperactivity disorder (ADHD) may actually be manifesting symptoms of sleep fragmentation with the consequent daytime behaviour problems secondary to rhythmic movements during sleep.[55] Sleep-related rhythmic movements, seen most frequently in childhood, comprise motor activity characterised by repetitive body movements such as head banging, head rolling and body rocking.[56]

COMMON SLEEP PROBLEMS BY AGE GROUP[56]

Infant/Toddler 1-2 yrs	Preschool 3-5 yrs	School age 6-12 yrs
Behavioural insomnia	Behavioural insomnia	Insufficient sleep
Rhythmic movements	Sleep terrors	Bedtime resistance
	Rhythmic movements	Sleep walking

Certain children are more vulnerable to acute or chronic sleep problems. These include children with medical problems such as chronic illnesses (cystic fibrosis, asthma, rheumatoid arthritis), acute illnesses (otitis media) and children taking stimulating medications (methylphenidate).[57]

Behavioural Insomnia (BI)

BI, as noted in the above table, is common in infants, toddlers and preschoolers. With this sleep problem the child learns to fall asleep under certain conditions or associations, such as being rocked, patted or fed. They do not develop the ability to self soothe.[57] If the child wakes during the night he or she cannot go back to sleep, except under the same conditions. Hence the problem can extend to prolonged night waking, impacting both child and parent.[57] The standard treatment approach is the gradual removal of parental presence. It is common for transitional objects, such as toys or blankets, to be used to help the child self soothe.[57]

Neurophysiology and Sleep

Sleep is described as a reversible state of perceptual disengagement and is a universal behaviour across the animal kingdom.[58] Until recently, the understanding of developmental progress has concentrated on the child's interaction with the environment, with little attention paid to the role of sleep. This was primarily due to the dramatic changes in skill development observed in the first few years of life that seemed to correspond with the increase in the time that the child spends awake.[59] However, recent evidence from school-age children points directly to a close association between a lack of sleep and impairment of learning and other cognitive functions.[60,61] Many researchers believe that a lack of sleep and sleep disorders amongst children can impair IQ as much as lead exposure.[61] One study amongst US sixth graders demonstrated that the loss of one hour of sleep per night was equivalent to the loss of two years of cognitive maturation and development.[62] Furthermore, a shorter sleep duration is associated with an increased risk for being overweight among 9- to 12-year-old children.[63] It appears that adequate sleep is as important as the learning process, in that it optimises the consolidation of newly acquired information.[64,65] The recommended time asleep for children of different ages is provided in the table below.

BEST REST GUIDE[66]

Age	Recommended hours of sleep
0-3 months	12-18 hours including naps
4-12 months	11-14 hours including naps
1-6 years	10-12 hours
7-13 years	9-11 hours
14-18 years	8-10 hours

Common symptoms of poor or inadequate sleep include:[66]
- Slow to get moving in the morning (sleep inertia)
- Daytime sleepiness
- Inattention
- Impaired memory and learning
- Hyperactivity
- Irritability
- Moodiness
- Temper tantrums
- Bedtime struggles

Herbal Treatment

There has been concern expressed over the pharmacological management of paediatric sleep disorders,[67] so herbal remedies seem to be ideally suited, due to their gentle nature and non-addictive properties. While some herbal authorities consider valerian to be a herbal sedative more suited to adults,[68] it has in fact been clinically evaluated in combination with lemon balm for restlessness and insomnia in children. The only real issue with valerian in children is taste and smell, with poor compliance a possible outcome. A total of 918 children less than 12 years of age suffering from restlessness and sleep onset insomnia were given a combined lemon balm/valerian tablet combination in an open, multicentre study. A distinct and convincing reduction in severity was found for all symptoms, as determined by both investigator and parent ratings.[69] Lemon balm seems ideally suited to sleep problems in children where cognitive function is impacted. It has been used for centuries to improve cognitive function and a recent study in healthy adults demonstrated cognition-enhancing properties.[70]

An example liquid formulation for sleep difficulties is as follows:

Chamomile	1:2	25 mL
Passionflower or Skullcap	1:2	25 mL
Lemon balm or Bacopa	1:2	25 mL
Lavender 1:2 or Withania	1:1	25 mL
	Total	100 mL

Dose: Calculate the standard dose according to the most appropriate guideline in Chapter 1, based on an adult dose of 5 mL and prescribe 1 to 3 doses with water before bed.

Chamomile is considered the archetypal children's remedy with a long history of use in folk medicine for whining, irritated infants.[48] It is an excellent herb for restlessness and nervous irritability in children.[46] Passionflower is another remedy with traditional indications for restlessness and insomnia in children.[46] Lemon balm is indicated for the reasons previously stated, supported by traditional indications for nervous sleeping disorders.[46] The formulation is rounded out with the "rescue remedy" of the herbal world, namely lavender. Lavender is a pleasant tasting, child-friendly herbal with traditional indications for restlessness and insomnia.[46] *Withania somnifera*, as the name implies, is a mild tonic with soporific properties.

Alternatives to the above liquid formulation are Nervous System Tonic tablets (adult dose 4 per day) or Sleep Anxiety Support tablets (adult dose 4 per day). See Appendix 1 for the suggested formulations. Calculate the child's tablet dose according to the most appropriate guideline in Chapter 1. For younger children the tablets can be crushed and mixed with honey or a suitable sweetener to improve compliance. The full daily dose can be taken about 1 hour before bed or as two doses, with the last 1 hour before bed.

Case History

A mother presented with a male child who was 18 months old but was not yet sleeping through the night. He exhibited behavioural insomnia that included the need to be patted before sleep and he woke frequently through the night when he could only be soothed by the sound of the clothes drier. The mother was exhausted through lack of sleep. The child was on solid foods supplemented with breast feeding.

The following formulation was prescribed:

Chamomile	1:2	35 mL
Lemon balm	1:2	35 mL
Lavender	1:2	30 mL
Total		100 mL

Dose: 1 mL in 5 mL of breast milk after the evening feed and 1 mL before bed.

It took several days before the child eventually responded to the herbal medicine. During that time the mother gave extra doses whenever the child awoke during the night. After 4 days the child slept through the night for the first time.

Attention Deficit/Hyperactivity Disorder (ADHD)

Historical Features

"Zappel Philip" or The Story of Fidgety Philip, is a poem in a children's book written by Dr Heinrich Hoffman, a German physician. Published in 1846, it described a child with the typical symptoms of ADHD. It is claimed that this description represents the first documented reference to the disorder now known as ADHD.[71] Later in 1902, Dr George Frederick Still (a renowned English paediatrician) described a group of children with an abnormal incapacity for sustained attention, coupled with restlessness and fidgetiness. He argued that these children had deficiencies in volitional inhibition and offered no treatment other than discipline.[72] In the 1920s, hyperactivity and poor attention came to be viewed as involving a small degree of brain damage, as it was observed that following epidemics of encephalitis children often presented with restlessness, personality changes and learning difficulties. Following this, the term minimal brain damage (MBD) was coined to describe the condition.[72] During the 1930s the chance discovery was made that psycho-stimulant medication could reduce these symptoms.[72] By the 1960s the term MBD had lost favour, as evidence for brain damage could not be established. It was during this time that interest grew in behavioural factors.[72]

By the mid-1960s the American Psychiatric Association expanded the second edition of the Diagnostic Statistical Manual (DSM-2) and the term "hyperkinetic reaction of children" was introduced to describe the condition. The DSM-3 in the early 1980s renamed the disorder attention deficit disorder (ADD).[72] A further descriptive name change came with the latest edition of the DSM, the DSM-IV, with the condition defined as ADHD.[5] The DSM-IV defines over 300 mental illnesses, most of which have been "identified" in the last 20 years.[5] In this context it has been suggested that the DSM has inappropriately become a guidebook telling us how we should think about manifestations of the human condition such as sadness, anxiety, sexual activity and alcohol and substance abuse. The concern is that it has the potential to influence our thinking about important social matters, creating medical issues where they may not in fact exist.[5] This is certainly a relevant perspective for ADHD (see later).

ADHD is defined behaviourally in the DSM-IV, since there are no biological markers. It is diagnosed using a number of steps. The symptoms detailed below in relation to inattention and distractibility must appear before the age of 7. They must also occur in two settings, the home and school (or work in the case of an adult). There must also be clear evidence of a clinically significant impairment of social, academic or occupational functioning, and the diagnostician must ensure the symptoms are not secondary to some other disorder or life event.[73]

Symptoms of inattention include:

- Failure to give close attention to detail
- Difficulty sustaining attention in tasks or play
- Often not listening when spoken to
- Often not following through on instructions and failure to finish tasks
- Difficulty in organising tasks and activities
- Avoiding, disliking or being reluctant to engage in tasks requiring sustained mental effort
- Often losing things necessary for a task
- Easily distracted
- Forgetful in everyday activities

Six or more of these must be present, persisting for 6 months or more.

Symptoms of hyperactivity-impulsivity include:

- Fidgets with hands or feet, squirms in seat
- Leaves seat when remaining in seat is the expectation
- Runs about or climbs excessively or inappropriately
- Often "on the go"
- Talks excessively
- Blurts out answers before the question is completed
- Difficulty waiting turn
- Interrupts or intrudes on others

Six or more of these must be present, persisting for 6 months or more.

The DSM-IV defines 3 patterns:

- Predominantly inattentive

- Predominantly hyperactive-impulsive
- A combined pattern

A key premise of the DSM-IV is that a syndrome occurs in an individual, which implies the fault lies within the individual.[74,75] Despite the fact the diagnostician must ensure the symptoms are not secondary to some other disorder or life event, the focus on the individual often inadvertently excludes the possibility that the symptoms may be a response to external events.[5,72,74] The priority of defining, naming and diagnosing the disorder overrides an understanding of the context of the individual's life and their interaction with the social world.[5,72,74]

This has perhaps led to a medicalisation of the condition. In other words a biological cause is emphasised, ignoring social and other factors.[76] Another prominent criticism is the highly subjective nature of the DSM-IV definition, which allows for a liberal interpretation, perhaps making ADHD a convenient dumping ground for a host of difficult problems.[5,72,76] As an example of the inconsistency and subjectivity in the diagnosis of ADHD, it has been shown that only 30% of already-diagnosed ADHD children met the diagnostic criteria when it is based on home and school reports.[76]

The rating of hyperactivity, inattention and disruptiveness can be highly culturally dependent, with different cultures being more tolerant of child-like behaviour.[5,72] All of the symptoms are open to subjective interpretation and can be influenced by the rater's cultural influences.[5,72] The fact is that inattention, impulsivity and motor restlessness is found in all children (and adults) to some degree.[5,72] The diagnosis is therefore based on what is felt to be an inappropriate intensity, frequency and duration of such behaviours. It is cultural norms that define "inappropriate" and non-specific terms such as "often" and "excessive".[5,72]

Recently, Dr Robert Spitzer, who was an architect of the DSM-IV, was quoted in the British press as saying: "30% of children diagnosed with ADHD, as defined by the DSM-IV, don't actually have ADHD but are instead showing normal signs of being happy or sad and many of these conditions might be normal reactions which are not really disorders".[77]

Despite investigations over the last 20 years or more endeavouring to establish ADHD as a neurological disorder, no concrete relationship has been established. The US National Institute of Health stated in 1998 that there was no evidence to support the proposition that ADHD is a biological brain disorder and that the proposed causes are speculative. However, they suggested that evidence supporting the validity of the disorder can be found.[78]

An area of influence that often escapes attention in the diagnosis and pharmacological control of children is the school. The school completes an influential triangle of power: namely medicine, psychology and the school.[79] If "problem" children have not been identified within the family realm, they are soon identified once enrolled at school, with teachers taking on the role of "disease spotters".[79] Teachers are often the first to suggest the diagnosis of ADHD to parents.[80] Pharmaceutical companies exploit the Internet to inform teachers and influence their disease spotting role. For example, Novartis (manufacturers of Ritalin) has an educational website separate from their industry site that contains ADHD resources for teachers.[81]

Epidemiology, Co-morbidity and Genetics

Depending on the source of information, the prevalence of ADHD is between 2 and 12% of children worldwide, with a male to female ratio of about 3:1 and an association with a low socioeconomic status.[82] A probable reason for the wide range in stated occurrence is that studies have used either one of two slightly differing diagnostic criteria: the DSM-IV or instead the European diagnostic criteria for hyperkinetic disorder (HKD), as defined by the International Classification of Diseases 10th Ed (ICD-10).[82] The ICD-10 is more restrictive, demanding a greater degree of symptom expression, possibly explaining why European studies report lower percentages than US and Australian studies where the DSM-IV is used.

The US Center for Disease Control and Prevention (CDC) estimates 4.4 million children aged 4 to 17 years have been diagnosed with ADHD by healthcare professionals. As of 2003, 2.5 million children aged 4 to 17 were receiving medication for the disorder and 7.8% of school-aged children were reported to have an ADHD diagnosis by their parents.[83] Australian statistics are equally alarming. The 1997 National Mental Health and Wellbeing Survey estimated a prevalence rate of 19.3% in boys aged between 6 and 12 years and 13% in children between 6 and 14 years.[84] Research examining data from the US and Australia has shown that ADHD diagnosis and prescription rates are concentrated at two socioeconomic points, low income and high unemployment.[85]

ADHD is not a stand-alone condition and 75% of diagnosed children will have at least one other diagnosable psychiatric condition.[86] This high rate of co-morbidity strongly suggests that the current diagnostic framework does not adequately reflect boundaries between symptoms and conditions, nor a biological cause, and is the subject of great debate in the literature.[5,75,86] Up to 70% of ADHD children will continue to have symptoms into adulthood and the condition has been linked to adult substance abuse and impaired social and emotional development.[73]

Family aggregation, adoption and twin studies suggest that ADHD does have some hereditary influence. Molecular genetic studies conclude that ADHD is associated with the dopamine transporter gene (DAT1) and the dopamine receptor gene (D4).[73] A more recent study of 126 sibling pairs concluded that these two genes, if they are involved in ADHD aetiology at all, make only a minor contribution to overall genetic susceptibility.[87] Genetics most likely dictate vulnerability, not inevitability.

Medical Treatment

For 40 years the drugs of choice for the medical treatment of ADHD have been the stimulants methylphenidate (Ritalin) and amphetamine.[88] Methylphenidate causes an amplification of dopamine signals, which enhances neuronal signalling and thereby improves attention and reduces distractibility.[88] Usual doses range from 10 to 60 mg/day, depending on the age and the response of the child.[89]

A controlled study has raised concerns that methylphenidate may have a growth-suppressive effect in developing children.[90] It appears that the drug detrimentally influences growth hormone secretion, with a subsequent impairment of normal growth.[91] A recent study on the cytogenetic effects of methylphenidate raised further questions over the toxicity of the drug. Treatment with methylphenidate induced a significant increase in chromosomal aberrations and chromatid exchanges in peripheral lymphocytes after 3 months.[92] The chromosomal breaks shown in the study are known to be associated with increased cancer risk.[93] Other side effects of methylphenidate include insomnia, anorexia, dependence, tolerance, liver dysfunction and neuroleptic malignant syndrome.[94]

A 10-country study examining the prescription of psychostimulants for ADHD between 1994 and 2000 found that total use has increased by an average of 12% per year, with the highest increase occurring between 1998 to 2000. Canada and the USA ranked highest, followed by Australia and NZ , then the UK, Sweden, Spain, Netherlands, France and Denmark.[95] Australian prescriptions between 1991 to 1998 increased from 13,398 to 96,582, a jump of 620%. When Ritalin was added to the Australian Pharmaceutical Benefits Scheme in 2005, there was a further 10-fold increase in prescriptions.[96] Not only are more children being prescribed Ritalin, the amount being consumed is increasing.[97] This is presumably because of either a poor response or increased drug tolerance.

Neurochemistry and Neuroimaging

Several neurotransmitters have been implicated in ADHD, including dopamine and noradrenaline (norepinephrine). However, the studies examining this issue demonstrate either inconsistent or conflicting results.[73]

Neuroimaging studies are often cited as confirmation that ADHD is a brain disorder. A recent review of these studies entitled "Broken brains or flawed studies?" noted a number of methodological flaws. Most subjects used in the studies had a history of prior medication use, often for years.[98] Other studies using unmedicated ADHD subjects avoided the necessary use of matched controls.[98] Animal models suggest that any brain differences observed in the studies may well be due to medication.[99] This possibly invalidates any suggestion that ADHD displays a specific neuropathology.

ADHD as a Social Construct

Social/cultural constructionists argue that the medical model of ADHD is a simplistic view that leads to a disengagement from social responsibilities by parents, teachers and doctors. They further propose that it supports the profit motive of the pharmaceutical industry, is a means of social control that stifles diversity in children and promotes the attitude of a "pill for life's problems".[100]

The same group suggests that many modern western cultural factors adversely affect mental health. These include:[100]

- loss of extended family support and shared responsibility for child raising

- mother blame
- pressure on schools and overworked teachers
- breakdown in moral authority of parents in relation to discipline
- busy and hyperactive family life, with hyper-parenting common
- a market economy value system that emphasises individuality, competitiveness and independence, resulting in social inequality

In addition, the central role of an electronic media that is fast-paced, non-linguistic and visually distracting in influencing the minds of children needs to be considered. Sustained attention such as reading and listening may have consequently become less appealing. Exposure to television and computer games from a young age can lead to a sensory addiction, creating problems in less stimulating environments such as school.[5,72] This concept is supported by several cross-sectional studies demonstrating that higher levels of television viewing at a young age, particularly non-educational programmes, are associated with a reduced attention span.[101,102,103]

Is ADHD a Stress Response?

Could an increase in life stressors for children be causing a rise in ADHD-type behaviours? Research pursuing a neurobiological approach notes that the symptoms of ADHD closely parallel those that occur during trauma, such as:

- hyper-alertness
- the need to act quickly
- the need to be "on the go" all the time in the expectation of danger
- an inability to focus attention to anything other than physical safety

The hypothesis is that, in a critical period in infancy, some children experience trauma (whether perceived or actual) that initiates a habitual autonomic response, as though to some external threat. When older, these children have a greater sensitivity to threat perception and revert to a state of "red alert" very easily.[104] Therefore, as with post-traumatic stress, such children will react quickly and with overactivity. It is proposed that many children suffering multiple stressors display symptoms of post-traumatic stress disorder that is wrongly diagnosed as ADHD.[105]

Food Additives and Intolerances

It was not until the 1970s that Feingold broke through with the message that up to 50% of hyperactive children respond favourably to his diet (Kaiser-Permanente) that removes artificial flavours, colours, preservatives and salicylates.[106] His conclusions fell largely on deaf ears among the medical community, possibly because his results were based on clinical observation and not rigorous scientific evidence.

However, a recent review of 23 double blind studies examining the impact of foods or food additives on behaviour in ADHD children has increased the understanding of this issue. In 8 of 9 studies using ADHD subjects, behaviour was worsened by the consumption of additives or improved by a diet free of additives. The other 14 studies looked at ADHD children who also had asthma, eczema or more severe behavioural/neurological disorders. In 10 out of the 14 trials, most children improved on diets free of additives or certain foods such as corn, wheat, milk, oranges, eggs and chocolate.[107]

Bateman and co-workers observed a significant reduction in hyperactivity in 3-year-old children on a diet free from artificial colourings or benzoate preservatives, with an increase in hyperactivity during active challenge.[108] More recently, artificial colours or a sodium benzoate preservative, or both, in the diet resulted in increased hyperactivity in 3-, 8- and 9-year-old children in the general population.[109]

Allergy and Sleep

A small study demonstrated that many children with ADHD also suffer from allergic rhinitis, with 83% reporting allergic rhinitis symptoms, 43% showing signs of allergic rhinitis and 53% noting other atopic disorders.[110] It is recognised that respiratory allergies reduce the time spent asleep.[111] This may well be an important issue, given the previous discussion on sleep and behaviour patterns in children.

Many children diagnosed with ADHD but not taking medication exhibited chronic sleep problems including:[112]

- reluctance or inability to settle into sleep
- difficulties in sleep onset and maintenance
- frequent awakenings
- higher incidence of restless sleep
- nightmares and night terrors
- insufficient daytime alertness

Refined Sugar

In a study involving 261 hyperactive children administered a 5-hour glucose tolerance test, 74% had abnormal glucose tolerance curves. Half of the abnormal curves were low and flat, similar to those in individuals with hypoglycaemia. Hypoglycaemia is associated with an increased production of adrenaline (epinephrine), which in turn can stimulate a nervous or restless reaction.[113] Despite these results, other studies have consistently failed to demonstrate a clear link between sugar intake and behaviour. However many of the studies used aspartame as the placebo and, given the recent link between aspartame and behavioural and neurological effects,[114] this might invalidate these studies. Another limitation of the refined sugar studies is the dose of sucrose used in comparison to the children's normal daily intake. It is estimated that the average US child consumes approximately 40 to 50 teaspoons of sugar per day.[113] Children who drink 3 to 4 carbonated beverages per day can easily achieve this intake, especially if they are also consuming sugar-coated cereals, ice cream and biscuits. The dosage used in the studies falls way below this intake.

Environmental Exposures

Recent investigations have identified several environmental factors associated with ADHD. Several research groups have shown that lead toxicity leads to distractibility, hyperactivity, restlessness and lower intellectual functioning. Such signs and symptoms are very similar to the profile of ADHD. For example, a study of 501 children showed a significant relationship between blood lead levels and aggressive/antisocial and hyperactive behaviour.[115] A striking dose-response relationship was found between hair lead levels and ADHD symptoms, as rated by teachers, in 277 first grade children.[116] An even stronger relationship was evident for physician ratings.[116] Raised blood lead levels were associated with a small but statistically significant increase in hyperactivity and inattention in children in general.[117]

Mercury and manganese are considered to be other neurodevelopmental toxins that might be linked to ADHD symptomatology. As mentioned previously mercury is commonly encountered as dietary MeHg. The New Zealand and Faroe Island studies noted earlier clearly demonstrated that maternal exposure to MeHg adversely affects offspring IQ, language development, visual-spatial skills, gross motor skills, memory and attention.[26] The developmental neurotoxicity of manganese has recently emerged as a significant public health concern. In several small epidemiological studies manganese hair levels in children were associated with ADHD symptoms.[118] The concern appears to be infant formulas (breast milk contains about 6 µg/L while infant formulas can contain up to 77-100 µg/L) as well as manganese-containing fuel octane enhancers.[118]

The neurodevelopmental effects of PCBs have been extensively studied. Most of the cohort studies have concentrated on prenatal PCB exposure and demonstrate that this is associated with poor concentration or attention, less accurate performance and slower reaction times.[119]

Foetal exposure to a high maternal intake of alcohol results in foetal alcohol spectrum disorder (FASD).[120] FASD is an umbrella term that includes foetal alcohol syndrome (FAS), alcohol-related birth defects and alcohol-related neurodevelopment disorder (ARND).[120] With ARND the child is exposed to alcohol during pregnancy and, while not displaying the full features of FAS, suffers a range of cognitive, emotional and behavioural problems.[120] The relationship between ARND and ADHD is not known at this time, however it has been established that ARND is often misdiagnosed as ADHD in indigenous communities.[121]

Essential Fatty Acids (EFAs)

Omega-3 fatty acids have been specifically implicated in nervous system function and, in animal models, a deficiency is associated with behavioural and neurological dysfunction.[122] A reliable symptom of EFA deficiency is polydipsia without polyuria and it was reported as early as 1981 that hyperactive children were significantly thirstier than controls.[123] Colquhoun and Bunday have proposed that hyperactive children are either unable to absorb or metabolise, or have a greater requirement for EFAs, and this is particularly relevant to boys.[123] These researchers have suggested that many of the foods that ADHD children are allergic to inhibit the conversion of EFAs to eicosanoids.[123] Many hyperactive children have allergies which are relieved by EFAs and many are zinc deficient, which is needed for EFA conversion.[123] Further research has established that plasma levels of docosahexaenoic acid (DHA), arachidonic acid (AA) and dihomo-gamma linolenic acid (DGLA) in ADHD boys were consistently and significantly lower than controls. Such children also manifested other symptoms of EFA deficiency, such as dry hair, dandruff and dry skin.[124] Preliminary data strongly suggest that ADHD children have higher rates of oxidative breakdown of omega-3 fatty acids than controls, as measured by exhaled ethane levels.[125]

The clinical evidence supporting the use of EFA supplements in ADHD patients is far from conclusive, possibly because of the complexities of the disorder. However, a recent double blind, placebo-controlled study concluded that unsaturated fatty acid supplementation appeared to reduce ADHD-related symptoms.[126] These results are further supported by a randomised, placebo-controlled crossover study of 6 months duration. In this study 117 children from 5 to 12 years with developmental coordination disorder were given a capsule containing 80% fish oil and 20% evening primrose oil at a dose of 6 capsules per day for 3 months treatment. There was no effect on motor skills, but a significant improvement was observed in reading, spelling and behaviour.[127]

Minerals

Iron (Fe) deficiency is the most common of all nutritional deficiencies in US school-age children.[107] It is associated with significant decreases in attentiveness and a narrower attention span, possibly due to abnormal dopaminergic transmission.[128] One recent study showed that 84% of the 53 children with ADHD had lower serum ferritin levels compared to 27 controls, with very low levels correlating to more severe symptoms.[128] More recently Fe supplementation improved ADHD symptoms in nonanaemic children with low serum ferritin levels.[129] It was recently reported that Fe protected the integrity of the blood/brain barrier against lead insults in an animal model.[130] It has been further shown that Fe deficiency could lead to an increased toxic effect of lead, and there is possibly a neuroprotective effect for Fe in relation to dopaminergic dysfunction from lead exposure.[131,132]

Zinc (Zn) deficiency has been demonstrated in ADHD children. Zn is an important element in the conversion of EFAs to eicosanoids and low serum Zn has been correlated with parent and teacher ratings of inattention.[133] A more recent study found that plasma Zn was low in ADHD children, which was thought to be relevant to brain information processing.[134] Two recent double blind, placebo-controlled randomised studies established the efficacy of improved Zn intake in children with diagnosed ADHD.[135,136]

A research team reported reduced magnesium (Mg) levels in 95% of a group of 116 children with diagnosed ADHD.[137] Two subsequent controlled studies using a Mg supplement reported an improvement in symptoms for a small group of ADHD children.[138,139]

Leaky Gut

A controversial causal relationship has been proposed between behavioural disorders such as autism, Asperger's syndrome, ADHD and dyslexia and an increased intestinal permeability brought about by gut pathogens, infections and/or inflammation. The onset of behavioural symptoms was associated by parents with the measles, mumps and rubella (MMR) vaccination which may trigger the leaky gut.[140]

Clinical Evidence for Herbs in ADHD

In modern phytotherapy, Bacopa is considered to be the specific herbal remedy for ADHD, due to its cognition enhancing, nervine tonic, mild sedative, mild anticonvulsant, anxiolytic and possibly adaptogenic properties.[46] Its specificity for ADHD is possibly explained by its beneficial effects on concentration and information processing, as evidenced by a study in children (1 g/day for 3 months) that demonstrated improved intellectual functions such as visual motor function, short-term memory and mental reaction times.[46]

Bacopa has been assessed in children via several clinical trials conducted in India. For example, one open-label trial found that Bacopa given to 110 normal boys aged 10 to 13 years for 9 months improved intelligence and memory.[141] In a placebo-controlled trial involving 41 children of normal intelligence, 1050 mg/day of Bacopa leaf for 3 months improved speed, accuracy and short-term memory.[142]

BR-16A or Mentat is a polyherbal Ayurvedic formulation containing Bacopa as the main ingredient. A double blind, placebo-controlled clinical trial was conducted to evaluate the efficacy of Mentat in children with learning disability. The study was carried out in 100 students with learning disability aged between 11 to 16 years who had secured <45% marks at the annual examination, had potential for performing better academically and had IQ >90 and also who did not have any visual or auditory problems. The assessment of cognitive function was done with Malin's intelligence scale of Indian children and the Bender visual motor Gestalt test. Mentat was administered orally for 6 months and results were then evaluated. Children receiving Mentat performed significantly better than placebo. An improvement in attention and concentration as well as an increase in their attention span was seen.[143] In another placebo-controlled study, the efficacy of Mentat in controlling behavioural and cognitive deficits in 40 mentally disadvantaged children was assessed. The efficacy of this remedy was further evaluated in 19 such children with epilepsy. Twelve patients had generalised seizure, 4 had partial and 3 had a mixed seizure pattern. In spite of the usual antiepileptic treatment, the frequency of seizures ranged from 1 to 7 attacks in periods from 1 week to 1 year. With Mentat it was possible to note a reduction in seizure frequency. Patients with higher frequency responded better and there was no further increase in the dosage of antiepileptic drugs. There was also significantly improved control of other abnormal behaviour as shown by a reduction in the rating score on the Children's Behavioural Inventory test. The authors concluded that Mentat was effective in controlling abnormal behaviour, especially hyperactivity and inappropriate behaviour, in mentally disadvantaged children with and without epilepsy.[144]

Mentat was evaluated for its efficacy in 25 children having hyperkinetic behavioural problems aged between 4 to 14 years in an open-label trial. The duration of illness ranged from 6 months to 3 years. Fifteen children were mentally disadvantaged and amongst them ten had a history of brain damage. Mentat syrup brought about "marked improvement" in 5 children as judged by both parents and doctors. No side effects were noted.[145]

In terms of controlled trials in ADHD, two have been conducted: one on Mentat and the other on Bacopa alone. A randomised, double blind, placebo-controlled trial was conducted to evaluate the efficacy of Mentat in school-going children with ADHD. A total of 195 children were screened, out of which 60 satisfied the DSM-IV criteria for ADHD. Among those enrolled in the study, 30 received Mentat and 30 received placebo. An assessment of academic functioning along with psychological tests was done before and after the treatment. Malin's Intelligence Scale for Indian Children, Conner's 10 point rating scale, Kaufman Assessment Battery for Children (KABC) and brain SPECT (Simple Photon Emission Computed Tomography) scans and subtests were assessed. Six children were dropped from the study as they were lost to follow-up and another 4 children showed variable results. Statistical analysis was carried out in only 50 children. The Conner's test and Gestalt closure subtest of KABC showed an improvement in the Mentat group as compared to the placebo group. Pre- and post-SPECT scan observations showed improvement in three children in the Mentat group as compared to one child in the placebo group. However, none of these differences achieved statistical significance because of the low number of trial participants.[146]

The study of Bacopa in ADHD was a small pilot study that has only been published in abstract form. In this trial, a double blind, randomised, placebo-controlled design was employed. A total of 36 patients were selected as per the DSM-IV criteria for ADHD. Of these, 19 patients received Bacopa extract 100 mg/day for 12 weeks and 17 were given placebo. The active herbal treatment was followed by a 4-week placebo administration, making the total duration of the trial 16 weeks in both groups. One patient in the Bacopa group and 6 in the placebo group dropped out. The mean ages were 8.3 years and 9.3 years in the Bacopa and placebo groups respectively. The children were evaluated on a battery of tests: personal information, mental control, sentence repetition, logical memory, word recall, digit span test, delayed response learning, picture recall and paired associate learning. Evaluation was undertaken before, during and at the end of the study. Data analysis revealed a significant improvement on sentence repetition, logical memory and paired associate learning following 12 weeks administration of Bacopa. This improvement was maintained at 16 weeks. During the clinical trial Bacopa exhibited excellent tolerability and no treatment-related adverse effects were reported.[147]

Mexican valerian has demonstrated efficacy in a small double blind, placebo-controlled, crossover, single case methodology study. Five children with intellectual deficits, including two with ADHD and one with moderate intellectual disability and hyperactivity, showed marked improvement in sleep latency and maintenance with a single nightly dose of valerian root (500 mg). This in turn led to an improvement in daytime behaviour and better sleep for parents.[148]

The preliminary data cited above, indicating that ADHD children have higher rates of oxidative breakdown of omega-3 fatty acids than controls, suggests that oxidative stress might play a role. Since 2002, 5 clinical trials have been published on Pycnogenol (a proprietary pine bark extract standardised for oligomeric procyanidins) in ADHD. Four trials were in children and one in adults, making it the most thoroughly investigated herbal extract for ADHD. In one pilot trial, 61 children were supplemented with 1 mg/kg/day Pycnogenol or placebo over a period of 4 weeks in a randomised, placebo-controlled, double blind study. Patients were examined at baseline, after 1 month of treatment and 1 month after the end of treatment period via standard questionnaires. Results showed that 4 weeks of Pycnogenol administration significantly reduced hyperactivity, improved attention and enhanced visual-motoric coordination and concentration in children with ADHD. No positive effects were found in the placebo group. One month after termination of Pycnogenol administration a relapse of symptoms was noted.[149]

The next trial was a randomised, double blind, placebo-controlled design investigating the influence of Pycnogenol or placebo on antioxidant status and the level of oxidised glutathione in children suffering from ADHD. This was the first investigation of glutathione redox status in relation to ADHD. One month of Pycnogenol administration (1 mg/kg/day) caused a significant decrease in oxidised glutathione and a highly significant increase in glutathione levels, compared to a group of patients taking a placebo. Total antioxidant status was also decreased compared to reference levels.[150] Glutathione is the brain's most important endogenous antioxidant and plays a key role in protecting proteins, lipids and nucleic acids against free radical damage.[151]

Following on from the previous trial was a randomised, double blind and placebo-controlled study examining the effect of Pycnogenol on the level of oxidised purines, as represented by 8-oxo-7,8-dihydroguanine (a marker of DNA oxidative damage), in children with ADHD. The study found a significantly increased baseline damage to DNA in ADHD children compared to controls. Levels of 8-oxo-7,8-dihydroguanine were significantly lower after 1 month of treatment in comparison to both baseline and the placebo group. Like the previous study, total antioxidant status was lower in comparison to controls at baseline and significantly increased after one month of pine bark treatment. These changes were also associated with improvements in attention.[152]

Finally, the most recent randomised, double blind, placebo-controlled study tested the hypothesis that one month of treatment with Pycnogenol would reduce hyperactivity in ADHD children. Urinary catecholamine excretion and oxidative stress were also assessed. At baseline, concentrations of catecholamines were higher in the urine of ADHD children compared to controls. Moreover, noradrenaline (norepinephrine) concentrations were positively correlated with the degree of hyperactivity. Both adrenaline (epinephrine) and noradrenaline concentrations were also positively correlated with plasma levels of oxidised glutathione. The pine bark treatment caused a significant decrease in dopamine and a trend to an adrenaline and noradrenaline decrease. The glutathione/oxidised glutathione ratio was significantly increased. The authors suggested that the treatment normalised catecholamine concentrations, leading to less hyperactivity and reduced oxidative stress.[153] Note that if pine bark extract is not available, grape seed extract is chemically very similar and should provide a suitable alternative.

To complete this review of the herbal evidence, a pilot study using a combination of a standardised extract of Ginkgo and American ginseng was tested for its ability to improve ADHD symptoms.[154] The results suggested a positive effect, however their significance is weaker due to a poor study design, such as no blinding or control group, assessment by parents only and the short treatment duration of 4 weeks.

In this context it is interesting to note that a combination of Ginkgo and Korean ginseng (*Panax ginseng*) significantly enhanced mental performance in healthy volunteers.[155] When Ginkgo extract (360 mg equivalent to 18 g of leaf) and Korean ginseng extract (600 mg equivalent to 3 g of root) were combined as a single treatment, results were remarkable. Not only was the effect on cognitive function more pronounced than treatment with either herb on its own, it was immediately evident when the volunteers were first tested. The lead researcher, Dr Andrew Scholey was quoted as saying: "The results were incredible in terms of improvements in speed and accuracy – usually there is a trade-off and you improve one at the expense of the other."

Ginkgo is often present in herbal remedies for ADHD, although reports of benefit are said to be anecdotal.[156] A recent survey found that its use in ADHD was relatively high.[157] Ginkgo has also shown benefit in dyslexia, which is again suggestive of a possible beneficial role in ADHD. Fifteen children (5 to 16 years) with dyslexia participated in a preliminary, unblinded trial of standardised Ginkgo extract given as a single morning dose of 80 mg.[158] Ginkgo was administered for a mean of 34.4 days, and on a weekly basis, parents and children were asked about possible side effects. Ginkgo was associated with an improvement in dyslexia as measured by efficacy (the capacity to read a list of words) and effectiveness (the capacity to read text). The improvement observed from Ginkgo administration was in terms of accuracy for the reading text, word list and non-word list, and the results were statistically significant. There was no significant difference in terms of speed. Treatment with Ginkgo was generally well tolerated. The authors recommended that a follow-up randomised, double blind trial should be carried out with a greater number of volunteers and with a repeat afternoon dose of Ginkgo.

Finally, St John's wort is sometimes considered in herbal treatments for ADHD. But it should be used cautiously if the person is also taking methylphenidate. Recently a case report was published of a potential interaction with this drug.[159]

The report describes a patient (male, 22 years) suffering from ADHD without any concomitant neurological/psychiatric disorder, diagnosed according to the DSM-IV criteria, medicated with methylphenidate. Six months after initiating methylphenidate therapy (20 mg/day), with an improvement of ADHD symptomatology (improvement from 75.3

to 68.4 measured by the Conner's score), he then started additional self-medication with St John's wort extract (600 mg/day). According to the authors this addition for 4 months had a significant impact on diminishing methylphenidate's efficacy: he became more disattentive according to the Conner's score (changed from 68.4 to 74.9). Three weeks after discontinuation of St John's wort the Conner's score dropped again to 70.3. There were no apparent adverse side effects, neither of methylphenidate nor of St John's wort.

Herbal Treatment

Given the biochemical and sociological complexities of ADHD, a thorough history will guide treatment and identify which factors are relevant.

The key treatment goals and associated actions and herbs are as follows:

- Cognitive enhancing herbs such as Schisandra, white peony, Bacopa, gotu kola, Ginkgo and rosemary. Gotu kola has recently been shown to enhance cognitive function in a clinical trial[160]

- Herbs to support the HPA axis and modify the stress response including adrenal tonics, adaptogens and nervine tonics such as licorice, Rehmannia, Rhodiola, Siberian ginseng, Withania, St John's wort, Korean ginseng and skullcap

- Use anxiolytic (eg valerian) and nervine tonic herbs with caution as clinical experience has demonstrated that sedative herbs can occasionally worsen ADHD symptoms. It is preferable to confine use of such herbs to the evening

- Improve digestion to decrease food reactivity and improve nutritional absorption with herbs such as chamomile, meadowsweet, St Mary's thistle and chen pi. Antiallergic herbs such as Albizia and Baical skullcap may be useful (see also below)

- Treat allergies if present. For upper respiratory allergy (hayfever), consider eyebright, golden rod, golden seal, Echinacea and Andrographis and the antiallergic herbs above. For lower respiratory allergy (ie asthma) consider turmeric, Ginkgo, Adhatoda, Baical skullcap, Grindelia and immune modulators (see also Chapter 6)

- Treat sleep disturbances with calming herbs given just before bed such as valerian, skullcap, lemon balm and lavender

- Use antioxidant herbs to improve oxidation status. Pine bark is clinically proven (as noted above), but grape seed, turmeric, rosemary and green tea can also be considered

- Heal the gut wall if indicated with herbs such as golden seal and Calendula

- Chelate heavy metals if indicated. Milk thistle and garlic are the most important herbs. Improve xenobiotic clearance with Schisandra, garlic, rosemary, turmeric and green tea

- Evening primrose oil as a source of EFAs

Example Liquid Formulations

For mornings and during the day:

Ginkgo	2:1	20 mL
Bacopa	1:2	30 mL
St John's wort	1:2	25 mL
Korean ginseng	1:2	15 mL
Gotu kola	1:1	20 mL
	Total	110 mL

Dose: Calculate the standard dose according to the most appropriate guideline in Chapter 1, based on an adult dose of 8 mL. To be taken with water twice a day in the morning and around midday.

For the evening (avoid if causes aggravation)

Valerian	1:2	25 mL
Skullcap	1:2	25 mL
St John's wort	1:2	25 mL
Bacopa	1:2	25 mL
	Total	100 mL

Dose: Calculate the standard dose according to the most appropriate guideline in Chapter 1, based on an adult dose of 8 mL. To be taken with water once or twice a day before dinner and/or 1 hour before bedtime.

Example Tablet or Capsule Formulations

For the older child or the younger one who will not take liquids, herbal tablets or capsules may prove a useful alternative for ADHD.

Key herbal formulations (examples provided in Appendix 1) which should be considered in ADHD are Memory/Brain Tonic tablets (adult dose 4 per day), Ginkgo tablets (adult dose 4 per day), Gotu Kola Combination tablets (adult dose 3 per day) and Herbal Antioxidant tablets (adult dose 2 to 3 per day). Other formulations to be considered as appropriate are Stress Control tablets (adult dose 4 per day) to support the HPA axis, High Allicin Releasing Garlic tablets (adult dose 2 per day) for heavy metal clearance and Liver Detox Assist tablets (adult dose 4 per day) to support hepatic clearance of toxins. A calming formulation in the evening such as Sleep Anxiety Support tablets (adult dose 4 per day) or Nervous System Tonic tablets (adult dose 4 per day) may be useful, but should be tried with caution. In general, no more than 3 or 4 different formulations should be prescribed at the one time.

Calculate the child's tablet dose according to the most appropriate guideline in Chapter 1. For younger children the tablets can be crushed and mixed with honey or a suitable sweetener to improve compliance. See Appendix 1 for the suggested formulations for these tablets.

Case History

A male aged 16 years presented with his mother. Had been diagnosed with ADHD at 13 years of age and his mother was seeking an alternative to Ritalin. His history included a parental separation when he was 12 years of age and cannabis use also from this age. The school difficulties included many clashes with teachers, truancy, poor concentration and being unable to complete homework and other tasks. His diet was poor with a high intake of sugar, cola drinks and so on. He had left school and was working at a local supermarket and had several work-related problems.

The following herbal liquid formulation was prescribed:

Bacopa	1:2	35 mL
Rosemary	1:2	15 mL
Withania	1:2	35 mL
Gymnema	1:1	25 mL
	Total	110 mL

Dose: 10 mL with water twice a day

Fish oil and evening primrose oil (2 1000 mg capsules of each per day) were prescribed.

Dietary recommendations included reducing sugar, cola drinks, refined foods and eating more fruits, vegetables and meat at home if possible. He was also guided to reduce or eliminate his cannabis use.

The patient was followed for 10 months during which time he slowly but steadily improved in concentration and task completion. At the 4-month mark, after his perceived dysglycaemia was under control, the Gymnema was replaced with Schisandra. At 10 months he was no longer taking cannabis and had been appointed a section manager in the supermarket.

The following is the rationale for the above herbal treatment:

- Bacopa to improve cognition and concentration
- Rosemary as a choleretic, antioxidant and memory tonic
- Withania as an adaptogen and general tonic
- Gymnema to improve his glucose tolerance and sugar craving
- Schisandra as an adaptogen, to support liver detoxification and for cognition enhancement

Autism Spectrum Disorder

Autism spectrum disorder (ASD) has received considerable attention from the media, the general public and health professionals. Stories of savants who excel in mathematical calculations have fascinated the public and this interest is exemplified in Dustin Hoffman's portrayal of a young man with autism in the movie *Rainman*.[161] More recently, public anxiety has increased as a result of reports linking the measles, mumps and rubella (MMR) vaccine with a type of inflammatory bowel disorder and autism.[140]

ASD is a complex neurodevelopmental disorder that results in social, behavioural and language impairment.[162] In terms of morbidity, outcome and impact on the family, it is among the most devastating disorders of childhood.[163] ASD actually comprises several different disorders, as defined by deficits in social behaviour and interactions, that prevent the development of normal interpersonal relationships with parents, siblings and other children.[163] These include the prototypic autistic disorder (AuD), Asperger's syndrome (AS) and pervasive developmental disorder (PDD).[163] AuD has three core symptom domains: deficits in communication, abnormal social interaction and restrictive and/or repetitive interest and behaviour.[163] Neonates normally have a remarkable interest in social interaction, however for the child with AuD facial expressions show little interest.[164] Social interest may increase over time, but even the highest functioning individuals remain socially impaired.[164] Delay in the development of language is the most common presenting issue with parents.[165] Many children with AuD never speak at all. The speech of those who do is different in several ways, with unusual intonation, severe difficulties in the social use of language, repetition of what is said and pronoun reversal.[164] Difficulties in imaginative play are also evident, where the child with AuD is often preoccupied by the non-functional features of play materials, such as taste and smell.[166] The child has difficulty coping with changes in circumstances and routine. Even a trivial change can trigger distress, with such difficulties becoming more prominent after infancy.[164]

AS also involves social symptoms, but language and non-verbal intelligence are nearly normal.[163] Therefore AS may not become apparent until the child is older, whereas AuD is usually identified during the first or second year of life.[163] PDD differs from AuD by either the absence of repetitive behaviour or communication deficits, or the presence of more subtle deficits in all three core symptom domains.[163]

Diagnosis of ASD

As is the case for ADHD, AuD is a behaviourally-defined disorder, with the criteria for diagnosis set out in both the ICD-10 and DSM-IV.[161] Both manuals use the terminology "pervasive developmental disorders", not ASD, to describe the condition. However, the two terms are used synonymously and parents find it easier to understand the term ASD.[161]

Epidemiology

The prevalence of AuD is now considered to be around 10 per 10,000 and the prevalence of PDD is around 27.5 per 10,000.[167] However, a recent US survey estimated 60 per 10,000.[168] An increase in the prevalence has been observed over time. The reasons for this are unclear, but may include changes in study methodology, a genuine rise in risk factors, an increase in available diagnostic services, increased awareness of the condition and a growing acceptance that AuD can co-exist with a range of other conditions.[167]

Aetiology

AuD has a complex aetiology involving genetic susceptibility, general health and nutritional status, the gastrointestinal and immune systems, vaccines and environmental exposures.[169] The question still remains as to whether AuD is fundamentally a brain disorder or a disease that affects the brain.[170]

Genetic Factors

Autism has been associated with several disorders with genetic causes, notably tuberous sclerosis, fragile X syndrome and neurofibromatosis. However, they represent a very small proportion of all AuD cases.[164] Based on twin and family studies it appears that AuD does have a genetic basis, however the mode of genetic transmission is unknown at this time.[171]

Environmental Exposure

Because of an observed increase in autism in recent decades, which parallels cumulative mercury exposure, it has been proposed that autism may be in part caused by mercury.[172] Several epidemiological studies have failed to find a correlation between mercury exposure through thimerosal and the risk of autism.[173,174] But recently it was found that autistic children had a higher mercury exposure during pregnancy due to maternal dental amalgam, fish consumption and thimerosal-containing vaccines.[175] Furthermore it has been demonstrated that children with autism have a decreased detoxification capacity for mercury due to genetic polymorphism.[172] An *in vitro* study found that mercury and thimerosal at levels typical of those found several days after vaccination inhibit methionine synthetase (MS) by 50%.[176] Normal functioning of MS is crucial in the biochemical steps necessary for brain development, attention and production of glutathione, an important antioxidant and detoxifying agent.[172] Additionally, repetitive doses of thimerosal lead to neurobehavioural deteriorations in autoimmune susceptible mice, and increased oxidative stress and decreased intracellular levels of glutathione *in vitro*.[172] It has been shown that AuD children have significantly decreased levels of reduced glutathione.[172] Furthermore, it appears that children with ASD have reduced levels of metallothioneins, endogenous proteins that naturally chelate metals and therefore have a buffering and detoxifying effect.[177]

Delayed detoxification of mercury can severely impair methylation reactions, which are required for the correct expression of DNA, RNA and neurotransmitters. This can further adversely affects brain development and attention abilities.[172] Phospholipid methylation, crucial for attention, is impaired in both AuD and ADHD children.[178] Mercury levels seen ten days after vaccination (and at levels lower than those infants received during the 1990s) produced a greater than 50% inhibition of methylation.[178]

Interestingly, despite thimerosal receiving the official all clear, it has been removed from the MMR vaccine. But it is still used in the diphtheria-tetanus-acellular pertussis (DTaP), hepatitis B and *Haemophilus influenzae* vaccines, depending on the country.[179,180] Infants who receive all three may have been exposed to a cumulative dose of mercury as high as 187.5 μg by 6 months of age.[179] This value exceeds the guidelines recommended by the

US EPA.[179] The US CDC has admitted that cumulative mercury exposure to children through vaccination exceeds known "safe" levels.[177] In 2001, the prestigious Institute of Medicine, which advises the US on health issues, conceded an autism link with mercury is "biologically plausible" and recommended that thimerosal be removed from vaccines.[177] According to the Australian Standard Vaccination Schedule, if a child was to receive the full schedule by the age of 4, he or she would have received 25 vaccinations![181]

An alarming discovery was revealed by a recent study on pesticide drift to residences near agricultural fields. The investigational group set out to examine a combination of three factors: the mother's distance from the site of pesticide application, the type of pesticide and the stage of gestation at the time of pesticide use in terms of AuD incidence. Two pesticides stood out: the organochlorides dicofol and endosulfan were found to be associated with AuD incidence.[182] These pesticides are commonly used in the production of cotton, fruit, vegetables, beans and nuts and accounted for 98% of the pesticide use in the study area.[182] Another similar study identified mercury, cadmium, nickel, trichloroethylene and vinyl chloride as hazardous air pollutants associated with AuD.[183]

It has been observed that AuD children have increased pica.[184] With this in mind, one study evaluated lead levels in AuD children. In this investigation of 18 AuD children and 26 controls it was established that the AuD children had significantly elevated lead blood levels compared to the controls. However, none displayed any signs of acute lead toxicity.[185]

Impaired Metabolism

The phase II detoxification system, mostly found in the liver, uses sulphation as a key pathway for the elimination of endogenous and exogenous substances.[177] Sulphation capacity is known to vary widely amongst individuals and is highly genetically determined.[177] In a study that examined 60 AuD children, 55 had marked sulphation impairment.[186] It has been suggested that these findings might explain why many AuD children are worsened by foods with a high phenolamine content such as bananas, chocolate, cheese and other fermented products. The sulphation pathway is largely responsible for the detoxification of these phenolics.[177]

Gastrointestinal Factors

Children with ASD tend to suffer from severe gastrointestinal problems. Common symptoms include diarrhoea and/or constipation, abdominal pain, flatulence, bloating, burping and gastro-oesophageal reflux.[184] Stool culture is often abnormal and it has been repeatedly demonstrated that the microflora of AuD children is characterised by the marked presence of the *Clostridium histolyticum* group of bacteria.[187,188]

The histopathological findings of the controversial Wakefield study[140] have been further explored. One study which examined the lactulose and mannitol recovery rates of 21 AuD children and 40 controls found that 43% of the AuD children had an altered lactulose to mannitol recovery, indicative of a leaky gut.[189] The measles virus (from the MMR vaccine) was implicated as a causative factor for this in the Wakefield study. One study found measles RNA in 82% of ileal tissue taken from AuD subjects and in only 5% of controls.[190] However, other studies have failed to identify the presence of measles RNA.[184]

Opioid Excess Theory

As early as 1979, it was hypothesised that autism may arise from an opioid peptide excess.[177,191] It had been demonstrated that enhancement of the endogenous opioid system, or administration of the opiates to infant animals, results in autistic-like symptoms.[191] The exogenous opioid peptides implicated are particularly those derived from dietary proteins, predominantly gliadin and casein.[192,193] Abnormal peptide components have been detected in the urine of AuD subjects.[193,194,195] The theory proposes that AuD children develop an enteropathy from gluten (and/or perhaps dairy) sensitivity which then allows opioid-like peptides, and particularly those derived from casein in milk, to enter the system. These then affect opioid receptors in the brain to produce ASD symptoms.[191,192] As a consequence, a gluten-free and casein-free (GFCF) diet has become popular, with many parents reporting an improvement in symptoms when such a diet has been implemented.

Three studies have been recently published examining various hypotheses relative to the GFCF diet in autism. Researchers measured the IgG, IgM, IgA antibodies against gliadin, casein and ethyl mercury in 50 children diagnosed with autism. Analysis of blood samples revealed a significant number of the children expressed antibodies against casein and gliadin. In addition, gliadin, casein and ethyl mercury (thimerosal) were shown to bind to lymphocytes and perhaps trigger inflammatory and immune reactions.[196]

Further to this, a randomised, single blind study involving 20 children assessed the effect of a GFCF diet on ASD. The children in the control and experimental groups were matched according to the severity of their autistic symptoms, age and cognitive level. Changes were observed in both the control and experimental groups. However, the experimental group showed more significant changes, demonstrating an improvement in autistic behaviour, non-verbal cognitive level, and motor problems.[197]

In a comparative study, amino acid patterns were evaluated in 26 children with autism on a regular diet, 10 on a GFCF diet, and 26 children with developmental delays who served as controls. The children with autism had higher deficiencies in essential amino acids, especially tryptophan and tyrosine, compared to the control group. Although preliminary, these findings suggest that children with autism are at a high risk for amino acid deficiencies and may benefit from a more structured diet in terms of protein intake.[198]

During the 1990s a hypothesis was developed that a protein in the milk of some cows, and not others, is an important risk factor for type 1 diabetes, coronary heart disease, schizophrenia and autism.[199,200,201] The protein implicated is the A1 variant of β-casein, the second most abundant protein found in milk. Other genetic variants include A2 and B β-casein.[199,200,201] Cows milk β-casein contains 209 amino acids, with the A1 and A2 variants differing only at position 67. There is a histidine in A1 and a proline in A2 milk at this position. A bioactive 7 amino acid peptide, β-casomorphin-7 (BCM-7), can be produced by digestion of A1 β-casein. But the alternative A-2 protein with proline at position 67 does not exhibit this particular split.[199,200,201] BCM-7 has been noted to have opioid and cytomodulatory properties. Through various lines of evidence it is postulated that BCM-7 reaches the brain and leads to susceptibility to schizophrenia, autism and sudden infant death syndrome.[202,203,204] The A1 variant of β-casein is common in dairy cows of European origin including Friesian, Ayrshire, British Shorthorn and Holstein, while the predominantly A2 β-casein is found in the milk of Channel Island cows, Guernsey, Jersey and the Southern French breeds, Charolais and Limousin.[201]

Immune Dysfunction

There is substantial evidence suggesting that the immune system plays an important role in the pathogenesis of ASD. All of the arms of immunity are often abnormal in these children, with some abnormalities having a genetic basis.[177] Natural killer (NK) cell numbers are decreased. There can also be abnormalities in macrophages, B cells and T cells, including decreased CD_4^+ cells and a shift away from Th1 towards Th2 responses, suggestive of autoimmunity.[205,206] It is interesting to note that mercury (with implications for thimerosal) is known for immunological effects that include the shifting of the cytokine profile from Th1 to Th2 and the induction of autoimmunity.[205] A high incidence of autoimmune alterations has been found in AuD children, such as increased antibody titres against myelin basic protein, neuron-axon filament protein, brain endothelial cells and cerebellar neuro-filaments.[207] AuD is also associated with an activation of the inflammatory response, as indicated by increased urinary neopterin, elevated plasma IFN-a and IL-12 and increased production of IL-6, TNF-a and IFN-γ.[205,206,207] The origin of the leaky gut, as noted earlier, could have an autoimmune basis.

Neurokines

Numerous neurotransmitter systems have been studied in ASD including acetylcholine, serotonin, dopamine, adrenaline, noradrenaline, glutamate and γ-aminobutyric acid (GABA). It has been found that there is a significant decrease in glutamic acid decarboxylase, the enzyme that converts glutamate to GABA in the brains of ASD patients.[208] This may result in abnormal brain development.[209] Increased serotonin has also been described in one third of AuD subjects.[210] Proinflammatory cytokines such as TNF-a and IFN-γ can increase serotonin levels in the brain.[206]

Fever Suppression

It has been proposed that maternal fever suppression during pregnancy may be linked to the aetiology of AuD. It has been demonstrated that treatment with paracetamol (acetaminophen) significantly decreases maternal and foetal serum IL-6.[211] This may be significant, as it appears that the foetus is incapable of producing IL-6 at the time of birth and is dependent on maternal IL-6. There is evidence that IL-6 is important in the development, differentiation, regeneration and degeneration of neurons in the central nervous system.[212] Furthermore, it has been shown that 43% of mothers with an autistic child have experienced either upper respiratory tract, influenza-like, urinary or vaginal infections during pregnancy, compared to only 26% of controls.[213]

In utero Hypothyroxinaemia

The current surge of autism and ADHD could also be related to transient maternal hypothyroxinaemia resulting from dietary and/or environmental exposure to antithyroid agents.[214] Alterations of cortical neuronal migration and cerebellar Purkinje cells have been observed in autism.[215] Neuronal migration requires triiodothyronine (T3), produced by deiodination of thyroxine (T4) by foetal brain deiodinases. Experimental models have shown that transient intrauterine deficits of thyroid hormones, as brief as 3 days, can result in permanent alterations of cerebral cortical architecture, reminiscent of those observed in the brains of patients with autism.[216] Common causes could include inhibition of deiodinases D2 or D3 from the maternal ingestion of dietary goitrogens or from antithyroid environmental contaminants such as PCBs.[214]

ASD and Complementary and Alternative Medicine (CAM)

In a recent survey of 112 families of ASD children it was reported that 74% used CAM for their child.[217] This observed usage was higher than the 30% rate seen in another published study, which used medical record reviews.[218] Of the biologically-based therapies, only 11% used herbal remedies. However, 74% of this 11% thought the herbal therapy was helpful. Dietary modification was used by 38%, of which 41% found it to be helpful, with similar results for vitamin/mineral therapy at 30% usage and 41% satisfaction.[218]

While a large number of clinical trials have been published using biologically-based CAM therapies on ASD children, no herbal studies could be found. A brief review of the more significant work follows. Of the vitamin regimens studied in the treatment of ASD the most successful and best studied is supplementation with pyridoxine (vitamin B6), usually in combination with magnesium (Mg).[219] Several well-designed studies using B6/Mg combination have demonstrated benefit in terms of improved social behaviour, improved language, reduced aggression and increased interest in the environment.[219,220] Pyridoxine is an important cofactor in the conversion of dopamine to noradrenaline and tryptophan to serotonin, thus raising serotonin.[221] Both folic acid and vitamin B12 have also attracted research attention, presumably due to their methyl donor properties and the impaired methylation seen in ASD subjects.[178] However the evidence is not as promising as for B6/Mg. Folic acid has been reported to decrease hyperactivity and increase attention and social behaviour in ASD subjects with fragile X syndrome.[219]

In an open-label study, the diets of 46 ASD patients aged between 5 and 31 years were supplemented with a digestive enzyme formulation for a period of 12 weeks. The enzyme product safely improved all 13 of the parameters measured, such as socialisation, mood and speech. Improvements at weeks 11 to 12 ranged from 50-90%, depending on the parameter.[222]

Herbal Treatment for AuD

There is a strong consensus that modifying the diet and addressing the gastrointestinal symptoms as initial treatment goals set the stage for the success of other treatments.[223] This makes sense in light of the enteropathy that most ASD children apparently suffer, which leads to poor digestive capacity and nutrient absorption. ASD children are also very difficult to treat with oral therapies.

The dietary modifications suggested include the removal of food additives, colourings, sweeteners, preservatives, dairy products (casein) and gluten. There may be sensitivities to other foods such as meat and members of the *Solanaceae* family of plants (eggplant, tomatoes, capsicum and potatoes) which need to be considered. AuD children are very often picky eaters and will only accept a small range of foods, so the practitioner should anticipate difficulties with the new dietary restrictions.

Herbal treatment should be first directed at reducing gastrointestinal inflammation and a leaky gut (Calendula, chamomile), relieving the diarrhoea and/or constipation, reducing abdominal pain (chamomile, wild yam) and easing the flatulence and gastro-oesophageal reflux. Keep in mind that the modified diet should bring about considerable relief of gastrointestinal symptoms. See also Chapter 5 and other relevant chapters. The autoimmune aspects of the leaky gut would suggest a role for Rehmannia, Hemidesmus and Bupleurum.

The next phase of treatment is similar to that recommended for ADHD, particularly as it relates to increasing cognition, supporting the HPA axis, chelating heavy metals and improving hepatic detoxification.

Example Liquid Formulation for AuD

Echinacea root blend	1:2	25 mL
Rehmannia	1:2	20 mL
Calendula	1:2	20 mL
Bacopa	1:2	25 mL
Schisandra	1:2	20 mL
	Total	110 mL

Dose: Calculate the standard dose based on an adult dose of 5 mL according to the most appropriate guideline in Chapter 1. Three to four doses can be taken with water during the day.

Example Tablet or Capsule Formulations

For the older child or the younger one who will not take liquids, herbal tablets or capsules may prove a useful alternative for AuD.

Key herbal formulations (examples provided in Appendix 1) which should be considered in AuD are Autoimmune Formula tablets (adult dose 4 per day) for the autoimmune/gut inflammation aspects, Upper Digestive Formula tablets (adult dose one tablet sucked for 30 to 60 seconds before meals) to promote digestive function and help heal a leaky gut, Echinacea Formula tablets (adult dose 2 per day) for immune support and High Allicin Releasing Garlic tablets (adult dose 2 per day) for heavy metal detoxification. Other formulations to be considered as appropriate are Boswellia Combination tablets (adult dose 4 per day) for the gut inflammation, Liver Detox Assist tablets (adult dose 4 per day), Memory/Brain Tonic tablets (adult dose 4 per day) or Nervous System Tonic tablets (adult dose 4 per day). In general no more than 3 or 4 different formulations should be prescribed at the one time.

Calculate the child's tablet dose according to the most appropriate guideline in Chapter 1. For younger children the tablets can be crushed and mixed with honey or a suitable sweetener to improve compliance. See Appendix 1 for the suggested formulations for these tablets.

Case History

This patient is currently in the initial phase of treatment. He is a 4-year-old male with a history of irritable-bowel-type symptoms, particularly fluctuating constipation and diarrhoea, and chronic upper respiratory tract infections including otitis media treated with antibiotics. The boy is a special needs child at preschool kindergarten and has been diagnosed as autistic. He has received one MMR, three Hepatitis B and three DTP (diphtheria/tetanus/acellular pertussis) vaccinations. The parents were aware of the need for dietary modification and the child was already largely on a GFCF diet, with a small degree of improvement in gastrointestinal symptoms.

Aside from the GFCF diet, it was recommended that he be gradually introduced to a simple miso soup and organic brown rice porridge. The miso (organic, unpasteurised) soup was prepared by boiling a small strip of kombu in spring water for 10 minutes. The decoction was turned to low heat before adding a ¼ teaspoon of miso and some chopped shallots and simmered for 5 minutes. A ½ a cup of miso soup was to be consumed with a ½ a cup of brown rice porridge, eventually twice a day.

The following herbal formulation was prescribed:

Echinacea root blend	1:2	20 mL
Chamomile high in bisabolol	1:2	20 mL
Calendula (low alcohol)	1:2	20 mL
Rhodiola	2:1	20 mL
Bacopa	1:2	20 mL
	Total	100 mL

Dose: 3 mL with water morning and night

There has been a significant improvement in the gastrointestinal symptoms and behaviour in the first 6 months of treatment. Since beginning the treatment he has not had a RTI and for the first time he was able to engage in the kindergarten Christmas concert at the end of 2007.

Rationale for the Treatment

The approach taken is based on using foods as medicines. The miso used was brown rice miso, which is the sweetest, and was suggested based on its ability to improve digestion and to provide a range of nutrients including iron.[224,225] The kombu provides minerals including iodine and is useful in detoxifying heavy metals.[225] Echinacea was prescribed in order to modulate the immune system and also to prevent the chronic respiratory infections. Both chamomile and Calendula were used to a treat leaky gut. The Rhodiola and Bacopa were used as adaptogens and to normalise cognitive function.

References

1 Porth CM. *Pathophysiology* 7th Ed, Lippincott Williams & Wilkins, 2005.
2 Kleigman RM, Behrman RE, Jenson HB, Stanton BF. *Nelson Textbook of Pediatrics* 18th Ed, Saunders Elsevier, Philadelphia, 2007.
3 Schott JM, Rossor MN. *J Neurol Neurosurg Psychiatry* 2003; **74**(5): 558-560
4 Kail R, Cavanaugh J. *Human Development: A Life-Span View.* Wadsworth, Belmont CA, 2004.
5 Timimi S. *Pathological Child Psychiatry and the Medicalization of Childhood,* Brunner-Routledge, New York, 2002.
6 Timimi S. *BMJ* 2005; **331**(7507): 37-39
7 Mackay H. *Advance Australia…Where?* Hachette Australia, Sydney, 2007.
8 Jenkins H. *Children's Culture Reader,* New York University Press, New York, 1998.
9 Timimi S. *BMJ* 2004; **394**(7479): 1394-1396
10 Grigg J. *Arch Dis Child* 2004; **89**(3): 244-250
11 Bearer CF. *Environ Health Perspect* 1995; **103**(Suppl 6): 7-12
12 Abelsohn A, Gibson BL, Sanborn MD, Weir E. *CMAJ* 2002; **166**(12): 1549-1554
13 Adachi J, Mori Y, Matsui S et al. *J Biol Chem* 2001; **276**(34): 31475-31478
14 Denison MS, Nagy SR. *Annu Rev Pharmacol Toxicol* 2003; **43**: 309-334
15 Koopman-Esseboom C, Weisglas-Kuperus N, de Ridder MA et al. *Pediatrics* 1996; **97**(5): 700-706
16 Patandin S, Lanting CI, Mulder PG et al. *J Pediatr* 1999; **134**(1): 33-41
17 Vreugdenhil HJ, Slijper FM, Mulder PG et al. *Environ Health Perspect* 2002; **110**(10): A593-598
18 Lidsky TI, Schneider JS. *Brain* 2003; **126**(1): 5-19
19 Kerper LE, Auderisk G. *Toxicol Appl Pharmacol* 1997; **146**(1): 127-133
20 Kerper LE, Hinkle PM. *J Biol Chem* 1997; **272**(13): 8346-8352
21 Lamphear BP, Hornung R, Koury J et al. *Environ Health Perspect* 2005; **113**(7): 894-899
22 Chen A, Cai B, Dietrich KN et al. *Pediatrics* 2007; **119**(3): e650-e658
23 Bellinger DC. *Altern Ther Health Med* 2007; **13**(2): S140-S144
24 Wilson MA, Johnston MV, Goldstein GW, Blue ME. *Proc Natl Acad Sci* 2000; **97**(10): 5540-5545
25 *Mercury Study Report to Congress.* Washington: Office of Air Quality Planning and Standards and Office of Research and Development, US Environmental Protection Agency, 2002, http://www.epa.gov/ttn/oarpg/t3/reports/volume 1.pdf.
26 Debes F, Budtz-Jorgensen E, Weihe P et al. *Neurotoxicol Teratol* 2006; **26**(3): 363-375
27 Corbett SJ, Poon CCS. *MJA* 2008; **188**(1): 59-60
28 Palmer RF, Blanchard S, Stein Z et al. *Health Place* **12**(2): 203-209
29 Advisory committee on hazardous substances. Department of Environment, Food and Rural Affairs. Sixth Annual Report 2001-2002, http://www.defra.gove.uk/environment/chemicals/achs/pdf/achs_annrpt01.pdf.
30 Carpenter DO, Arcaro K, Spink D. *Environ Health Persp,* 2002; **110**(1): 25-42
31 Environmental Working Group and Commonweal. Body Burden: the Pollution in Newborns. 2005, http://archive.ewg.org/reports_content/bodyburden2/pdf/bodyburden2_final-r2.pdf.
32 Welshons WV, Thayer KA, Judy BM et al. *Environ Health Perspect* 2003; **111**(8): 994-1006
33 Cha CW. *J Korean Med Sci* 1987; **2**(4): 213-224
34 Hanafy MS, Shalaby SM, el-Fouly MA et al. *Dtsch Tierarztl Wochenchr* 1994; **101**(4): 157-158
35 Morgan M, Andrews C. *Nutritional Perspective* 2006; #19: 1-4
36 Bone K. *Townsend Letter for Doctors and Patients* 2003; #245: 108-112
37 Rozanski A, Blumenthal JA, Davidson KW et al. *J Am Coll Cardiol* 2005; **45**(5): 637-651
38 Cohen S, Tyrrell DA, Smith AP. *NEJM* 1991; **325**(9): 606-612
39 Boyce WT, Chesterman EA, Martin M et al. *J Dev Behav Pediatr* 1993; **14**(5): 296-303
40 Boyce WT, Chesney M, Alkon A et al. *Psychosom Med* 1995; **57**(5): 411-422
41 Wright RJ, Finn P, Contreras JP et al. *J Allergy Clin Immunol* 2004; **113**(6): 1051-1057
42 Wright RJ, Cohen S, Carey V et al. *Am J Respir Crit Care Med* 2002; **165**(3): 358-365
43 Chen E, Fisher EB, Bacharier LB, Strunk RC. *Psychosom Med* 2003; **65**(6): 984-992
44 Wyman PA, Moynihan J, Eberly S et al. *Arch Pediatr Adolesc Med* 2007; **161**(3): 228-234
45 Ben-Eliyahu S, Page GG, Schleifer SJ. *Brain Behav Immunol* 2007; **21**(7): 881-887
46 Bone K. *A Clinical Guide to Blending Liquid Herbs.* Churchill Livingstone, Edinburgh, 2000.
47 Bone K. *Clinical Applications of Ayurvedic and Chinese Herbs.* Phytotherapy Press, Warwick, 1996, p.88.
48 Wood M. *The Book of Herbal Wisdom,* North Atlantic Books, Berkeley, 1997.

49   Sadeh A. *Pediatrics* 2004; **113**(6): e570
50   Anders TF, Halpern LF, Hua J. *Pediatrics* 1992; **90**(4): 554-560
51   Armstrong KL, Quinn RA, Dadds MR. *Med J Aust* 1994; **161**(3): 202-206
52   Anders TF, Carskadon MA, Dement WC, Harvey K. *Child Psychiatry Hum Dev* 1978; **9**(1): 56-63
53   Richman N, Douglas J, Hunt H et al. *J Child Psychol Psychiatry* 1985; **26**(4): 581-590
54   Gibson ES, Powles AC, Thabane L et al. *BMC Public Health* 2006; **6**: 116
55   Walters As, Mandelbaum DE, Lewin DS et al. *Pediatr Neurol* 2000; **22**(3): 182-186
56   Moore M, Allison D, Rosen CL. *Chest* 2006; **130**(4): 1252-1262
57   Kleigman RM, Behrman RE, Jenson HB, Stanton BF. *Nelson Textbook of Pediatrics* 18th Ed, Saunders Elsevier, Philadelphia, 2007.
58   Hill CM, Hogan AM, Karmiloff-Smith A. *Arch Dis Child* 2007; **92**(7): 637-643
59   Dan B, Boyd SG. *Devel Med Child Neurol* 2006; **48**(9): 773-779
60   Randazzo AC, Muehlbach MJ, Schweitzer PK, Walsh JK. *Sleep* 1998; **21**(8): 861-868
61   Suratt PM, Barth JT, Diamond R et al. *Pediatrics* 2007; **119**(2): 320-329
62   Sadeh A, Gruber R, Raviv A. *Child Dev* 2003; **74**(2): 444-455
63   Lumeng JC, Somashekar D, Appugliese D et al. *Pediatrics* 2007; **120**(5): 1020-1029
64   Blissit PA. *J Neurosci Nurs* 2001; **33**(4): 208-215
65   Born J, Rasch B, Gais S. *Neuroscientist* 2006; **12**(5): 410-424
66   Sparrow J. *Scolastic Par Child* 2007; **15**(3): 48-49
67   Mindell JA, Emslie G, Blumer J et al. *Pediatrics* 2006; **117**(6): e1223-e1232
68   Weiss RF, Fintelmann V. *Herbal Medicine* 2nd Ed, Thieme, Stuttgart, 2000.
69   Muller SF, Klement S. *Phytomedicine* 2006; **13**(6): 383-387
70   Braun L, Cohen M. *Herbs & Natural Supplements* 2nd Ed, Churchill Livingstone, Sydney, 2007.
71   Thome J, Jacobs KA. *European Psychiatry,* 2005; **19**(5): 303-306
72   Timimi, S. *Naughty boys, anti-social behaviour, ADHD and the role of culture*, Palgrave Macmillan, New York, 2005.
73   Dey F, Bone K. *Townsend Letter for Doctors and Patients*. 2003; **243**: 64-71
74   Crowe M. J *Psychiatr Mental Health Nurs* 2000; **7**(1): 69-77
75   Timimi S, Moncrieff J, Jureidini J et al. *Clin Child Fam Psychol Rev* 2004; **7**(1): 59-63
76   Wolraich ML, et al. *Pediatrics* 1990: **86**(1): 95-101
77   Kamper A. Changing minds on ADHD. *Daily Telegraph,* 2007, March 12th.
78   NIH *Consensus Statement: Diagnosis and Treatment of Attention Deficit Hyperactivity Disorders* http:consensus.nih. gov/1998/1998AttentionDeficitHyperactivityDisorder110Program.pdf
79   Phillips CB. *PLoS Med* 2006; **3**(4): 433-435
80   Sax L, Kautz KJ. *Ann Fam Med* 2003; **1**(3): 171-173
81   http://www.adhdinfo.com/info/school/caring/sch_if_parents_ask_jsp
82   Biedermann J, Faraone SV. *Lancet* 2005; **366**(9481): 239-248
83   CDC http://www.cdc.gov/ncbddd/adhd
84   Sawyer M, Arney F, Baghurst P et al. The mental health of young people in Australia: child and adolescent component of the National Survey of Mental Health and Well-being. *Mental Health and Special Programs Branch, Commonwealth Department of Health and Aged Care*, Canberra, 2000.
85   Prosser B, Reid R, Shute R, Atkinson I. *Aust J Edu* 2002; **46**(1): 65-78
86   Hazell P. *J Paediatr Child Health,* 1997; **33**(2): 131-137
87   Fisher SE, Francks C, McCracken JT et al. *Am J Hum Genetics,* 2002; **70**(5): 1183-1196
88   Volkow ND, Fowler JS, Wang G et al. *J Atten Disord,* 2002; **6**(1): S31-43
89   Morton WA, Stockton GG. *Prim Care Companion J Clin Psychiatry* 2000; **2**(2): 159-164
90   Lisska MC, Rivkees SA. *J Pediatr Endocrinol Metab*, 2003; **16**(5): 711-718
91   Holtkamp K, Peters-Wallraf B, Wuller S et al. *J Child Adolesc Psychopharmacol* 2002; **12**(1): 55-61
92   El-Zein RA, Abdel-Rahman SZ, Hay MJ et al. *Cancer Lett* 2005; **230**(2): 284-291
93   Drug News. *Nursing,* 2005; **35**(5): 30
94   Ross RG. *Am J Psychiatry* 2006; **163**(7): 1149-1152
95   Berbatis CG, Sunderland BV, Bulsara M. *MJA,* 2002; **177**(10): 539-543
96   Pirani, C. Dark side of a wonder drug. *The Australian*, 2006, Sydney, Tuesday March 28th p. 13.
97   Davis E, Beer J, Gligora C, Thorn A. Accounting for Change in Disability and Severe Restriction. *Working Paper in Social and Labour Statistics (No. 2001/1),* 1981-1998, Belconnen, ACT, Australian Bureau of Statistics.
98   Leo JL, Cohen DA. *J Mind Behavior,* 2003; **24**(1): 29-56
99   Moll GH, Hause S, Ruther E et al. *J Child Adolesc Psychopharmacol,* 2001; **11**(1): 15-24
100 Timimi S, Taylor E. *Br J Psychiatry,* 2004; **184**: 8-9
101 Ozmert E, Toyran M, Yurdakok K. *Arch Pediatr Adolesc Med* 2002; **156**(9): 910-914
102 Christakis DA, Zimmerman FJ, DiGiuseppe DL, McCarty CA. *Pediatrics* 2004; **113**(4): 708-713
103 Zimmerman FJ, Christakis DA. *Pediatrics* 2007; **120**(5): 986-992
104 Perry BD. *Infant Ment Health J,* 1995; **16**(4): 271-291
105 Thomas JM. *Infant Ment Health J,* 1995; **16**(4): 306-317

106 Schnoll R, Burshteyn D, Cea-Aravena J. *Appl Psych Biofeedback,* 2003; **28**(1): 63-75
107 Kidd PM. *Altern Med Rev,* 2000; **5**(5): 402-428
108 Bateman B, Warner JO, Hutchinson E et al. *Arch Dis Child,* 2004; **89**(8): 506-511
109 McCann D, Barrett A, Cooper A et al. *Lancet* 2007; **370**(9598): 1560-1567
110 Brawley A, Silverman B, Kearney S et al. *Ann Allergy Asthma Immunol,* 2004; **92**(6): 663-667
111 Krouse HJ, Krouse JH. *J Asthma* 2007; **44**(9): 759-763
112 Kirov R, Kinkelbur J, Heipke S et al. *J Sleep Res* 2004; **13**(1): 87-93
113 Schnoll R, Burshteyn D, Cea-Aravena J. *Appl Psych Biofeedback,* 2003; **28**(1): 63-75
114 Maher TJ, Wurtman RJ. *Environ Health Perspect* 1987; **75**: 53-57
115 Thomson GO, Raab GM, Hepburn WS et al. *J Child Psychol Psychiatry,* 1989; **30**(4): 515-528
116 Tuthill RW. *Arch Environ Health,* 1996; **51**(3): 214-220
117 Silva P A, Hughes P, Williams S, Faed FM. *J Child Psychol Psychiatry,* 1988; **29**(1): 43-52
118 Schettler, T. *Environ Health Perspect* 2001; **109**(6): 813-816
119 Banerjee TD, Middleton F, Faraone SV. *Acta Paediatr* 2007; **96**(9): 1269-1274
120 Peadon E, O'Leary C, Bower C, Elliott E. *Aust Fam Physician* 2007; **36**(11): 935-939
121 Baydala L, Sherman J, Rasmussen C et al. *J Atten Disord* 2006; **9**(4): 642-647
122 Burgess JR, Stevens L, Zhang W, Peck L. *Am J Clin Nutr* 2000; **71**(1 suppl): 327S-330S
123 Colquhoun I, Bunday S. *Med Hypotheses,* 1981; **7**(5): 673-679
124 Stevens LJ, Zentall SS, Abate ML et al. *Physiol Behav,* 1996; **59**(4-5): 915-920
125 Ross BM, McKenzie I, Glen I, Bennett CP. *Nutrl Neurosci,* 2003; **6**(5): 277-281
126 Richardson AJ, Puri BK. *Prog Neuropsychopharmacol Biol Psychiatry,* 2002; **26**(2): 233-239
127 Richardson AJ, Montgomery P. *Pediatrics* 2005; **115**(5): 1360-1366
128 Konofal E, Lecendreux M, Arnulf I, Mouren MC. *Arch Pediatr Adolesc Med,* 2004; **158**(12): 1113-1115
129 Konofal E, Lecendreux M, Deron J et al. *Pediatr Neurol* 2007; **38**(1): 20-26
130 Wang Q, Luo W, Zheng W et al. *Toxicol Appl Pharmacol* 2007; **219**(1): 33-41
131 Wright RO. *Curr Opin Pediatr* 1999; **11**(3): 255-258
132 Wright RO, Tsaih SW, Schwartz J et al *J Pediatr* 2003; **142**(2): 9-14
133 Arnold LE, Bozzolo H, Hollway J et al, *J Child Adolesc Psychopharmacol,* 2005; **154**: 628-636
134 Yorbik O, Ozdag MF, Olgun A et al. *Prog Neuropsychopharmacol Bio Psychiatry* 2007; **17** [Epub ahead of print]
135 Bilici M, Yildirim F, Kandil S et al. *Prog Neuropsychopharmacol Biol Psychiatry* 2004; **28**(1): 181-190
136 Akhondzadeh S, Mohammadi MR, Khademi M. *BMC Psychiatry* 2004; **8**(4): 9
137 Kozielec T, Starobrat-Hermelin B. *Magnes Res* 1997; **10**(2): 143-148
138 Starobrat-Hermelin B, Kozielec T. *Magnes Res* 1997; **10**(2): 149-156
139 Nogovitsina OR, Levitina EV. *Eksp Klin Farmacol* 2006; **69**(1): 74-77
140 Wakefield AJ, Murch SH, Anthony A, et al. *Lancet* 1998; **351**(9103): 637-641
141 Abhang R. *J Res Ayurveda Siddha* 1993; **14**(1-2): 10-24
142 Sharma R, Chaturvedi C, Tewari PV. *J Res Educ Indian Med* 1987; **6**: 1-10
143 Upadhyay SK, Bhatia BD, Kulkarni KS. *Neurosciences Today* 2002; **4**(3): 184-188
144 Dave UP, Chauvan V, Dalvi J. *Indian J Pediatr* 1993; **60**(3): 423-428
145 Shah LP, Seth GS. *Probe* 1992; **31**(2): 125-129
146 Kalra V, Hina Z, Pandey RM, Kulkarni KS. *Neurosciences Today* 2002; **6**(4): 223-227
147 Negi KS, Singh YD, Kushwaha KP et al. *Indian J Psychiatry* 2000; **42**(2 Suppl): Abstract Only, http://www.aor.ca/int/abstracts/bacopa_monniera_linn.php
148 Francis AJP, Dempster RJW. *Phytomedicine,* 2002; **9**(4): 273-279
149 Trebaticka J, Kopasova S, Hradecna Z et al. *Eur Child Adolesc Psychiatry* 2006; **15**(6): 329-335
150 Dvorakova M, Sivonova M, Trebaticka J et al. *Redox Rep* 2006; **11**(4): 163-172
151 Chinta SJ, Kumar MJ, Hsu M et al. *J Neurosci* 2007; **27**(51): 13997-14006
152 Chovanova Z, Muchova J, Sivonova M et al. *Free Radic Res* 2006; **40**(9): 1003-1010
153 Dvorakova M, Jezova D, Blazicek P et al. *Nutri Neurosci* 2007; **10**(3-4): 151-157
154 Lyon MR, Cline JC, Totosy de Zepetnek J et al. *J Psych Neurosci* 2001; **26**(3): 221-228
155 Kennedy D, Scholey A, Wesnes K. *Nutritional Neuroscience* 2001; **4**(5): 399-412
156 Baumgaertel A. *Pediatric Clinics of North America,* 1999; **46**(5), 977-992
157 Cala S, Crismon ML, Baumgartner J. *Pharmacotherapy* 2003; **23**(2): 222-230
158 Donfrancesco R, Ferrante L. *Phytomed* 2007; **14**(6): 367-370
159 Niederhofer H. *Med Hypotheses* 2007; **68**(5): 1189
160 Wattanathorn J, Mator L, Muchimapura S et al. *J Ethnopharmacol* 2008; **116**(2): 325-332
161 Baird G, Cass H, Slonims V. *BMJ* 2003; **327**(7413): 488-493
162 Axelrod FB, Chelimsky GG, Weese-Mayer DE. *Pediatrics* 2006; **118**(1): 309-321
163 DiCicco-Bloom E, Lord C, Zwaigenbaum L et al. *J Neurosci* 2006; **26**(26): 6897-6906
164 Volkmar FR, Pauls D. *Lancet* 2003; **362**(9390): 1133-1141
165 De Giacomom A, Fombonne E. *Eur Child Adolesc Psychiatry* 1998; **7**(3): 131-136

166 Sigman M, Ruskin E, Arbeile S et al. *Mongr Soc Res Child Dev* 1999; **64**(1): 1-114
167 Williams JG, Higgins JPT, Brayne CEG. *Arch Dis Child* 2006; **91**(1): 8-15
168 Fombonne E. *JAMA* 2003; **289**(1): 87-89
169 Angley M, Young R, Ellis D et al. *Aust Fam Physician* 2007; **36**(9): 741-744
170 Herbert MR. *Clin Neuropsychiatry* 2005; **2**(6): 354-379
171 Hoekstra RA, Bartels M, Verweij CJH, Boomsma DI. *Arch Pediatr Adolesc Med* 2007; **161**(4): 372-377
172 Mutter J, Naumann J, Schneider R et al. *Neuroendocrinol Lett* 2005; **26**(5): 439-446
173 Hviid A, Stellfeld M, Wohlfahrt J, Melbye M. *JAMA* 2003; **290**(13): 1763-1766
174 Andrews N, Miller E, Grant A et al. *Pediatrics* 2004; **114**(3): 584-591
175 Holmes AS, Blaxill MF, Haley BE. *Int J Toxicol* 2003; **22**(4): 277-285
176 Waly M, Olteanu H, Banerjee R et al. *Mol Psychiatry* 2004; **9**(4): 358-370
177 Kidd PM. *Alt Med Rev* 2002; **7**(4): 292-316
178 Pichichero ME, Cernichiari E, Lopreiato J, Treanor J. *Lancet* 2002; **360**(9347): 1737-1741
179 Offit PA, Jew RK. *Pediatrics* 2003; **112**(6): 1394-1397
180 Eldred BE, Dean AJ, McGuire TM, Nash AL. *MJA* 2006; **184**(4): 170-175
181 http://www9.health.gov.au/immhandbook/pdf
182 Roberts EM, English PB, Grether JK et al. *Environ Health Perspect* 2007; **115**(10): 1482-1489
183 Windham GC, Zhang L, Gunier R et al. *Environ Health Perspect* 2006; **114**(9): 1438-1444
184 Erikson CA, Stigler KA, Corkins MR et al. *J Autism Develop Dis* 2005; **35**(6): 713-727
185 Cohen DJ, Johnson WT, Caparulo BK. *Am J Dis Child* 1976; **130**(1): 47-48
186 Alberti A, Pirrone P, Elia M et al. *Biol Psychiatry* 1999; **46**(3): 420-424
187 Finegold SM, Molitoris D, Song Y et al. *Clin Infect Dis* 2002; **35**(Suppl 1): S6-S16
188 Parracho HM, Bingham MO, Gibson GR, McCartney AL. *J Med Microbiol* 2005; **54**(10): 987-991
189 D'Eufemia P, Celli M, Finocchiaro R et al. *Acta Paediatr* 1996; **85**(9): 1076-1079
190 Uhlmann V, Martin CM, Sheils O et al. *Mol Pathol* 2002; **55**(2): 84-90
191 Hunter LC, O'Hare A, Herron WJ et al. *Dev Med Child Neurol* 2003; **45**(2): 121-128
192 Wakefield AJ, Puleston JM, Montgomery SM et al. *Aliment Pharmacol Ther* 2002; **16**(4): 663-674
193 Shattock P, Whiteley P. *Expert Opin Ther Targets* 2002; **6**(2): 175-183
194 Gilberg C, Trygstad O, Foss I. *J Autism Dev Disord* 1982; **12**(3): 229-241
195 Reichelt KL, Hole K, Hamberger A et al. *Adv Biochem Psychopharmacol* 1981; **28**: 627-643
196 Vojdani A, Pangborn JB, Vojdani E, Cooper EL. *Int J Immunopathol Pharmacol* 2003; **16**(3): 189-199
197 Knivsberg AM, REichelt KL, Hoien T, Nodland M. *Nutr Neurosci* 2002; **5**(4): 251-261
198 Arnold GL, Hyman SL, Mooney RA, Kirby RS. *J Autism Dev Disord* 2003; **33**(4): 449-454
199 Kaminski S, Cieslinska A, Kostyra E. *J Appl Genet* 2007; **48**(3): 189-198
200 Bell SJ, Grochoski GT, Clarke AJ. *Crit Rev Food Sci Nutr* 2006; **46**(1): 93-100
201 Truswell AS. *Eur J Clin Nutr* 2005; **59**(5): 623-631
202 Sun Z, Cade JR, Fregly M, Privette RM. *Autism* 1999; **3**(1): 67-83
203 Sun Z, Cade JR. *Autism* 1999; **3**(1): 85-95
204 Sun Z, Zhang Z, Wang X et al. *Peptides* 2003; **24**(6): 937-943
205 Krause I, He XS, Gershwin ME, Shoenfeld Y. *J Aut Dev Disord* 2002; **32**(4): 337-345
206 Ashwood P, Wills S, Van de Water J. *J Leukoc Biol* 2006; **80**(1): 1-15
207 Croonenberghs J, Wauters A, Devreese K et al. *Psychological Med* 2002; **32**(8): 1457-1463
208 Fatemi SH, Halt AR, Stary JM et al. *Biol Psychiatry* 2002; **52**(8): 805-810
209 Bittigau P, Ikonomidou C. *J Child Neurol* 1997; **12**(8): 471-485
210 Anderson GM, Horne WC, Chatterjee D, Cohen DJ. *Ann NY Acad Sci* 1990; **600**: 331-340
211 Goetzl L, Evans T, Rivers J et al. *Am J Obstet Gynecol* 2002; **187**(4): 834-838
212 Marz P, Heese K, Dimitriades-Schmutz B et al. *Glia* 1999; **26**: 191-200
213 Comi AM, Zimmerman AW, Frye VH et al. *J Child Neurol* 1999; **14**(6): 388-394
214 Roman GC. *J NeurolSci* 2007; **262**(1-2): 15-26
215 Mazur-Kolecka B, Cohen IL, Jenkins EC et al. *Brain Res* 2007; **1168**: 11-20
216 Sadamatsu M, Kanai H, Xu X et al. *Congenit Anom (Kyoto)* 2006; **46**(1): 1-9
217 Hanson E, Kalish LA, Bunce E et al. *J Autism Dev Disord* 2007; **37**(4): 628-636
218 Levy SE, Mandell DS, Merhar S et al. *J Dev Behav Pediatr* 2003; **24**(6): 418-423
219 Page T. *J Autism Dev Disord* 2007; **30**(5): 463-469
220 Levy SE, Hyman SL. *Ment Retard Dev Disabil Res Rev* 2005; **11**(2): 131-142
221 Bernstein AL. *Ann NY Acad Sci* 1990; **585**: 250-260
222 Brudnak MA, Rimland B, Kerry RE et al. *Med Hypotheses* 2002; **58**(5): 422-428
223 Kidd PM. *Alt Med Rev* 2002; **7**(4): 472-499
224 Kataoka S. *J Biosci Bioeng* 2005; **100**(3): 227-234
225 Kushi M, Kushi A. *Macrobiotic Diet* 2nd Ed, Japan Publications, Tokyo, 1993.

CHAPTER 8

Common Urinary Tract Disorders in Children

URINARY TRACT PROBLEMS IN infants are often of great concern to parents. However, most voiding problems are transient in nature, being part of a developmental process.[1] They usually have no organic basis and do not represent a behavioural problem. Almost all children have wetting and/or soiling accidents at one time or another and, as with other developmental milestones, transient disturbances in toilet training can be expected.[1] That said, untreated issues can indeed spiral into physical, behavioural and developmental problems that may disrupt toilet training and the maintenance of bladder and bowel continence.[1]

Normal Voiding and Toilet Training

The foetus voids by reflex bladder contraction in combination with simultaneous relaxation of the sphincter.[2] Urine storage is promoted by sympathetic and pubendal nerve-mediated inhibition of detrusor muscle contraction, accompanied by closure of the bladder neck and proximal urethra with increased activity of the external sphincter.[2] The young infant has a coordinated reflex voiding as often as 15 to 20 times a day.[2,3] Over time the bladder capacity increases. The first period of increased volume is around birth and represents a four fold increase over that of the foetus. The second period occurs at toilet training, when control over voiding is gained.[3] At an age of 2 to 4 years the child is usually ready to begin toilet training.[4] It is thought that overnight storage of urine in the bladder rather than daytime continence, is the stimulus for bladder growth.[3]

Urine production decreases with age in terms of production per kg of body weight per hour, but increases in total volume over 24 hours.[3] A newborn will have a median urine production of 5 mL/kg per hour, whilst a 1-year-old will produce 3.5 mL/kg per hour.[3] The number of voids per hour is still around one per hour for this age group, but only when awake and usually not at night due to the response to the circadian rhythm of antidiuretic hormone (ADH).[5] The number of voids from the age of one until after toilet training is reduced to 4 to 7 per 24 hours, due to the increase in bladder capacity.[3]

To achieve conscious control over the bladder several conditions need to be met. These are an awareness of bladder filling, cortical inhibition of reflex bladder contraction, the ability to consciously tighten the external sphincter to prevent incontinence, normal bladder growth and the motivation to stay dry.[2] Girls typically acquire bladder control before boys and bowel control generally precedes urinary control.[2]

Toilet training is approached differently in different cultures. Cultures that depend on disposable nappies (diapers) tend to toilet train infants at a later age.[6] It has been suggested that the increased use of disposable nappies has led to a delay in the timing of toilet training.[7] The Digo people of East Africa begin toilet training within the first few weeks of life and expect the infant to be well trained between the ages of four to six months.[6] Compared to other groups, African-American children begin and complete training at an early age.[6] When surveyed, 50% of African-American parents felt it was important that their child be toilet trained by the age of 2. In contrast only 4% of Caucasian parents agreed with this statement.[6]

Key Herbal Actions

Before considering the therapeutics of some common urinary tract disorders in children, it is worthwhile to review the key herbal actions.

Diuretics

Although the term diuretic denotes all substances which increase urine flow (and in this sense water itself is a diuretic agent), modern diuretic drugs are designed to increase sodium excretion, since cardiac oedema largely results through sodium retention. In contrast, in herbal texts the term diuretic is often loosely or inaccurately applied.

In particular, when a herb was taken as a decoction or infusion, as it often was traditionally, the water consumed in conjunction with the herb would have produced an observable diuresis which might have had little to do with any diuretic action of the herb itself. Hence, many herbs have been mistakenly classified as diuretics. Those herbs which did exhibit a mild diuretic activity might have done so because of their mineral (electrolyte) content (see below).

Confounding the issue, the term diuretic is often used in quite a different context in herbal writings. Herbs which are said to enhance the excretion of metabolic waste from the kidneys are also often described as diuretics. However, a more accurate description is encompassed by the terminology "diuretic depurative". Examples of diuretic depuratives include celery and clivers. Any frank diuretic action of these herbs is probably variable, depending on the individual, and unlikely to be outside normal physiological limits.

In Europe, phytotherapists have proposed that the term aquaretic might more accurately describe some herbs which genuinely do increase urine output. The thinking here is that these herbs act on the glomerulus (unlike conventional diuretic drugs which act further along the nephron) to increase water excretion from the body, but their effect on electrolytes such as sodium and potassium is largely neutral. In other words, aquaretics act by increasing fluid loss from the body in a physiological manner, by increasing the formation of primary urine.[8] The herb combination which has been most studied in this context is asparagus root (*Asparagus officinalis*) with parsley herb (*Petroselinum crispum*).[9] In uncontrolled trials, this combination caused significant weight loss in overweight patients and significantly lowered blood pressure in patients with hypertension, without changing other biochemical parameters.[9] Aquaretics have potential for the treatment of excessive weight, hypertension, congestive heart failure, kidney stones and premenstrual syndrome.

The mineral (electrolyte) content of herbs can often underpin any observed diuretic activity. The ratio of potassium to sodium was found to be higher in decoctions of herbs which are traditionally regarded as diuretics, compared to other herbs.[10] A pharmacological study concluded that the high potassium content of dandelion leaf is the agent responsible for any diuretic activity.[11]

The rationale for using diuretic herbs is sometimes misguided in herbal texts. In particular, herbs with a reputation for acting as diuretics are often recommended for the treatment of cystitis. The obvious basis for this approach is to flush the infecting bacteria from the bladder. However, in this context, the cheapest, safest, best and most certain flushing agent is water. Any action of herbal diuretics will be marginal compared to the flushing effect of a copious intake of water and cannot be justified. Key diuretic or aquaretic herbs include dandelion (especially the leaf), golden rod (probably), asparagus root, parsley, juniper and horsetail. The evidence for the diuretic activity of herbal medicines has been recently reviewed.[12]

Urinary Tract Antiseptics

Metabolites of the phytochemicals in certain herbs are excreted in the urine where they exert an antiseptic effect. This activity should be regarded as mild and in acute infections such as cystitis these herbs should be taken often and in high doses. The most important urinary tract antiseptics are buchu, bearberry and juniper.

Urinary Tract Demulcents

These agents will exert a soothing effect on the lining of the urinary tract and are indicated for inflammation and infections such as urethritis and cystitis. They may also be of value for inflammation higher up the urinary tract and the irritation of kidney stones. Some urinary tract demulcents such as marshmallow leaf act by a reflex effect (reflex demulcents). Others, specifically couch grass and corn silk probably have a direct effect.

Bladder Tonics

These herbs have a toning effect on the smooth muscle of the bladder. They are therefore useful in the treatment of hypotonic bladder, as can occur with the urinary outlet obstruction caused by benign prostatic hyperplasia, and other neurological conditions of the bladder. During bladder infection, bacteria may remain with the residual urine which stays in the bladder after each voiding. Bladder tonics decrease this residual volume and therefore assist greatly with the flushing of the bladder. In this context they can be particularly valuable in the resolution of recurrent cystitis. The best established bladder tonic is Crataeva bark. Golden rod also appears to have a regulatory effect on bladder function.[13,14]

Nocturnal Enuresis (NE) or Bedwetting

In societies using disposable nappies, 90-95% of 5 year olds are continent during the day and 80-85% are continent at night.[2] Nocturnal enuresis (NE) refers to the occurrence of involuntary voiding at night after 5 years of age, when volitional control over micturition is expected.[2] New theories have recently been proposed regarding the pathophysiology of NE. It is now divided into primary nocturnal enuresis (PNE) and secondary nocturnal enuresis (SNE).[15] PNE is considered to be related to a problem with poor arousal from sleep, overproduction of urine at night, small nocturnal bladder capacity or a combination of these.[15] The common reported causes of SNE include urinary tract infection (UTI), constipation, urge syndrome/dysfunctional voiding, psychological stress, disturbed circadian rhythm of ADH, diabetes and obstructive sleep apnoea.[15] Further to this, a general classification of bladder control problems has been developed by the International Children's Continence Society and is described in the table below.[16] This classification can help in accurately defining the problem.

LOWER URINARY TRACT DYSFUNCTION IN CHILDREN

Classification	Symptoms
Nocturnal Enuresis	Involuntary passage of urine at night in the absence of physical disease, beyond the age of 5
Primary Nocturnal Enuresis	The child has never been dry at night for more than 6 months. This is more common than secondary enuresis
Secondary Nocturnal Enuresis	Bedwetting after a period of at least 6 months of night dryness. This is more likely to be associated with a psychological or organic cause
Monosymptomatic Nocturnal Enuresis	Bedwetting without daytime symptoms. This is the most common form
Non-monosymptomatic Nocturnal Enuresis	Bedwetting with daytime voiding symptoms, such as urgency and frequency, with or without daytime incontinence. This suggests underlying bladder dysfunction
Urinary Incontinence	Daytime wetting with or without bedwetting

Epidemiology of NE

Bedwetting is more common in boys and occurs in up to 20% of school age children, with up to 2.4% wetting at least nightly.[5] The prevalence ranges from about 20% in 5 year olds to 10% in 10 year olds and 3% in 15 year olds.[5] Children tend to outgrow bedwetting, with an annual spontaneous remission rate of about 14%.

Impact of NE

The impact of bedwetting can be significant, as it can affect self esteem, relationships with friends and family and schooling.[5] Children are often teased by siblings and friends and are reluctant to participate in school trips requiring an overnight stay or sleepovers.[5] In contrast, a 1996 Australian survey found that only 34% of families seek professional help and others surprisingly did not express a high level of concern about NE.[17]

Assessment of Children with NE

Taking a thorough case history is most important in order to differentiate PNE from SNE and monosymptomatic NE from non-monosymptomatic NE.[5] Daytime symptoms may be caused by detrusor overactivity, with involuntary detrusor contraction during bladder filling resulting in symptoms of urgency and/or frequency. This may occur with or without urge incontinence, which is often associated with a small functional bladder capacity.[5] Other relevant information includes medication, sleep history, developmental history and past medical history including UTIs and family history.[5]

Conventional Management of Monosymptomatic NE

The initial treatment of choice for children with monosymptomatic NE is an enuresis alarm. There are two types of alarms typically available: a pad-and-bell alarm where the child lies on a large pad placed in the bed and any liquid triggers the alarm, and a personal alarm clipped either onto the child's underpants or a continence pad placed inside the child's underpants.[5] Children generally use the alarm until they achieve 14 consecutive dry nights. Treatment beyond 16 weeks is unlikely to produce a positive result.[5]

Herbal Management of Monosymptomatic NE

The Eclectics considered sweet sumach (*Rhus aromatica*) as a specific for NE especially when associated with sphincter weakness.[18] Ellingwood also cites kava as useful for NE,[19] while others considered ribwort to be indicated[20] which is also the remedy of choice in macrobiotic medicine.[21] Weiss on the other hand suggested both sweet sumach and St John's wort as the remedies of choice.[22] Pumpkin seeds may also be useful in the treatment of NE, particularly with an irritated bladder.[23] The spasmolytic properties of cramp bark will also be useful.[24]

Example Liquid Formulation for Monosymptomatic NE

St John's wort	1:2	40 mL
Ribwort or Cramp bark	1:2	40 mL
Flavouring mix		20 mL
	Total	100 mL

Dose: Calculate the standard dose (based on an adult dose of 5 mL) according to the most appropriate guideline in Chapter 1. To be taken before each meal with water or juice.

Herbal Management of Non-Monosymptomatic NE

The management of non-monosymptomatic NE is similar to the above. However, treatments for bladder dysfunction such as Crataeva and corn silk should be considered. For secondary NE the cause needs to be identified and addressed.

Urinary Tract Infections (UTIs)

UTI is defined by the presence of organisms in the normally sterile urinary tract.[2] Clinically evident infections are typically due to bacteria, although several viruses, fungi and parasites can also cause infection.[25] Over recent decades UTI has been increasingly recognised as an important occult cause of febrile illness in children.[25]

Epidemiology

The occurrence of UTIs during childhood varies with gender and age. In girls the first UTI usually occurs by the age of 5 years and the incidence peaks during infancy and toilet training.[2] After the first UTI, 60-80% of girls will develop a second UTI within 18 months. In boys, most UTIs occur during the first year of life and are more common in uncircumcised infants.[2] During the first year of life, the male:female incidence ratio for UTIs is about 1:2, beyond this age the ratio is 1:10.[2]

Pathophysiology

In general, bacteria infect the urinary tract by ascending from the urethra, although haematogenous infections may occur in rare instances.[25] The most common bacterial pathogens associated with UTI include gram-negative species such as *Escherichia coli*, *Klebsiella, Proteus, Enterobacter, Pseudomonas* and *Serratia* spp.[2,25] Common non-bacterial causes of UTI include haemorrhagic cystitis from adenovirus and *Candida albicans* infection in immunocompromised individuals.[2,25]

UTIs can be subdivided according to location. Those localised to the bladder and urethra are termed cystitis and urethritis respectively, whilst those impacting the ureter, collecting system and renal parenchyma are termed pyelonephritis.[25] Ascending infection of the urinary tract is a complex process that is associated with bacterial adhesion, bacterial virulence and motility in combination with host anatomic, immune and genetic factors.[25] The bacteria arise from faecal microflora, colonise the perineum and enter the bladder via the urethra. In uncircumcised boys, the bacterial pathogen can also arise from the flora beneath the foreskin.[2]

Immunology

UTIs activate a mucosal inflammatory response with neutrophils dominating the acute cellular infiltrate after rapidly migrating through the tissues into the urine.[26] This response is initiated when bacteria reach epithelial cells and stimulate the secretion of chemokines such as IL-8 and expression of chemokine receptors.[26] Antibiotic treatment blocks neutrophil passage into the urine and causes them to accumulate under the kidney and bladder epithelium.[26] One possible immunological reason for the observed infant susceptibility to UTIs is a developmental weakness in neutrophils (see Chapter 2). As noted previously, infants have a transient reduced capacity to increase neutrophil production in response to infection. Their neutrophils have a reduced capacity for adhesion and to induce a respiratory burst, thus phagocytosis is deficient.[27]

Uropathogens achieve tissue specific attachment through the expression of surface fimbriae, a key event in the activation of the inflammatory response.[26] There are two types of fimbriae, type I and type II. Type I are found on most strains of *E. coli* and their attachment to target cells can be blocked by D-mannose.[2] These fimbriae are referred to as mannose sensitive and organisms expressing them appear to have no role in pylonephritis.[2] Type II fimbriae are not inhibited by D-mannose and are only expressed on certain strains of *E. coli*. Because they can agglutinate P blood group erythrocytes, they are also known as P fimbriae.[2] Bacteria with P or Type II fimbriae are more likely to cause pylonephritis.[2]

Risk Factors

In girls UTIs often occur at the onset of toilet training because voiding dysfunction can occur at that stage. The child is trying to stay dry by retaining urine, yet the bladder may still have uninhibited contractions forcing urine out. The result may be a high pressure, turbulent urine flow or incomplete bladder emptying, both of which increase the likelihood of bacteriuria.[2] Voiding dysfunction can also occur when the child voids infrequently. This occurs most often with school age children who refuse to use the school toilet.[2] Obstructive uropathy results in hydronephrosis, which increases the risk of UTIs from urinary stasis.[2] Constipation can increase the risk of UTIs because of its association with voiding dysfunction.[2] The bubble bath is a controversial risk factor for UTI in children, presumably because of a perceived irritant effect or a change in skin pH. Most paediatricians recommend the avoidance of bubble baths[28] and this advice is reflected on many websites, including that of the National Kidney Foundation, UK.[29] However, there appears to be little evidence for these recommendations.[28] Anatomical abnormalities such as labial adhesion are associated with UTIs, and neuropathic bladder may cause UTI if there is incomplete bladder emptying or detrusor/sphincter dyssynergia or both.[2] Frequent UTIs in a young boy suggest an anatomical or functional abnormality.

Clinical Manifestations

Symptoms of cystitis include dysuria, urgency, frequency, suprapubic pain, incontinence and malodorous urine (which is specific for a UTI). Cystitis does not cause fever and does not result in renal injury.[2] Clinical pylonephritis is characterised by any or all of the following: abdominal or flank pain, fever, malaise, nausea, vomiting and occasionally diarrhoea.[2] Pylonephritis is the most common serious bacterial infection in infants under 24 months of age who have fever without focus.[2]

Herbal Treatment of Cystitis

No clinical evidence supporting the use of herbal medicines in childhood cystitis could be found, therefore reliance will be placed on adult studies and traditional information. There is no known safety or efficacy reason why a herb that may be indicated for an adult with cystitis is not also suitable for a child with cystitis, with the possible exception of kava.

Owing to its safety and tolerability, cranberry is ideally suited to the management and prevention of UTIs in children. It has been found to exert anti-adhesion activity against uropathogenic *E. coli* strains for both antibiotic-susceptible and resistant bacteria.[30] A recent systematic review of the clinical evidence for cranberry in UTI prevention concluded that there is evidence from four good quality randomised controlled trials that cranberry juice may decrease the number of symptomatic UTIs over a 12-month period, particularly in women with recurrent UTIs.[31]

Example Herbal Formulation for Childhood Cystitis

Echinacea root blend	1:2	35 mL
Buchu or Uva ursi	1:2	25 mL
Licorice (high in glycyrrhizin)	1:1	15 mL
Golden rod 1:2 or Marshmallow root	1:5	25 mL
	Total	100 mL

Dose: Calculate the standard dose according to the most appropriate guideline in Chapter 1, based on an adult dose of 5 mL and administer 5 to 6 times a day in juice or water until symptoms are relieved.

An alternative to the above liquid formulation is the Urinary Tract Support tablets containing cranberry, Crataeva, bearberry and buchu essential oil (see Appendix 1). Calculate the child's dose (based on an acute adult dose of 6 tablets per day) according to the most appropriate guideline in Chapter 1. These can be supplemented with extra Short Term Immune Support tablets (see Appendix 1) based on an adult dose of 4 per day. For younger children the tablets (or part thereof) can be crushed and mixed with honey or a suitable sweetener to improve compliance.

Rationale

Echinacea is included to positively modulate the immune system in the face of infection and has demonstrated an ability to increase the number of neutrophils in humans.[32] Buchu is a pleasant tasting child-friendly urinary tract antiseptic with traditional indications for cystitis, urethritis and dysuria.[24] Uva ursi is an alternative urinary tract antiseptic. Licorice provides the demulcency necessary to soothe an irritated bladder and also has anti-adhesion properties.[33] Marshmallow root is also an excellent reflex demulcent. The formulation is rounded off with golden rod which possesses anti-inflammatory activity relevant to the urinary system and is indicted for cystitis and urinary disorders.[24]

Case History

A 5-year-old female presented with a 12-month history of UTIs. She suffered spasm and pain with every UTI and most were treated with antibiotics. The mother was unaware of any particular toilet training issue that may be a factor. The child was otherwise well and the diet was fine. The following liquid formulation was prescribed:

Echinacea root blend	1:2	30 mL
Buchu	1:2	20 mL
Marshmallow root glycetract	1:5	20 mL
Golden rod	1:2	30 mL
	Total	100 mL

Dose: 3 mL twice a day in juice. In the event of a UTI, 6 doses to be taken per day until symptoms are relieved.

The marshmallow was prescribed for its urinary demulcent activity.

The child took the medicine for 6 months, during which time there was not one single episode of a UTI. She remained UTI-free once the herbal treatment was stopped.

References

1   Issenman RM, Filmer RB, Gorski PA. *Pediatrics* 1999; **103**(6): 1346-1352
2   Kleigman RM, Behrman RE, Jenson HB, Stanton BF. *Nelson Textbook of Pediatrics* 18th Ed, Saunders Elsevier, Philadelphia, 2007.
3   Sillen U. *J Urol* 2001; **166**(6): 2376-2381
4   Brazelton TB, Christophersen ER, Frauman AC et al. *Pediatrics* 1999; **103**(6): 1353-1358
5   Caldwell PHY, Edgar D, Hodson E, Craig JC. *MJA* 2005; **182**(4): 190-195
6   Klassen TP, Kiddoo D, Lang ME et al. *Evid Rep Technol Assess (Full Rep)* 2006; **147**: 1-57
7   Bakker E, Wyndaele JJ. *BJU Int* 2000; **86**(3): 248-252
8   Werk W. *Erfahrungsheilkunde*, 1994; **11**: 712-714
9   Beitz G, Hippe SK, Schremmer D. *Naturheilpraxis* 1996; **2**: 247-252
10 Szentmihályi K, Kéry A, Then M et al. *Phytother Res* 1998; **12**: 163-166
11 Hook I, McGee A, Henman M. *Intl J Pharmacog* 1993; **31**(1): 29-34
12 Wright CI, Van-Buren L, Kroner CI et al. *J Ethnopharmacol* 2007; **114**: 1-31
13 Bauer HW, Wiedemann A. *Zeitschrift für Phytotherapie*, 2003; **24**(5): 218-221
14 Pfannkuch A, Stammwitz U. *Zeitschrift für Phytotherapie* 2002; **23**(1): 20-25
15 Robson LM, Leung AK, Van Howe R. *Pediatrics* 2005; **115**(4): 956-959
16 Norgaard JP, van Gool JD, Hjalmas K et al. *Br J Urol* 1998; **81**(Suppl 3): 1-16
17 Bower WF, Moore KH, Shepherd RB, Adams RD. *Br J Urol* 1996; **78**(4): 602-606
18 Felter HW. *The Eclectic Materia Medica, Pharmacology and Therapeutics,* Eclectic Medical Publications, Portland Oregon 1983, First Published Cincinnati, Ohio, 1922.
19 Ellingwood F. *American Materia Medica, Therapeutics and Pharmacognosy,* Reprint Eclectic Medical Publications, Portland Oregon 1983.
20 Burgess N. *Mod Phytother* 1995; **1**(2): 6-7
21 Kushi M, Van Cauwenberghe M. *Macrobiotic Home Remedies* Japan Publications, Tokyo, 1989.
22 Weiss RF. *Herbal Medicine,* Beaconsfield Publishers, Beaconsfield, England, 1991.
23 Schilcher H. *Phytotherapy in Paediatrics,* Medpharm, Stuttgart, 1997.
24 Bone K. *A Clinical Guide to Blending Liquid Herbs. Herbal Formulations for the Individual Patient.* Churchill Livingstone, Edinburgh, 2003.
25 Zore JJ, Kiddoo DA, Shaw KN. *Clin Microbiol Rev* 2005; **18**(2): 417-422
26 Godaly G, Bergsten G, Hang L et al. *J Leukoc Biol* 2001; **69**(6): 899-906
27 Petrova A, Mehta R. *Indian J Pediatr* 2007; **74**(2): 185-191
28 Modgil G, Baverstock A. *Arch Dis Child* 2006; **91**(10): 863-865
29 National Kidney Foundation. *Urinary Tract Infections in children* http:www.kidney.org.uk/kids/uti_in_kids/page06.html
30 Lavigne JP, Bourg G, Botto H, Sotto A. *Pathol Biol (Paris)* 2007; **55**(8-9): 460-464
31 Jepson RG, Craig JC. *Mol Nutr Food Res* 2007; **51**(6): 738-745
32 Goel V, Lovlin R, Chang C et al. *Phytother Res* 2005; **19**(8): 689-694
33 Mills S, Bone K. *Principles and Practice of Phytotherapy: Modern Herbal Medicine.* Churchill Livingstone, Edinburgh, 2000, pp. 465-478.

CHAPTER 9

Common Skin Disorders in Children

THE SKIN IS THE LARGEST organ of the body and serves as a primary defence, a sensory and excretory organ and a critical regulator of body temperature.[1,2] Its barrier properties extend to protection against ultraviolet (UV) radiation, oxidants, micro-organisms and toxic agents.[2] A critical function is the regulation of water loss, with the permeability barrier residing within the stratum corneum (SC), the wafer-thin superficial layer of the skin.[1,2]

The skin is not a static barrier, but a complex organ able to maintain internal homeostasis through multidirectional communication. The endocrine, immune and central nervous systems share a common language of neuropeptides, cytokines, hormones and other effector molecules, creating a neuro-immuno-cutaneous-endocrine system (NICE).[3] It can be assumed that the NICE system in infants and children undergoes a developmental process and is subject to both genetic and environmental influences. The connection between mind and the skin is obvious, with facial blushing associated with strong emotions, or pallor and sweating from fear or anxiety.[3] The pathological results of the link between the skin and nervous system perturbations are commonly seen in clinical practice: it is often noted that stressful life events may cause or exacerbate eczema, acne, urticaria and psoriasis.[4]

The skin is also important for the manufacture of vitamin D.[5,6] Vitamin D or the sunshine vitamin is essential for the maintenance of health and the prevention of skeletal problems, cancer and cardiovascular and autoimmune disease.[5,6,7] Dietary sources of vitamin D include fatty fish, orange juice and cows milk.[5,6] Each of these foods carries certain risks: fatty fish and methyl mercury toxicity, orange juice with its high glycaemic index and milk with allergy. Regular sun exposure is essential to prevent vitamin D deficiency and is a safer means of adequate intake.

Vitamin D deficiency has become increasingly recognised as a problem in many populations worldwide.[7] It has been suggested that the increasing publicity over sun exposure and skin cancer has led to many children not receiving adequate sunlight.[5,6,7] Chronic severe vitamin D deficiency in infancy and children causes a bone deformation known as rickets, a consequence of poor mineralisation.[7] A large Australian prospective study is a good example of the current issue. There has been a steady increase observed in the incidence of rickets, with a doubling of the number of cases between 2002 to 2003. The median age of presentation was 15.1 months, with 25% of cases detected at less than 6 months of age. The most common presenting features were hypocalcaemic seizures and bowed legs.[8] Australia has adequate sunshine and should not suffer the risk of vitamin D deficiency known in those areas subject to long freezing winters and inadequate sunshine. On the other hand, it is a common practice in these regions for the children to be given cod liver oil as a good source of vitamins A and D.[6] It is estimated that just 5 to 15 minutes per day between 10am and 3 pm on the arms, legs and face during spring, summer and autumn (fall) provides the body with 1000IU of cholecalciferol.[6]

The skin is an important organ in terms of food and environmental hypersensitivities.[9] The clinical manifestations of hypersensitivities on the skin range from the symptoms of atopic dermatitis to urticaria and angioedema. For the most part, pruritis is a prominent feature.[9]

A recent review could find no specific studies on skin vulnerability in the paediatric population, particularly in terms of the possible differing sensitivities between adults and children.[10] This also appears to be the case at the time of writing. Ethical considerations have probably imposed a limitation on this type of research.[10] However, as noted previously, children are at an increased risk of toxicity via the skin due to the immaturity of their epidermal barrier, underdeveloped xenobiotic metabolising systems and a higher surface area to weight ratio.[10] Toxic exposure has a bimodal age distribution in childhood. The first peak occurs between 9 months and 3 years (the risk being mainly from oral exposure as a result of oral exploration) and the second peak is in late childhood and early adolescence.[10] Toxic agents which can be absorbed through the skin include insecticides and solvents. Paediatric poisonings from cleaning agents (dishwashing liquids, degreasers, bleach, glass cleaners, furniture cleaners, oven cleaners) are usually the result of oral ingestion. However, absorption via the skin and conjunctiva are possible, although considerably less common.[10]

The skin is also a general indicator of health status, with skin disease traditionally linked to vicarious elimination.[11] From a traditional western herbal perspective the most distinctive feature of stagnation or "bad blood" is a skin lesion, usually accompanied by digestive, liver and lymphatic sluggishness.[11] The skin is at the periphery of the body and therefore reflects the state of the inner compartments. When the internal organs, glands, blood and lymph become disordered, the symptoms almost always appear on the skin.[12] Since one of the primary functions of the skin is the balance between the external environment and internal body conditions, the skin will also reflect environmental change.[12] Traditional medical systems rely on the condition of the skin as a diagnostic tool, where the condition, colour and marks are indicators of inner disharmony. The details of skin diagnosis are beyond the scope of this text, however a normal healthy skin should be clear, smooth, slightly shiny and slightly moist.[12] It is not uncommon to observe these qualities in healthy robust children.

Viral Warts

Cutaneous viral warts are discrete benign epithelial proliferations caused by the human papillomavirus (HPV). The incidence is highest in children and during adolescence.[13,14] HPV is spread by direct contact and autoinoculation, as well as fomite transmission. The clinical manifestations of infection appear after approximately 4 weeks, depending on the type of HPV (there are over 200), the site of inoculation and the immune status of the host.[14]

Clinical Manifestations and Pathophysiology

Cutaneous warts develop in 5 to 10% of children. Common warts (verruca vulgaris), typically caused by HPV types 2 and 4, occur mainly on the fingers, dorsum of the hands, the tissue surrounding the finger and toe nails and on the face, knees and elbows.[14] The lesions are well circumscribed papules with an irregular, roughened, keratotic surface.[14] Plantar warts, although similar to the common wart, are caused by HPV type 1 and occur on the soles of the feet. They are usually flush with the surface of the sole because of the constant weight-bearing pressure.[14] Genital HPV infection can occur in sexually active adolescents, most often as a result of HPV types 6 or 11.[14]

The various types of warts all share the basic tissue characteristics of hyperplasia of the epidermal cells and vacuolation of the spinous keratinocytes, which may contain viral particles.[14] Children with impaired cell-mediated immunity are particularly susceptible to HPV infection.[14]

Herbal Treatment of Warts

There are many folk treatments for warts, mostly involving the application of a keratolytic latex from the stems of various plants, such as greater celandine, petty spurge, fig tree and dandelion.[15,16] Interestingly, a prospective, open right/left comparative trial of fig tree latex therapy versus local standard cryotherapy was recently undertaken. Twenty-five adult patients with common warts were recruited into the study from an outpatient clinic. They were instructed in the self-application of fig tree latex which was applied to warts on one side of the body. Warts on the opposite side were treated using standard cryotherapy. At the 6-month follow-up, 11 (44%) of the 25 patients experienced a complete resolution for the warts treated with the latex. Fourteen patients (56%) had a complete cure following cryotherapy. Two patients had complete remission on both sides (and so were included in both groups above) and another two failed to respond to either cryotherapy or fig tree latex. It was therefore found that fig tree latex therapy was marginally less effective than the current standard of cryotherapy. Of note, adverse effects were only observed for the cryo-treated warts.[17]

Covering warts with an occlusive tape is another folk treatment that has attracted some research attention. A prospective, randomised, controlled trial was initiated in 61 children. Patients were randomised to receive either cryotherapy (liquid nitrogen applied to each wart for 10 seconds) every 2 to 3 weeks for a maximum of 6 treatments or duct tape occlusion (applied directly to the wart) for a maximum of 2 months. Patients had their warts measured at baseline and on return visits. Of the 51 patients completing the study, 26 (51%) were treated with duct tape, and 25 (49%) were treated with cryotherapy. Twenty-two patients (85%) in the duct tape arm experienced complete resolution of their warts, versus 15 patients (60%) enrolled in the cryotherapy arm. The majority of warts that responded to either therapy did so within the first month of treatment.[18]

Two herbal extracts have been traditionally used as a topical application for the treatment of common warts: greater celandine and thuja.[19] Oral treatment involves the prescription of immunomodulatory remedies such as Echinacea or Andrographis.[19] Thuja can also be prescribed internally, but this is best avoided in younger children.

Example Treatments for Common Warts

As suggested above, the treatment of warts best involves a topical application and internal immunomodulators. The following cream is recommended.

Thuja	1:5	5 mL
Greater celandine	1:2	5 mL
Natural cream base		40 g

Apply to wart/s morning and night and cover with an occlusive dressing.

Echinacea extract or tablets at appropriate doses can provide the required immunomodulation. For an adult the dose for an Echinacea 1:2 root blend would be 5 mL twice a day. For Echinacea Formula or Short Term Immune Support tablets (see Appendix 1) the adult dose should be 4 per day. Calculate the dose for the child according to the most appropriate guideline in Chapter 1. For younger children the tablets can be crushed and mixed with honey or a suitable sweetener to improve compliance. See Appendix 1 for the suggested formulations for these tablets.

The above topical approach has been used in clinical practice for over 25 years by one of the authors (RS). Countless children have been successfully treated, occasionally with additional Echinacea. Plantar warts in adults are a little more difficult to treat and require a more concentrated cream (but based on the same ingredients).

Herpes Simplex Viral Infections

The two closely-related herpes simplex viruses (HSVs), HSV-1 and HSV-2, cause a variety of illnesses depending on the anatomical site where infection is initiated, the immune status of the host and whether the infection is primary or recurrent.[14] HSV-1 mostly infects the gingivae, the dermis, the upper respiratory tract and central nervous system. HSV-2 mostly infects the genitals and perineum.[14,20] Infection tends to be mild and self-limiting, except in the immunocompromised patient and newborn infant, where it can be severe and life threatening.[14]

Primary infection occurs in those who have not been previously exposed to either HSV-1 or HSV-2. Because they are HSV seronegative and have no pre-existing immunity, infection can be severe. Nonprimary first infection is said to occur in individuals previously infected with one type of HSV who become infected for the first time with the other type. Because immunity to one type infers some cross-protection against the other, nonprimary first infections tend to be less severe than true primary infections. During primary and nonprimary initial infections, HSV establishes a latent infection in the regional sensory ganglion neurons.[14] It is maintained in this latent state for the life of the host and can periodically reactivate, thereby causing recurrent infection.

Symptomatic recurrent infections tend to be less severe and are of shorter duration than the first infection. Asymptomatic recurrent infections are common.[14]

Epidemiology, Pathogenesis and Clinical Features

HSV infection is ubiquitous and there is no seasonal variation in risk. The only natural host is humans. The mode of transmission is direct contact between mucocutaneous surfaces and there is no evidence for incidental transmission from inanimate objects such as toilet seats.[14]

All infected individuals harbour a latent infection and the subsequent recurrent infections may be symptomatic or go unrecognised. They are periodically contagious, which helps explain the widespread prevalence of HSV.[14]

HSV-1 and HSV-2 are equally capable of causing initial infection at any anatomical site, but differ in their capacity to cause recurrent infection. HSV-1 has a greater propensity to cause recurrent oral infection while HSV-2 causes recurrent genital infection. For this reason HSV-1 infections typically result from contact with contaminated oral secretions, whereas HSV-2 infections most commonly result from anogenital contact.[14]

HSV seroprevalence rates are highest in developing nations and among lower socioeconomic groups. However, high rates are still found in developed nations and amongst persons of high socioeconomic advantage. The incidence of HSV-1 infection is more common in childhood and adolescence.[14]

Viral infection typically begins at a cutaneous portal of entry such as the oral cavity, genital mucosa, ocular conjunctiva or breaks in keratinised epithelia.[14,21] HSV replicates locally, resulting in the death of the host cell which sometimes produces a clinically apparent inflammatory response. This facilitates the development of the characteristic herpes vesicles.[14,21] The virus also enters nerve endings and spreads to sensory ganglia via intraneuronal transport. HSV replicates in some sensory neurons as well. The progeny are sent back to the periphery where they are released from nerve endings and replicate further in the skin or mucosal surfaces.[14,21]

The hallmarks of HSV infection are the skin vesicles and shallow ulcers. Classical infections present with small, 2 to 4 mm vesicles that may be surrounded by an erythematous base. These may persist for a few days before evolving into shallow, minimally erythematous ulcers.[14]

Herbal Treatment of HSV

Several topical herbal applications have attracted research attention. A double blind, placebo-controlled, randomised trial using a high potency lemon balm cream (1% of a 70:1 lemon balm concentrate) for HSV-1 yielded positive results. The active cream shortened the healing period, prevented the spread of the infection and exerted a beneficial effect on the typical symptoms of herpes such as itching, tingling, burning, stabbing pain, swelling, tautness and erythema.[22] Several other studies using the concentrated lemon balm cream have demonstrated similar results.[19]

Ninety men and women with recurrent genital HSV-2 participated in a randomised, single blind, masked investigator, controlled, multicentre study. The efficacy of a propolis ointment was compared with topical acyclovir and placebo. Thirty patients were randomised to each group and treatment was commenced in the blister phase. In the case of women with vaginal or cervical lesions, a tampon with the appropriate ointment was inserted four times daily for 10 days. The propolis ointment was observed to be more effective than both the acyclovir and placebo ointments in terms of healing the lesions and in reducing local symptoms.[23]

The efficacy of a topical preparation combining rhubarb and sage extracts was compared to sage extract alone or acyclovir in a double blind, randomised trial. A total of 145 patients (111 female, 34 male) with HSV-1 completed the trial, of whom 64 received the rhubarb-sage cream, 40 the sage cream and 41 the reference cream. The sage and rhubarb preparation proved to be as effective as the topical acyclovir cream and tended to be more active than the sage cream.[24]

Clinical experience of the authors strongly suggests that propolis is a most effective topical treatment for both HSV-1 and HSV-2. Calendula is also an effective topical treatment for HSV. Using lemon balm requires that the extract is concentrated over a water bath. This adds another dimension of difficulty in terms of extemporaneous prescribing.

In terms of oral herbal treatments, these are directed primarily at immune support and antiviral therapy. Both Echinacea and St John's wort have experimental evidence suggesting anti-HSV activity[25] and St John's wort was active in a clinical trial.[26]

In summary, the key aspects of herbal treatment are:

- Immune-enhancing herbs will assist the fight against the virus in acute outbreaks and prevent the reactivation of latent virus. Key herbs include Echinacea root, Andrographis and Astragalus. Astragalus should not be used during acute outbreaks

- Internal treatment with St John's wort preparations high in hypericin, which appears to exert a significant activity against the viruses (which are enveloped)

- Debilitated young patients suffering from recurrent outbreaks may benefit from adrenal tonics, tonics, adaptogenic herbs and nervine tonics between outbreaks. Key herbs in these categories include Rehmannia, licorice, Withania, Siberian ginseng and St John's wort

- Topical treatment of lesions includes Calendula extract (applied neat to the lesions) and lemon balm, propolis or licorice in ointment or cream form. Clinical studies have shown that use of lemon balm ointment on lesions also helps to prevent future outbreaks of herpes simplex (see above)

Example Treatments for both HSV-1 and HSV-2

Topical Cream

Propolis	1:5	
or Calendula	1:2	10 mL
Natural cream base		40 g

Apply to lesions at least 4 times a day.

Example Formulations

The following liquid formulation could be used:

Echinacea root blend	1:2	35 mL
St John's wort high in hypericin	1:2	35 mL
Flavouring mixture		30 mL
	Total	100 mL

Dose: Calculate the standard dose according to the most appropriate guideline in Chapter 1, using the adult dose of 5 mL. About 2 to 3 doses can be taken with water throughout the day as a preventative and this can be increased to 4 to 5 doses during acute outbreaks.

An alternative to the above liquid formulation is the combination of Echinacea Formula tablets (adult dose 2 per day as a preventative and 4 per day during acute outbreaks) and St John's Wort tablets (adult dose 2 to 3 per day as a preventative and 4 to 6 per day during acute outbreaks). See Appendix 1 for the suggested formulations for these tablets. Calculate the child's tablet dose according to the most appropriate guideline in Chapter 1. For younger children the tablets can be crushed and mixed with honey or a suitable sweetener to improve compliance.

Impetigo

Impetigo is a highly contagious bacterial infection of the superficial epidermis that most often affects children in the 2 to 5 year age group.[27] It is the most common epidermal bacterial infection amongst children and the third most common skin disease, following eczema and viral warts.[13,27] *Staphylococcus aureus* is the most important organism involved. However, *Streptococcus pyogenes* is implicated in a smaller number of patients, either alone or in combination with *S. aureus.*[14,27]

There are two types of impetigo: nonbullous (impetigo contagiosa) and bullous. Nonbullous is the most common, accounting for 70% of cases and is a host response to infection following an insect bite, abrasion, chicken pox or burn.[14] Bullous impetigo is the manifestation of a localised *S. aureus* infection that develops on intact skin.[14]

Epidemiology and Clinical Manifestations

Impetigo is usually transmitted through direct contact. Patients can further spread the infection to themselves or to others after excoriating an infected area.[27] Infections often spread rapidly through schools and day care centres, with a greater incidence in the summer months. Poor personal hygiene and crowded living conditions are also predisposing factors.[27]

Nonbullous impetigo begins as a single red macule or papule that quickly becomes a vesicle. The vesicle ruptures readily to form an erosion and the contents dry to form a characteristic honey or golden-coloured crust that may be pruritic.[14,27]

Herbal Treatment for Impetigo

A number of lines of evidence point to topical herbal treatments for impetigo. A total of 104 patients aged from 1 month to 40 years (median age 4 years) with impetigo contagiosa were included in a clinical study. The study was divided into two parts. The first consisted of an *in vitro* examination of the antibacterial properties of tea (*Camellia sinensis*) on 33 isolates of *S. aureus* and a combination of *S. aureus* and *Streptococcus pyogenes* taken from the patients. The antibacterial activity of a tea lotion against *S. aureus* proved to be very effective. The second part of the study looked at the antibacterial effects of the tea lotion and ointment by treating 64 patients with impetigo contagiosa. Another 40 patients served as controls and were divided into two groups. For the first group given an ointment containing framycetin and gramicidin (soframycin), the cure rate was 72.2%. The second group was given oral cephalexin with a cure rate of 78.6%. Tea ointment proved to be very effective with a cure rate of 81.3%.[28]

The combination of a 4% tea tree oil nasal ointment and 5% tea tree oil body wash was compared with a standard 2% mupirocin nasal ointment and triclosan body wash for the eradication of methicillin-resistant *Staphylococcus aureus* carriage. The tea tree oil combination appeared to perform better than the standard combination, although the difference was not statistically significant due to the small number of patients.[29]

The internal and external application of Echinacea for the treatment of impetigo is supported by traditional indications.[30] Calendula and wild indigo are also candidates for topical treatments, based on traditional prescribing.[31]

Example Treatments for Impetigo

Topical Cream

Calendula	1:2	2 mL
Echinacea root blend	1:2	2 mL
Cranesbill	1:2	4 mL
Natural cream base		40 g

Apply to lesions at least 4 times a day. Tea tree (1 to 2 mL) oil can also be added to the cream for stubborn cases.

Internal Herbal Treatment

Echinacea root either in liquid extract or tablet form at appropriate doses is often all that is necessary in terms of internal herbal treatment. However, acute (higher) doses should be used. For an adult the dose for an Echinacea 1:2 root blend would be 5 mL 3 to 4 times a day. For Echinacea Formula tablets (see Appendix 1) the dose should be 6 to 8 per day. Calculate the child's tablet dose according to the most appropriate guideline in Chapter 1. For younger children the tablets can be crushed and mixed with honey or a suitable sweetener to improve compliance. See Appendix 1 for the suggested formulations for these tablets.

The use of the ingredients of the topical preparation is based on the previously cited evidence. The cranesbill duplicates the research on tea, as cranesbill is rich in polyphenols similar to those found in tea that were presumably responsible for the antibacterial effect.

Case History

A 4-year-old preschool male child with several impetigo lesions on the forearms presented with his mother.

The following treatments were prescribed:

St John's wort high in hypericin	1:2	2 mL
Calendula	1:2	2 mL
Echinacea angustifolia	1:2	2 mL
Witch hazel	1:2	4 mL
Natural cream base		40 g

Apply to lesions at least 4 times a day.

Echinacea purpurea glycetract	1:3	100 mL

Dose: 3 mL in water twice a day.

The lesions resolved without scarring within 5 days.

Dermatophytoses (Ringworm or Tinea)

Dermatophytoses are caused by a group of closely related filamentous fungi with a propensity for invading the stratum corneum, hair and nails.[14] The three principle genera responsible for infection are *Trichophyton, Microsporum* and *Epidermophyton*.[14] Ringworm is classified according to the affected part, with tinea capitis affecting the scalp, tinea corporis the body, tinea cruris the groin and upper thighs, tinea pedis the foot and tinea unguium the nails.[14,32]

Host immune defence has an important bearing on the severity of infection. Ringworm tends to be more severe in individuals with diabetes, lymphoid malignancies, immune suppression and conditions with high plasma cortisol such as Cushing's syndrome.[14] The most common form affecting children is tinea capitis, which is seen mainly in urban pre-school and school-aged children.[32] The spread of infection is caused by contact with either an infected individual or animal, or fomites such as infected combs, brushes, hats and furniture.[32] Tinea capitis can cause patchy alopecia and six main patterns are recognised.[13]

Herbal Treatment for Ringworm

A number of herbal remedies have been clinically evaluated in the treatment of dermatophytoses. Sixty patients participated in a study with three treatment arms, with 20 patients each. All groups had comparable numbers of patients with tinea corporis, cruris and pedis. Group 1 was treated with a 25% emulsion of oil of bitter orange (OBO; *Citrus aurantium*) three times daily; group 2 was treated with 20% OBO in alcohol three times daily and group 3 was treated with pure OBO, once daily. Clinical and mycologic examinations were performed before therapy and every week until a complete cure had occurred. In group 1, 80% of patients were cured in 1 to 2 weeks and 20% in 2 to 3 weeks. In group 2, 50% were cured in 1 to 2 weeks, 30% in 2 to 3 weeks and 20% in 3 to 4 weeks. In group 3, 25% of patients did not continue with the trial. Of the remaining patients, 33.3% were cured in one week, 60% in 1 to 2 weeks, and 6.7% in 2 to 3 weeks. The OBO produced no side effects except for a mild irritation seen with the use of the pure form.[33] From this trial, the emulsion of OBO was the most effective, although a control or placebo group would have strengthened the results.

Tea tree oil has been shown to have activity against dermatophytes *in vitro* and in clinical studies. A randomised, controlled, double blind study was conducted to determine the efficacy and safety of topical tea tree oil in the treatment of interdigital tinea pedis. One hundred and fifty-eight patients with a confirmed dermatophyte infection were randomised to receive either placebo, 25% or 50% tea tree oil solution. Patients applied the solution twice daily to affected areas for 4 weeks and were reviewed after 2 and 4 weeks of treatment. There was a marked clinical response seen for 68% of patients in the 50% tea tree oil group and 72% in the 25% tea tree oil group, compared to only 39% in the placebo group. Mycological cure was assessed by the culture of skin scrapings taken both at baseline and after 4 weeks of treatment. The mycological cure rate was 64% for the 50% tea tree oil group, compared to 31% in the placebo group. Four (3.8%) patients applying tea tree oil developed moderate to severe dermatitis that improved quickly on stopping the study medication.[34]

Garlic is reported to have antifungal properties and three clinical trials described the use of ajoene, derived from garlic, as a successful topical treatment for tinea pedis, cruris and corporis.[35]

Example Treatment for Ringworm

Topical Cream

Tea tree oil	2 mL
Bitter orange oil	2 mL
Natural cream base	46 g

Apply to affected areas three times a day. Pau d'arco 1:2 can be added at around 5 mL.

Internal Herbal Treatments

Echinacea root either in liquid extract or tablet form at appropriate doses is all that is necessary in terms of internal herbal treatments. However, acute (higher) doses should be used. For an adult the dose for an Echinacea 1:2 root blend would be 5 mL 3 to 4 times a day. For Echinacea Formula tablets (see Appendix 1) the dose should be 6 to 8 per day. Calculate the child's tablet dose according to the most appropriate guideline in Chapter 1. For younger children the tablets can be crushed and mixed with honey or a suitable sweetener to improve compliance. See Appendix 1 for the suggested formulations for these tablets. Internal doses of Pau d'arco 1:2 should also be considered, based on an adult dose of 10 mL per day.

Acne Vulgaris

In western societies acne vulgaris is the most common and nearly universal skin disease, afflicting 79 to 95% of the adolescent population to some degree. Even 40 to 54% of men and women older than 25 years will have some degree of facial acne. Facial acne persists into middle age in 12% of women and 3% of men. Acne affects between 40 and 50 million individuals in the US alone.[36]

Acne is the inflammation of the pilosebaceous unit. This is the sebaceous gland (that produces the sebum) and the sebaceous duct that runs from it to the keratinocyte-lined follicular canal that opens to the skin surface.[37]

There are four necessary sequential stages in the development of acne:[37]

- The sebaceous gland increases sebum production
- A keratin plug develops within the follicular canal, resulting from an alteration in the pattern of keratinisation within the pilosebaceous unit
- The resulting rich keratin and sebum environment allows for the proliferation of the Gram-positive bacteria *Propionibacterium acnes*
- With the continued accumulation of the follicular contents and increased bacterial presence, the follicular contents leak into surrounding tissues inducing an inflammatory response

Notwithstanding the above process, the following quote represents the current status regarding acne's ultimate cause: "despite years of research, the basic cause of acne remains unknown".[38]

Clinical Manifestation

The variety of lesions seen in acne can be divided into two primary categories: inflammatory and non-inflammatory.[37] Acne is defined as the presence of at least 5 to 10 comedomes (non-inflammatory lesions). All acne lesions result from the precursor lesion, the microcomedo. These are not visible to the naked eye and represent the follicular plug stage. The classification of acne is as follows:

- Mild: primarily non-inflammatory lesions with or without some inflammatory papules (pimples). Nodules, cysts and scars are not present

- Moderate: non-inflammatory lesions occurring with many more inflammatory lesions. A few nodules may be present and scarring is generally mild or not observed

- Severe: non-inflammatory lesions occurring with numerous, extensive inflammatory papules, pustules and nodules. Scarring is more prevalent. Increased scarring is seen with frequent manipulation of the acne lesion

Diet and Acne

Evidence now exists that diet-induced changes in hormonal and cytokine homeostasis are likely environmental factors underlying the development of acne.

A recent investigation has demonstrated that the hormonal cascade triggered by diet-induced hyperinsulinaemia elicits an endocrine response that simultaneously promotes unregulated tissue growth and enhances androgen secretion.[36] Hyperinsulinaemic diets may therefore represent a previously unrecognised environmental factor in the development of acne, via an influence on follicular epithelial growth and keratinisation and on androgen-mediated sebum secretion.[36]

In terms of a specific mechanism, chronic and acute hyperinsulinaemia initiates a hormonal cascade that favours unregulated tissue growth by simultaneously elevating levels of free insulin-like growth factor 1 (IGF-1) and reducing insulin-like growth factor binding protein 3 (IGFBP-3).[39] IGF-1 is a powerful mitogen that stimulates the growth of all tissues including the prostate and follicle.[39] It has also been demonstrated that IGF-1 is required for keratinocyte proliferation in humans.[40] Post-adolescent women with acne have elevated serum concentrations of IGF-1 and are mildly insulin resistant.[41]

IGFBP-3 is a potent proapoptotic factor in epithelial cells, including keratinocytes.[42] As keratinocytes differentiate into terminal corneocytes, only basal keratinocytes produce IGFBP-3. Serum-derived IGFBP-3 may influence localised concentrations of this hormone within differentiating corneocytes. Chronically elevated insulin concentrations result in lowered IGFBP-3 and ingestion of high glycaemic load meals results in acute depression of IGFBP-3. Hence the dietary lowering of IGFBP-3 represents a mechanism that could delay or impair apoptosis in corneocytes.[42]

IGFBP-3 is a ligand for the retinoid X nuclear receptor (RXR alpha) that, along with other endogenous RXR alpha ligands such as *trans* retinoic acid and 9-*cis* retinoic acid, operates in an additive manner to induce apoptosis. Hence the pharmaceutical retinoids may function in part by restoring the RXR signal reduced by diet/insulin-mediated lowering of IGFBP-3.[42]

Androgens, Inflammation and Acne

Sebum production is controlled by androgens.[43] Both insulin and IGF-1 stimulate the synthesis of androgens in ovarian[44] and testicular tissue.[45] Furthermore, insulin and IGF-1 inhibit the hepatic synthesis of sex hormone binding globulin (SHBG), thereby increasing the bioavailability to tissues of circulating androgens.[46] This is supported by cross-sectional studies that demonstrate an inverse relationship between serum SHBG and both insulin[47] and IGF-1.[48] Additionally sebum production is also directly stimulated by insulin[49] and IGF-1.[50] Taken together, these data suggest that the endocrine cascade induced by hyperinsulinaemia enhances sebum production and the development of acne.

A large scale dietary intervention demonstrated that diets based around low glycaemic load foods reduced serum testosterone, fasting glucose levels, improved insulin metabolism and increased SHBG concentrations.[51] These endocrine changes are consistent with those known to normalise follicular development and reduce sebum production.

The inflammation of the dermis characteristic of acne is thought to be caused by an interaction of the immune system with *P. acnes*, which colonises the sebum-rich closed comedo.[52] Peptidoglycans in the cell wall directly induce the expression of proinflammatory cytokines, such as TNF-α, IL-1β and IL-8 from peripheral blood monocytes. Increases in these cytokines stimulate the expression of other inflammatory mediators, including prostanoids and leukotrienes. Increased expression of IL-1α adversely affects keratinisation and promotes inflammation.[52]

Increased sebum production is associated with a decrease in linoleic acid in the sebaceous lipids.[53] As a result, the follicular epithelium is bathed in essential-fatty-acid-deficient lipids, resulting in hyperkeratosis. Linoleic acid is known to downregulate neutrophil oxygen metabolism and phagocytosis as well as inhibit the activity of 5-α-reductase (which governs the influence of androgens on sebum production).[54]

Stress and Acne

The skin is considered to be a peripheral endocrine gland. Recent studies have indicated that human sebaceous glands express functional receptors for numerous hormones, including corticotropin-releasing hormone (CRH).[55] Stress-sensing cutaneous signals lead to production and release of CRH from dermal nerves and sebocytes. After binding to these receptors, this modulates the production of inflammatory cytokines, lipogenesis and androgen metabolism.[55]

Numerous case control and cross-sectional studies have demonstrated that individuals with acne have a high incidence of depression, anxiety, embarrassment and social inhibition.[56] However, this might be an effect of acne, rather than a cause.

Herbal Treatment for Acne

Acne is an androgen-driven inflammation and a low-grade infection resulting from altered insulin metabolism. Therefore some key actions indicated are hypoglycaemic (goat's rue, Gymnema, fenugreek), anti-inflammatory (Rehmannia, Bupleurum) and immune modulating (Echinacea) herbs.

Other important herbs for acne include:

- Depurative herbs, which are a mainstay of treatment. In particular Calendula and burdock may reduce excess sebum production, but other important depuratives for acne include yellow dock, poke root and Oregon grape

- Chaste tree, which given to men and women has shown benefit in acne in early clinical trials, possibly due to its hormonal effects. Linseeds (flaxseeds) contain lignans which may raise SHBG. A recent observational study found that consumption of licorice could lower testosterone levels,[57] but high doses may be necessary

- Other herbs used to treat acne include garlic and golden seal. On the surface it might appear that these herbs are selected because of their antimicrobial properties. However, their oral use for acne could be better explained by depurative and immune-regulating effects

Example Liquid Formulation for Acne

Calendula	1:2	15 mL
Chaste tree	1:2	15 mL
Echinacea root blend	1:2	25 mL
Rehmannia	1:2	25 mL
Bupleurum or Burdock	1:2	20 mL
	Total	100 mL

Dose: Calculate the dose according to the most appropriate guideline from Chapter 1, based on an adult dose of 5 mL. This dose can be taken three times a day with water.

Glucose Metabolism Support tablets (adult dose 4 per day) should be included in the protocol. Calculate the child's tablet dose according to the most appropriate guideline in Chapter 1. For younger children the tablets can be crushed and mixed with honey or a suitable sweetener to improve compliance. See Appendix 1 for the suggested formulation for this tablet.

Rationale for the Liquid Formulation

Calendula is a specific for acne and has antimicrobial, lymphatic and vulnerary actions.[19] Chaste tree has been clinically validated for effectiveness in acne possibly reducing androgens.[19] Echinacea is to modify immunity and to aid with lymphatic drainage.[19] Rehmannia is prescribed to reduce inflammation, whilst Bupleurum is used to reduce inflammation and improve liver function.[19] Gymnema will aid with blood sugar control.[19] Burdock is an excellent traditional derpurative.[19]

Example Tablet or Capsule Formulations

For the older child or the younger one who will not take liquids, herbal tablets or capsules may prove a useful alternative for acne management.

Key herbal formulations (examples provided in Appendix 1) which should be considered in acne are Skin/Elimination Support tablets for depurative activity (adult dose 4 per day), Chaste Tree tablets (adult dose 2 per day) and Short Term Immune Support tablets (adult dose 4 per day). Other formulations to be considered as appropriate are Glucose Metabolism Support tablets (see above), Golden Seal tablets (adult dose 4 per day), Autoimmune Formula tablets for stress regulation and anti-inflammatory activity (adult dose 4 per day) or Long Term Immune Support tablets (adult dose 4 per day). In general no more than 3 different formulations should be prescribed at the one time. Calculate the child's tablet dose according to the most appropriate guideline in Chapter 1. For younger children the tablets can be crushed and mixed with honey or a suitable sweetener to improve compliance. See Appendix 1 for the suggested formulations for these tablets.

Case History

A 15-year-old male with a 12-month history of acne was treated with an identical protocol to that described above, as well as dietary modification and a tea tree oil wash. This was 50% tea tree oil with 50% essential oil emulsifier, 5 mL in 100 mL of warm water to use as a face wash morning and night. It was allowed to dry on the face. The acne was completely cleared after 3 months of treatment.

Atopic Dermatitis

Atopic dermatitis (AD) or eczema belongs to that familiar family of atopic diseases that include allergic rhinitis, allergic bronchial asthma and food allergies. Although well-described, there is no international agreement regarding the precise definition and diagnosis of AD.[58] The UK refinement of the Hanifin-Rajka Diagnostic Criteria is useful for diagnosis. This describes AD as an itchy skin condition occurring in the last 12 months, plus three or more of the following:[59]

- Onset below 2 years of age
- History of flexural involvement
- History of generally dry skin (xerosis)
- Personal history of other atopic disorders
- Visible flexural dermatitis

AD is "an itch that rashes" in contrast to contact dermatitis, where the rash appears before the itch and so is "a rash that itches".[59] The pruritus leads to scratching, which can result in changes to the skin including lichenification, excoriation and a breakdown of the skin barrier function with subsequent risk of infection.[59]

Epidemiology, Aetiology and Immunology

AD is frequently the first manifestation of atopic disease in infancy. As such it is often thought of as a condition of early childhood, with the prevalence falling substantially in the teenage years. Infants with AD are predisposed to develop allergic rhinitis and/or asthma later in childhood, the so-called "atopic march".[14,59] It is linked to socioeconomic advantage and smaller family size, key elements in the hygiene hypothesis.[59]

AD is a complex genetic disorder that leads to chronic skin inflammation.[14] It manifests as a defective skin barrier, reduced innate immune responses and exaggerated T cell responses to environmental allergens and microbes. The clinically unaffected skin of AD patients is not normal and is characterised by mild epidermal hyperplasia and a sparse perivascular T cell infiltrate.[14] Acute skin lesions are characterised by spongiosis, which is marked intercellular oedema of the epidermis.[14]

The major immunopathological abnormality in AD concerns T cells. Helper T cells (Th cells) recognise antigens and modulate immune responses such as inflammation, the defence against viral infection and the proliferation of specific T and B cell clones.[60,61] Cytotoxic T cells (Tc cells) are responsible for the destruction of host cells infected with intracellular pathogens.[60] There is a relative decrease in Tc cells in AD patients, which may contribute to an increased susceptibility to infections such as herpes.[61] As noted previously, helper T cells are further classified as either Th1 or Th2, depending on the cytokine profile expressed by the cell. Th1 are involved in cell-mediated inflammatory reactions and produce large quantities of IFN-γ, TNF-β and IL-2.[60] These cytokines activate cytotoxic, inflammatory and delayed hypersensitivity reactions and promote macrophage development. Th2 cells produce IL-4, IL-5, IL-6, IL-9, IL-10 and IL-13.[60] They encourage the production of antibodies, particularly IgE, and are therefore important regulators of antibody and allergic reactions.[60] Both Th1 and Th2 play a key role in the pathogenesis of AD and the immunoregulatory mix of cytokine expression is dependent on the phase of the AD.[61] Based on the cytokine milieu found in the skin of AD patients, the activation of Th2 predominates over Th1 in the acute phase and vice versa in the chronic phase.[14,61] The factors that control the Th1/Th2 balance are complex and possibly relate to a lack of microbial stimulation at certain stages in life (see a full discussion in Chapter 4).

There is a controversial concept that vaccination may promote the development of atopic disease. Although contrary data exist, some evidence supports this concept, providing some interesting connections. A random sample of 9,744 children was followed from birth to 3 to 15 years. The main finding was a significant increase in AD in children after the measles, mumps and rubella (MMR) vaccination.[62] The study also found a similar association with measles infection, which is inconsistent with the hygiene hypothesis. This might also be connected to thimerosal in vaccines, since a recent study demonstrated a Th2-skewing effect of mercury by promoting the expression of cytokines associated with Th2 cells.[63] It has been shown that thimerosal causes a depletion in intracellular glutathione in dendritic cells, which then leads to the expression of Th2 cytokines.[64]

AD and the Digestive Tract

The intestinal microflora (MF), gut epithelium and mucosal immune system constitute a highly integrated unit, often termed the gastrointestinal ecosystem.[65] Full morphological and functional maturity of the digestive system requires the presence of all three components functioning correctly.[66] It is clear that the MF plays a pivotal role in harmonising the gastrointestinal ecosystem. For instance, commensal MF and probiotics help to regulate intestinal barrier function,[67] modulate the function of intestinal epithelia and dendritic cells[68] and are critical to the development of oral tolerance.[65] As described in Chapter 4, exposure of the intestine to MF and "old friends" is necessary for a balanced maturation of the immune system. This issue is even more acute for newborns, who already have a tendency towards Th2 responses.

Targeted postnatal colonisation with probiotic strains is useful to reduce immune responses favouring Th2 cytokines. Several studies have demonstrated the benefit of probiotics for children with AD. A double blind, placebo-controlled study of the administration of whey enriched with *Bifidobacterium lactis* or *Lactobacillus GG* to children with AD for 2 months was followed by a significant improvement in the disease.[69] *Lactobacillus rhamnosus* and *L. reuteri* administered for 6 weeks improved AD in children aged from 1 to 13 years.[70]

Some early studies found a low gastric production of hydrochloric acid was correlated with incidence of atopic dermatitis, for example Ayers in 1929 and Brown and co-workers in 1935. Therapy with hydrochloric acid resulted in a dramatic improvement in some cases.[71] A Russian study found markedly reduced activity of membrane-bound small-intestinal enzymes in 346 patients with atopic dermatitis. Correction of this dysfunction resulted in improvements in both digestion and skin.[72] A related study found a similar problem in infants with atopic dermatitis and reduction of disaccharide intake (such as lactose, sucrose and maltose) was instituted.[73]

Abnormal Skin Microflora

Skin colonisation with *Staphylococcus aureus* is a feature of AD, with one study demonstrating that more than 90% of patients were affected in this way.[74] It was found that the degree of colonisation was in direct relationship to the severity of AD.[74] *S. aureus* influences inflammatory processes by secreting superantigens that stimulate a marked activation of T cells and macrophages.[75] Most patients make specific IgE antibodies directed against these superantigens. Superantigens also induce glucocorticoid resistance, which suggests that they could increase the severity of AD via several mechanisms. Scratching enhances *S. aureus* binding by disturbing the skin barrier and exposing the extracellular matrix adhesins to the micro-organism.[75]

Fatty Acids and AD

The metabolism of polyunsaturated fatty acids (PUFA) is highly active in the epidermis and it is widely accepted that a dietary deficiency of linoleic acid (LA) results in water loss and a dry scaly skin.[76] The main permeability barrier, the stratum corneum, is formed from extracellular lipids and corneocytes during epidermal differentiation of the skin.[77] Epidermal lipids are synthesised by keratinocytes and stored in epidermal lamellar bodies, which contain cholesterol, ceramides, phospholipids and hydrolytic enzymes including acid sphingomyelinase (A-SMase).[77] It has been found that both the affected and non-affected skin of AD patients have a defect in A-SMase not apparent in healthy controls. This leads to decreased ceramides, the primary factor leading to skin dryness through water loss (a similar process happens with ageing and wrinkling). The disturbed barrier function enables pathogens and allergens to penetrate the skin more easily. Ceramides are derived from LA and any disturbance in LA metabolism will impact the production of ceramides.[77]

The weight of evidence suggests that AD patients are not deficient in plasma LA in phospholipids compared to healthy controls.[78] However, there is suggested deficiency in the metabolites of LA, namely gamma linolenic acid (GLA), dihomogamma linolenic acid (DGLA) and arachidonic acid (AA).[76,78] It has therefore been suggested (but not as yet demonstrated) that a reduced activity of the enzyme Δ6-desaturase could be responsible. This enzyme converts LA to GLA and α-linolenic acid to stearidonic acid.[76,78] The reduction in activity may be due to a mutation, altered expression of the enzyme, a change in hormone regulation, a change in the cofactors required for the enzyme or the presence of enzyme inhibitors.[76] What is uncertain is whether the disturbance in LA metabolism is a causative factor or is a consequence of AD. However, some evidence suggests that this disturbance is indeed a causative factor.[76,78] It has also been demonstrated that as children age, the disturbance attenuates and often resolves.[76]

The above understanding has lead to the use of GLA supplements such as evening primrose oil (EPO), blackcurrant seed oil and borage oil in the treatment of AD. Studies demonstrate that such GLA supplementation increases DGLA without any changes in AA.[76,78,79] The DGLA can be subsequently converted to anti-inflammatory and antiproliferative prostaglandins and leukotrienes, thereby rendering a therapeutic effect.[79]

Although the weight of clinical evidence, as assessed by meta-analysis, slightly favours the use of GLA in the treatment of AD,[80,81] the controversy surrounding EPO in particular[82] and the negative studies have damaged the above case. However, it is important to note that a considerable number of the AD subjects participating in the clinical trials were using topical steroids as well.[76] This is because clinical trial ethics committees that oversee trial protocols have refused to allow such a treatment to be discontinued during the trials. In many cases the trials of GLA in AD have really been trials of whether GLA or placebo can produce improvements over and above that produced by topical steroids.[76]

Free Radical Activity and AD

The inflammatory process within the skin of children with AD is characterised by an intense infiltration of lymphocytes, monocytes and eosinophils that express cytokines and reactive oxygen species (ROS).[83] The urine of these patients has been shown to contain many metabolites indicative of ROS damage to DNA and lipids, significantly greater than controls.[83] Additionally, it has recently been demonstrated that the increase in ROS in AD patients causes the isomerisation of *cis* fatty acids into *trans* fatty acids, leading to loss of function in the cell membrane as well as immune activation.[84] It has also been proposed that dietary *trans* fatty acid consumption further complicates the problem.[84] Dietary antioxidants (A, C and E) can protect the naturally-occurring *cis* geometry of fatty acids in the cell membrane.[85]

Dietary Triggers of AD

A recent systematic review of 14 prospective studies of dietary intervention in childhood AD concluded that an elimination diet is efficacious, provided a specific diagnosis of food allergy had been made.[86] The studies in the review identified numerous foods as being problematic, including dairy products and in particular cows milk, eggs, tomatoes, peanuts and processed wheat products.[86] Other agents known to affect AD are sugar, chocolate, food additives, yeast extracts, pork, beef, members of the nightshade family and nuts.[31]

Manipulation of the diet of children with AD by their parents is apparently common and occurs mostly without a consultation with a health professional. In a study involving 100 children, 75% had certain foods excluded from their diets (dairy products, cows milk and eggs were the most common), with 39% of these reporting improvement.[87] The same study found that 41% had tried dietary supplements, with EPO the most common, of whom 13% of those who tried it felt that it had helped the skin.[87]

Clinical Evidence for Herbs in AD

Although not specifically involving children, three herbal extracts have been clinically evaluated as topical treatments for AD. In a partially double blind, randomised study, carried out as a half-side comparison, chamomile cream was tested against a 0.5% hydrocortisone cream, with the vehicle cream as placebo. The trial was conducted in patients suffering from medium-degree AD. After 2 weeks of treatment the chamomile cream showed a mild superiority over the 0.5% hydrocortisone cream and the placebo.[88] The effects of several concentrations of licorice extract as a topical preparation were evaluated in AD. A 2% licorice topical gel was found to be more effective than a 1% gel in reducing the scores for erythema, oedema and itching over two weeks. The results showed that licorice extract could be considered as a treatment of atopic dermatitis.[89] Recent investigations also support the use of St John's wort as a topical treatment for AD. Twenty-one patients suffering from mild to moderate AD were treated with either a topical preparation containing St John's wort extract standardised to 1.5% hyperforin or placebo applied randomly to either the right or left side of the body. Application was twice daily for 2 weeks and 18 patients completed the trial. The results indicated that the active cream was significantly superior to placebo, reducing both the inflammation and the *S. aureus* colonisation.[90]

Numerous traditional Chinese herbal formulations have been clinically evaluated for AD, however most are not relevant to the practice of western herbal medicine. Only one clinical study could be found with any relevance. In this open study, 121 patients with AD consumed oolong tea for 6 months. At this time point 8% had markedly improved, 47% had moderately improved, 24% slightly improved and 3% had worsened.[91] It was thought that the observed effects were due to tea polyphenolics such as epigallocatechin gallate, which is also the main component of green tea. Green tea polyphenolics have repeatedly demonstrated antioxidant and protective effects on dermocytes after exposure to UV-induced ROS.[92]

Herbal Treatment of AD

The treatment of AD in very young infants can be a considerable challenge to the herbal clinician, primarily because of the taste of the medicines and the poor compliance that might ensue. In these cases topical treatments are often most appropriate. This particular problem is not so evident when treating older children, particularly when parental partnership is encouraged and received or when tablets are used as an alternative. Tablets, if crushed, can of course be used with younger children.

Central to herbal treatment are immune modulators such as Echinacea that will aid in dampening an excessive Th2 response. Experience shows that it does not aggravate atopic dermatitis. Boosting the immune response with Echinacea, Andrographis and other immune herbs may help to control *Staph. aureus* infection. Antiallergic herbs such as Albizia, Baical skullcap and nettle leaf will help to control the production of histamine. Anti-inflammatory herbs such as Bupleurum, Rehmannia and Hemidesmus, in combination with antioxidants such as turmeric, green tea and grape seed, will aid in controlling inflammatory cytokines and ROS. Depurative remedies such as Oregon grape, sarsaparilla, yellow dock and burdock that reputedly improve the entire metabolic cycle should follow initial symptomatic treatment. Bitters and other digestive remedies may also be indicated as well as adaptogens and nervines if stress is a significant causative or exacerbating factor. Probiotics are also useful as previously described, as well as GLA supplements, especially EPO. Golden seal can also be useful for AD.

Example Topical Treatment for AD

Licorice	1:1	4 mL
St Johns wort	1:2	3 mL
Chamomile	1:2	3 mL
Natural cream base		40 g

Mix ingredients thoroughly. Apply generously at least twice a day

Example Herbal Formulations for AD[93]

The following is an example liquid formulation for AD:

Echinacea root blend	1:2	50 mL
Baical or Chinese skullcap	1:2	25 mL
Nettle leaf	1:2	25 mL
Total		100 mL

Dose: Calculate the dose according to the most appropriate guideline from Chapter 1, based on an adult dose of 5 mL and take three times a day with water.

For the older child or the one who will not take liquids, herbal tablets or capsules may provide a useful alternative for the management of atopic dermatitis.

Key herbal formulations (examples provided in Appendix 1) which should be considered in atopic dermatitis in children are Skin/Elimination Support tablets for depurative activity (adult dose 4 per day), Allergy Support tablets (adult dose 4 per day), Golden Seal tablets (adult dose 4 per day) and Echinacea Formula tablets (adult dose 3 per day). Other formulations to be considered as appropriate are Upper Digestive Formula (adult dose 1 tablet sucked for 30 to 60 seconds before each meal) to improve gastric acid production and upper digestive processes, Autoimmune Formula tablets (adult dose 4 per day) as a long-term treatment to rebalance T-lymphocyte responses and provide anti-inflammatory activity and Evening Primrose Oil capsules (adult dose 3 per day). In general, no more than 3 to 4 formulations should be prescribed at the one time. Calculate the child's tablet dose according to the most appropriate guideline in Chapter 1. For younger children the tablets can be crushed and mixed with honey or a suitable sweetener to improve compliance. See Appendix 1 for the suggested formulations for these tablets. The Evening Primrose Oil capsules can be cut and applied to the stomach.

Case History

An 8-year-old girl had AD which had begun 4 years ago. It was worse each summer, perhaps as a result of swimming in the local chlorinated pool. The mother had tried removing dairy products from her diet, without much success. The diet included excessive consumption of sweet biscuits and it was suggested that this should be reduced. She had been prescribed a topical steroid and examination of the skin showed signs of secondary infection.

The following formulation was prescribed:

Echinacea angustifolia root	1:2	50 mL
Baical or Chinese skullcap	1:2	25 mL
Nettle leaf	1:2	25 mL
Total		100 mL

Dose: 3 mL with water twice a day

In addition, the topical application of a chickweed cream was also recommended and one 500 mg capsule of EPO was to be either broken and taken internally or applied on the abdomen twice a day.

After 4 weeks the rash had improved substantially and the face was clear. Swimming in the pool no longer seemed to aggravate the condition. Further improvements in the condition came with an additional few months of treatment.

References

1   Porth CM. *Pathophysiology* 7th Ed, Lippincott Williams & Wilkins, 2005.
2   Harding CR. *Dermatol Ther* 2004; **17**(1): 6-15
3   O'Sullivan RL, Lipper G, Lerner EA. *Arch Dermatol* 1998; **134**(11): 1431-1435
4   Buske-Kirschbaum A, Hellhammer DH. *Ann NY Acad Sci* 2003; **992**: 231-240
5   Bandeira F, Griz L, Dreyer P et al. *Arq Bras Endocrinol Metab* 2006; **50**(4): 640-646
6   Holick MF. *J Nutr* 2005; **135**(11): 2739S-2748S
7   Holick MF. *Mayo Clin Proc* 2006; **81**(3): 353-373
8   Robinson PD, Hogler W, Craig ME et al. *Arch Dis Child* 2006; **91**(7): 564-568
9   Burks W. *Pediatrics* 2003; **111**(6): 1617-1624
10 Mancini AJ. *Pediatrics* 2004; **113**(4): 1114-1119

11 Scudder J. *Specific Diagnosis* 1874 Wilstach, Baldwin and Co, reprinted Eclectic Medical Publications, Portland, Oregon, 1985.

12 Kushi M. *Your Body Never Lies,* Square One Publisher, New York, 2007.

13 Sladden M, Johnston GA. *BMJ* 2004; **329**(7457): 95-99

14 Kleigman RM, Behrman RE, Jenson HB, Stanton BF. *Nelson Textbook of Pediatrics* 18th Ed, Saunders Elsevier, Philadelphia, 2007.

15 Meyer C. *American Folk Medicine* Plume Books, New York, 1973.

16 Messegue M. *Of Men and Plants* Corgi Books, Suffolk, 1972.

17 Bohlooli S, Mohebipoor A, Mohammadi S et al. *Int J Dermatol* 2007; **46**(5): 524-526

18 Focht DR, Spicer C, Fairchok MP. *Arch Pediatr Adolesc Med* 2002; **156**(10): 971-974

19 Bone K. *A Clinical Guide to Blending Liquid Herbs.* Churchill Livingstone, Edinburgh, 2000.

20 Whitly RJ. *Semin Pediatr Infect Dis* 2002; **13**(1): 6-11

21 Taylor JM, Lin E, Susmarski N et al. *Cell Host Microbe* 2007; **2**(1): 19-28

22 Koytchev R, Alken RG, Dundarov S. *Phytomedicine* 1999; **6**(4): 225-230

23 Vynograd N, Vynograd I, Sosnowski Z. *Phytomedicine* 2000; **7**(1): 1-6

24 Saller R, Buechi S, Meyrat R, Schmidhauser C. *Forsch Komplementarmed Klass Naturheilkd* 2001; **8**(6): 373-382

25 Mills S, Bone K. *Principles and Practice of Phytotherapy: Modern Herbal Medicine.* Churchill Livingstone, Edinburgh, 2000.

26 Mannel M, Koytchev R, Dundarov S. Oral hypericum extract LI 160 is an effective treatment of recurrent herpes genitalis and herpes labialis. Paper presented at the 3rd International Congress on Phytomedicine, Munich, October 11 to 13, 2000 (SL-25).

27 Cole C, Gazewood J. *Am Fam Physician* 2007; **75**(96): 859-864

28 Sharquie KE, al-Turfi IA, al-Salloum SM. *J Dermatol* 2000; **27**(11): 706-710

29 Caelli M, Porteous J, Carson CF et al. *J Hosp Infect* 2000; **46**(3): 236-237

30 Ellingwood F. *American Materia Medica, Therapeutics and Pharmacognosy,* Reprint Eclectic Medical Publications, Portland Oregon 1983.

31 McIntyre A. *Herbal Treatment of Children.* Elsevier Butterworth Heinemann, Edinburgh, 2005.

32 Sarkar R, Kanwar AJ. *Indian Pediatr* 2001; **38**(9): 995-1008

33 Ramadan W, Mourad B, Ibrahim S, Sonbol F. *Int J Dermatol* 1996; **35**(6): 448-449

34 Satchel AC, Saurajen A, Bell C, Barnetson RS. *Australas J Dermatol* 2002; **43**(3): 175-178

35 Martin KW, Ernst E. *Mycoses* 2004; **47**(3-4): 87-92

36 Cordain L, Lindeberg S, Hurtado M et al. *Arch Dermatol,* 2002; **138**(12): 1584-1590

37 Rudy SJ. *Pediatr Nurs* 2003; **29**(4): 287-293

38 Harper JC, Thiboutot DM. *Adv Dermatol,* 2003; **19**: 1-10

39 Nam SY, Lee EJ, Kim KR et al. *Int J Obes Relat Metab Disord* 1997; **21**(5): 355-359

40 Rudman SM, Philpott MP, Thomas GA, Kealy T. *J Invest Dermatol* 1997; **109**(6): 770-777

41 Aizawa H, Niimura M. *J Dermatol* 1995; **22**(4): 249-252

42 Cordain L. *Semin Cutan Med Surg* 2005; **24**(2): 84-91

43 Guyton AC, Hall JE. *Textbook of Medical Physiology,* 10th Ed, Saunders, Philadelphia, 2000.

44 Barbieri RL, Smith S, Ryan KJ. *Fertil Steril* 1988; **50**(2): 197-212

45 Bebakar WM, Honour JW, Foster D et al. *Steroids* 1990; **55**(6): 266-270

46 Singh A, Hamilton-Fairley D, Koistinen R et al. *J Endocrinol* 1990; **124**(2): R1-R3

47 Pugeat M, Crave JC, Elmidani M et al. *J Steroid Biochem Mol Biol* 1991; **40**(4-6): 841-849

48 Erfurth EM, Hagmar LE, Saaf M, Hall K. *Clin Endocrinol* 1996; **44**(6): 659-664

49 Zouboulis CC, Xia L, Akamatsu H et al. *Dermatology* 1998; **196**(1): 21-31

50 Deplewski D, Rosenfield RL. *Endocrinology* 1999; **140**(4): 4089-4094

51 Berrino F, Bellati C, Secrero G et al. *Cancer Epidemiol Biomarkers Prev* 2001; **10**(1): 25-33

52 Golick H. *Drugs* 2003; **63**(15): 1579-1596

53 Downing DT, Stewart ME, Wertz PW et al. *J Invest Dermatol* 1987; **88**(3): 2-6

54 Namazi MR. *Int J Dermatol* 2004; **43**(9): 701

55 Zouboulis CC, Bohm M. *Exper Dermatol* 2004; **13**(Suppl 4): 31-35

56 Tan JK. *Skin Therapy Lett* 2004; **9**(7): 1-3

57 Armanini D, Bonanni G, Palermo M. *NEJM* 1999; **341**(15): 1158

58 Lilja G, Wickman M. *Allergy* 1998; **53**(11): 1011-1012

59 Williams HC. *Clin Exp Dermatol* 2000; **25**(7): 522-529

60 Parkin J, Cohen B. *Lancet* 2001; **357**(9270): 1777-1789

61 Meagher LJ, Wines NY, Cooper AJ. *Aust J Dermatol* 2002; **43**(4): 247-254

62 Olesen AB, Juul S, Thestrup-Pedersen K. *Arch Derm Venereol* 2003; **83**(6): 445-450

63 de Vos G, Abotaga S, Liao Z et al. *Immunopharmacol Immunotoxicol* 2007; **29**(3): 537-548

64 Agrawal A, Kaushal P, Agrawal S et al. *J Leukoc Biol* 2007; **81**(2): 474-482

65 Fric P. *CEJ Med* 2007; **2**(3): 237-270

66 Bjorksten B. *Springer Semin Immunol* 2004; **25**(3-4): 257-270
67 Baumgart DC, Dignass AU. *Curr Opin Clin Nutr Metab Care* 2002; **5**(6): 685-694
68 Drakes M, Blanchard T, Czinn S. *Infect Immunol* 2004; **72**(6): 3299-3309
69 Isolauri E, Arvola T, Sutas Y et al. *Clin Exp Allergy* 2000; **30**(11): 1605-1610
70 Rosenfeldt V, Benfeldt E, Nielsen SD et al. *J Allergy Clin Immunol* 2003; **111**(2): 389-395
71 Ayers S. *Arch Derm Syphilol* 1929; **20**: 854-859
72 Nikitina LS, Shinsky GE, Trusov VV. *Vestn Dermatol Venerol* 1989; **2**: 4-7
73 Vasiliev YV. *Vestn Dermatol Venerol* 1984; **10**: 16-20
74 Abeck D, Mempel M. *Br J Dermatol* 1998; **139**(53): 13-16
75 Leung DY, Bieber T. *Lancet* 2003; **361**(9352): 151-160
76 Horrobin DF. *Am J Clin Nutr* 2000; **71**(1): 367S-372S
77 Jensen JM, Folster-Holst R, Baranowsky A et al. *J Invest Dermatol* 2004; **122**(6): 1423-1431
78 Calder PC. *Clin Exp Allergy* 2006; **36**(2): 138-141
79 Fan YY, Chapkin RS. *J Nutr* 1998; **128**(9): 1411-1414
80 Morse PF, Horrobin DF, Manku MS et al. *Br J Dermatol* 1989; **121**(1): 75-90
81 Morse NL, Clough PM. *Curr Pharmaceut Biotechnol* 2006; **7**(6): 503-524
82 Williams HC. *BMJ* 2003; **327**(7428): 1358-1359
83 Tsukahara H, Shibata R, Ohshima Y et al. *Life Sci* 2003; **72**(22): 2509-2516
84 Ferreri C, Angelini F, Chatgilialoglu C et al. *Lipids* 2005; **40**(7): 661-667
85 Chatgilialoglu C, Zambonin L, Altieri A et al. *Free Radic Biol Med* 2002; **33**(12): 1681-1692
86 Fiocchi A, Bouygue GR, Martelli A et al. *Allergy* 2004; **59**(78): 78-85
87 Johnston GA, Bilboa RM, Graham-Brown RA. *Br J Dermatol* 2004; **150**(6): 1186-1189
88 Patzelt-Wenczler R, Ponce-Poschl E. *Eur J Med Res* 2000; **5**(4): 171-175
89 Saeedi M, Morteza-Semnani K, Ghoreishi MR. *J Dermatolog Treat* 2003; **14**(3): 153-157
90 Schempp CM, Windeck T, Hazel S, Simon JC. *Phytomedicine* 2003; **10**(4): 31-37
91 Uechara M, Sugiura H, Sakurai K. *Arch Dermatol* 2001; **137**(1): 42-43
92 Levin C, Maibach H. *Arch Dermatol* 2002; **138**(2): 207-211
93 Bone K. *The Ultimate Herbal Compendium.* Phytotherapy Press, Warwick, Qld, 2007.

CHAPTER 10

Common Endocrine Disturbances in Children

THE HYPOTHALAMIC-PITUITARY-ADRENAL (HPA) axis and the maintenance of homeostasis and resistance to stress in adults are well researched and documented. In recent years a clearer picture has also emerged of a critical role the HPA axis plays in foetal and neonatal development. As a consequence, there are many ways that prenatal and early childhood stressors can have negative long-term health consequences. Following a discussion of the neonatal and early childhood development of the endocrine system, this chapter will examine three important childhood disorders involving the endocrine system, namely failure to thrive, childhood obesity and type I diabetes.

Factors Influencing Endocrine Development

The HPA Axis and the Foetus

During foetal development the hypothalamus, pituitary and adrenal glands behave as dynamic endocrine organs.[1] The progressive increase in the concentration of corticotropin releasing hormone (CRH) in the foetal and maternal circulation at late gestation suggests the pivotal role of this hormone in modulating the time of birth.[1,2] Adrenocorticotropin (ACTH) is the primary trophic hormone controlling foetal adrenal growth and development. It acts via local mediators or growth factors, such as vascular endothelial growth factor, in synchronising foetal adrenocortical growth and angiogenesis.[1] The adrenal glands exhibit a remarkable transformation in size, morphology and function during the prenatal and neonatal periods.[1] Cortisol is important for maintaining intrauterine homeostasis and impacts the structural and functional development of various organ systems, including the lungs, gastrointestinal tract, liver and central nervous system, all of which are vital for neonatal survival.[1,2] It is clear that the role of the HPA axis is pivotal in the preparation for birth and adaptation to life.

A considerable range of influences has been identified in foetal and early life that can permanently modify the development and subsequent functioning of the HPA axis.[3] For instance, stress can lead to numerous cardiovascular and endocrine changes in the mother, including increases in ACTH and glucocorticoid and catecholamine concentrations.[3,4] The placenta forms both a structural and biochemical barrier to many of these factors, although a number will still enter the foetal circulation.[4] There may also be indirect influences on the foetus via the modulation of placental function. For example, stress-induced increases in maternal catecholamine concentrations could lead to the constriction of placental blood vessels that might result in foetal hypoxia, an event demonstrated in several animal models.[5,6] However, the foetus does have several defence mechanisms against hypoxia, so any deleterious effects are likely to be subtle.[7]

In utero Programming of Adult Disease

The hypothesis known as the foetal origins of adult disease (FOAD) or the Barker hypothesis (named after the epidemiologist David Barker) states that environmental factors, particularly nutrition, act in early life to programme the risk for cardiovascular and metabolic disease in adult life. The ultimate consequence of this is early death.[8,9] Barker and colleagues observed that those regions in England and Wales that had the highest rates of infant mortality in the early 20th century also had the highest rates of mortality from coronary heart disease decades later.[10] As the most commonly registered cause of infant death at the time was low birth weight, these observations led to the hypothesis that low birth weight babies who survived infancy and childhood might be at a greater risk of coronary heart disease later in life.[11] It is important to stress that the cohort used in this study was full-term babies with low birth weight, not premature babies.

A proposed mechanism for this phenomenon is the well-recognised phenomenon of foetal undernutrition leading to increased glucocorticoid exposure. Low birth weight is possibly a surrogate marker for stress during foetal life. An extensive body of literature demonstrates that the lower the birth weight the higher the glucocorticoid levels in adults ranging from 20 to 70 years of age.[12,13,14] Furthermore, this relationship becomes even more pronounced when low birth weight is coupled with premature birth.[12] It is proposed that adverse prenatal environments lead to lifelong alterations in the activity of the HPA axis, as expressed through increased secretion of glucocorticoid hormones. It is well established that glucocorticoids can directly influence disease susceptibility through their adverse effects on endocrine metabolism and the vasculature.[12,13,14]

Postnatal Stress

Postnatal psychosocial stress and the risk of adult disease has not been well studied. However, a number of publications suggest that a similar mechanism is at play in infants and children exposed to this form of stress. For example, studies show that the stress of losing a parent or sibling places a child at a greater risk of adult depression.[15,16] Excessive glucocorticoids are increasingly linked to depression due to effects on the hypothalamus inducing an atrophic state and thereby altering feedback inhibition.[12] Additionally, a recent systematic review established that early life trauma is a significant risk factor for adult irritable bowel syndrome.[17]

Environmental Chemicals and Endocrine Disruption

Much of the early work in this area was driven by wildlife studies. These documented oestrogenic, androgenic, antiandrogenic and antithyroid effects in fish found below the outfalls of sewage or paper pulp mills. Exposure of alligators to agricultural chemicals and birds, fish and mammals to complex mixtures of chemicals in the Laurentian Great Lakes of North America or in the Baltic Sea of Northern Europe also demonstrated similar endocrine disruption.[18]

Numerous environmental pollutants have been shown to adversely affect the endocrine system, including diethylstilbestrol (DES), DDT, PCBs and dioxins.[19] Other chemicals are also suspected of possessing endocrine-disrupting effects, including a range of pesticides and plasticisers (phthalates).[20] It is widely acknowledged that many of these chemicals are capable of crossing the placental and blood-brain barriers to subsequently interfere with neurodevelopment and function.[19,20,21] Some chemicals can directly bind to or block hormone receptors, thereby initiating or blocking receptor-activated gene transcription.[22] Other exogenous chemicals act indirectly on hormonal homeostasis by either altering hormone transport on binding proteins, receptor numbers on target organs or hormone metabolism.[21]

Taking the example of PCBs, these molecules can interfere with thyroid function through a variety of mechanisms. These include the increased metabolism of thyroxine (T_4), interference with T_4 delivery to the developing brain by displacement from the carrier protein and interference with the conversion of T_4 to T_3.[23] It is well established that thyroid hormones are important regulators of neurodevelopment during foetal and neonatal life.[24] The emerging picture is that T_4 and T_3 enter the brain through specific transporters. T_4 is converted to the active hormone T_3 in glial cells and astrocytes, although the main target cells are neurons and maturing oligodendrocytes. Acting through nuclear receptors, T_3 controls the expression of genes involved in myelination, cell differentiation, migration and signalling.[25] Higher levels of PCBs in human breast milk have been correlated with higher thyroid stimulating (TSH) hormone levels in nursing infants.[26] In children aged from 7 to 10 years, blood levels of PCBs are positively correlated with TSH levels and negatively correlated with free T_4.[27] Studies have shown that higher levels of TSH are associated with hypotonia in infants.[28] Cohort studies involving children exposed to PCBs *in utero* through the maternal consumption of Great Lakes fish have revealed delayed psychomotor development and increased distractibility in those most highly exposed.[29,30] Further to the information provided for ADHD in Chapter 7, one study found that thyroid abnormalities were five times more frequent in children with ADHD.[31] More recent work has found that T_4 concentrations (either high or low) were associated with adverse mood symptoms and unusual behaviour in ADHD-diagnosed children.[32]

Adolescent Growth and Sexual Maturation

Observations of humans and wildlife over the past 40 years reveal a trend to increased adverse development of the reproductive system. As a result of these observations, environmental oestrogens have been prominent in the literature since the early 1990s. The research originated from an increased understanding following the legacy of diethylstilbestrol (DES) exposure during pregnancy. DES is a synthetic oestrogen that was prescribed to over 2 million pregnant women in the mid-20th century. In later years, it was found to be associated with the occurrence of vaginal clear cell adenocarcinoma.[33] Many of the contaminant-induced oestrogenic effects described to date appear to be due to receptor-mediated interactions. However, other responses are possible.[34] Several studies have provided support for the hypothesis that greater oestrogenic activity could result from an increase in aromatase activity. For example, the feminising effect of atrazine (a systemic triazine herbicide) on alligators and frogs has been linked to increased aromatase-modulated conversion of androgens to oestrogens.[35,36]

One form of dichlorodiphenyldichloroethene (DDE), a chemical similar to DDT that contaminates DDT preparations, has been shown to have antiandrogenic activity.[28] In women, DDE is known to reduce the duration of lactation and increase the chances of having a premature baby.[28]

The onset and development of puberty is regulated by the neuroendocrine system. Population-based studies worldwide have observed significant trends towards the earlier development of puberty.[37,38] These changes are apparently associated with environmental factors such as improved socioeconomic status, improved healthcare and nutrition.[39] However, they might also result from the increased presence of endocrine-disrupting chemicals in our environment. Epidemiological research on girls shows that higher prenatal exposure to polybrominated biphenyls (PBBs), as a result of contamination of the food chain in Michigan, was associated with an earlier age of menarche.[40] Higher prenatal exposure to DDE in the offspring of Michigan fish eaters was also linked to an earlier age of menarche,[41] as was higher pubertal exposure to phthalate esters in Puerto Rican girls.[42] Research on boys is not as extensive but nevertheless reveals some disturbing findings. A Taiwanese study of the effects of ingestion of rice oil contaminated with PCBs and their heat degradation products showed that the boys born after the contamination had reduced penile length compared to controls.[43] An Indian study of endosulfan (a pesticide used on cashew nut crops) and reproductive development in male children and adolescents suggested that endosulfan exposure delayed sexual maturity and interfered with sex hormone synthesis.[44]

Failure to Thrive

When viewing a growth chart, you will see a number of curves that follow the same pattern. Each one represents a different percentile, for example the 3rd, 5th, 10th, 25th, 50th, 75th, 90th and 95th percentiles. The 50th percentile represents the average for age. Percentiles are the most commonly used clinical indicator to assess the size and growth patterns of individual children. They rank the position of an individual by indicating what percent of the reference population the individual would equal or exceed. For example, on the weight-for-age growth chart, a 2-year-old girl whose weight is at the 25th percentile weighs the same or more than 25 percent of the reference population of 2-year-old girls, or weighs less than 75 percent.

Failure to thrive (FTT) is diagnosed in an infant or child when physical growth is significantly less than that of his or her peers. It is associated with poor development and cognitive functioning.[19] Severe FTT refers either to growth below the 3rd or 5th percentile or a change in growth rate that has crossed two major percentiles (from above the 75th percentile to below the 25th percentile) in a short period of time.[19] Thus a child whose growth is below the 3rd or 5th percentile is growing less than 97 or 95 percent of his or her peers, and is therefore considered to suffer FTT. The second category is the child whose growth is impeded over time and will drop from above the 75th to below the 25th percentile, meaning that they are not gaining weight over time as would be expected and are therefore classified as suffering FTT.

In 2000, the US Centers for Disease Control and Prevention (CDC) published revised growth charts, based on the data from five national surveys representative of the US population.[19] These charts are freely available at http://www.cdc.gov/growthcharts. The data are presented in five gender-specific charts: weight for age, height for age, head circumference for age, weight for height and body mass index (BMI) for children over two years of age. Most health professionals use the weight-for-age charts when assessing growth patterns.[45] The CDC charts represent observed, but not necessarily optimal, growth due to the incorporation of data from many bottle-fed infants.[19] For this reason the World Health Organisation (WHO) has developed charts based on optimal growth conditions, such as exclusive breast feeding. These charts are once again freely available at http://www.who.int/growthref/en/.

Epidemiology and Aetiology

The prevalence of FTT depends on the population sample and the assessment criteria. For instance, a recent Danish study found that 27% of infants met one or more criteria for FTT and concluded that no single measurement seemed to be adequate in identifying FTT.[46]

FTT is associated with poverty in developing countries, family dysfunction, maternal deprivation and subsequent low birth weight, as well as maternal depression.[19] It can be divided into organic FTT which is marked by an underlying medical condition or nonorganic or psychosocial FTT, which occurs in children under 5 years where no known medical condition is identified that may impair growth.[19] In developed countries, psychosocial FTT is far more common.[19] However many children have mixed aetiologies, for example small organic problems can often be magnified by psychosocial factors.[47]

Clinical Manifestation

The clinical presentation of FTT can range from failure to meet the expected age norms for height and weight to alopecia, loss of subcutaneous fat, reduced muscle mass, dermatitis, recurrent infections and malnutrition.[19] Depending on the severity, an infant with FTT may exhibit thin extremities, a narrow face, prominent ribs and wasted buttocks. Neglect of hygiene may be evidenced by nappy rash (diaper rash), unwashed skin, untreated impetigo, uncut and dirty fingernails or unwashed clothing.[19] The degree of FTT is usually measured by calculating each growth parameter (weight, height and weight/height ratio) as a percentage of the median value for age, based on appropriate growth charts. For weight, mild, moderate and severe FTT is equivalent to 75 to 90%, 60 to 74% and less than 60% the standard, respectively.[19]

The following table represents the many conditions that can cause or contribute to FTT.[45] These factors need to be assessed and addressed as appropriate.

DIFFERENTIAL DIAGNOSIS OF FAILURE TO THRIVE

Inadequate caloric intake

Incorrect preparation of formula (too diluted, too concentrated)

Unsuitable feeding habits (food fads, excessive juice)

Behaviour problems affecting feeding

Poverty and food shortages

Neglect

Disturbed parent/child relationship

Mechanical feeding difficulties (oromotor dysfunction, congenital abnormalities, central nervous system damage, severe reflux)

Inadequate absorption

Coeliac disease

Cystic fibrosis

Cows milk protein allergy

Liver disease

Short gut syndrome

Increased metabolism

Hyperthyroidism

Chronic infection (HIV, malignancy, renal disease)

Hypoxaemia (congenital heart defects, chronic lung disease)

Herbal Treatment of FTT

The management for FTT is likely to involve a two-tiered approach. Obviously any of the above factors and relevant food hypersensitivities need to be addressed, while psychosocial factors need to identified and counselled by an appropriate health professional. Understandably, there has been no clinical evaluation of the role that herbal medicines can play in the treatment of FTT. Given the complex nature of FTT, herbs may be useful for many of the associated issues, such as the functional gastrointestinal problems that impair feeding. In such cases the treatments discussed in Chapter 5 could be appropriate. Herbs indicated for emaciation and failure to thrive in children, such as Withania, are often useful.[48] Whole body tonics such as Siberian ginseng, Korean ginseng and Rhodiola may be indicated, as well as remedies for poor appetite such as Angelica and dandelion root.

Example Formulations for FTT

The following liquid formulation could be used:

Withania	1:1	30 mL
Siberian ginseng (Eleuthero)	1:2	20 mL
Angelica root or Cinnamon	1:2	10 mL
Dandelion root	1:2	20 mL
Korean ginseng	1:2	20 mL
	Total	100 mL

Dose: Calculate the standard dose according to the most appropriate guideline in Chapter 1, based on an adult dose of 5 mL. Give the calculated standard dose with water 3 to 4 times a day.

Alternatively, Stress Control tablets (adult dose 4 per day) can be prescribed, possibly with Upper Digestive Formula tablets (adult dose 1 tablet sucked for 30 to 60 seconds before each meal). See Appendix 1 for these formulations. Calculate the child's tablet dose according to the most appropriate guideline in Chapter 1. For younger children the tablets can be crushed and mixed with honey or a suitable sweetener to improve compliance.

Childhood Overweight and Obesity

Obesity and overweight are terms used interchangeably in children, however the term overweight is recommended by the CDC.[19,49] There has been a significant increase in overweight children in recent years, to such an extent that in 1998 the WHO declared it to be a "global epidemic".[50] With the recently documented increases, childhood obesity now represents one of the most challenging nutritional and sociological problems facing children today in the industrialised world. The sense of urgency in facing this problem has increased with recent publications, such as the one examining the change in the prevalence of overweight and obesity among young Australians between 1969 and 1997. Researchers from the University of Sydney analysed data from five independent surveys, revealing disturbing findings. From 1985 to 1997 the prevalence of overweight children increased by 60-70% and obesity increased 2- to 4-fold.[51] Similar data exist for the US. The National Health and Nutrition Examination Surveys found the prevalence of obesity in preschool (2 to 5 years) and older children (6 to 11 years) from 1999 to 2002 was double that between 1976 and 1980. It was triple for adolescents (12 to 19 years).[52,53] In general, the prevalence of overweight is high among the poor in developed nations and the rich in poorer nations.[19]

BMI (weight in kilograms divided by the square of height in metres) is the most widely accepted method used to screen for obesity in children and adolescents.[49] The CDC uses the term overweight to designate children (aged from 2 to 9 years) with a BMI at or above the 95th percentile for age and gender. The term 'at risk for overweight' is used for children with a BMI between the 85th and 95th percentile.[49]

Children who are overweight or obese are more likely to develop a range of health issues. These include gallstones due to increased biliary excretion of cholesterol, insulin resistance and metabolic syndrome which can lead to type 2 diabetes. Orthopaedic abnormalities can also result from increased weight and, in the longer term, cardiovascular disease.[54] The Harvard Growth Study found a doubling of the death rate from cardiovascular disease in males who were overweight during adolescence.[19] There is also increasing evidence that overweight is associated with delayed sexual maturity in boys.[19] The reverse seems to be true for girls, overweight is linked to early sexual maturity.[55]

Pathogenesis

Overweight and obesity are thought to be caused by an increase in the consumption of high fat, high energy foods, coupled with a lack of physical activity. This can be further complicated by genetic and other lifestyle/sociological factors.[19,56] Although the genetic component is widely acknowledged, the burgeoning rates of overweight in children during the past several decades have occurred within genetically stable populations.[57] It is therefore evident that an 'obesogenic environment' is the principle driving force in the current epidemic.

The Obesogenic Environment

Problematic Social Trends

A number of underlying social changes have been linked to the rising prevalence of childhood overweight. These issues are either a part of, or a consequence of, social development and urbanisation. For instance, increased consumption is generally regarded in a positive light, especially in developing nations as they emerge from poverty.[57] Examples of problematic social trends contributing to an excess energy intake and a low energy expenditure are:[57]

- Increased use of motorised transport
- Reduced opportunities for recreational physical activity
- Increased sedentary recreation (computer games, TV)
- Greater quantities and varieties of energy dense foods
- Greater promotion and marketing of energy dense foods
- More use of restaurants and fast food outlets
- Larger portions of food seen as representing better value for money
- Rising use of sweetened drinks at the expense of water
- Housing developments with reduced outside space for play

An Australian study revealed some interesting data on the topic of increased levels of promotion and marketing of energy dense foods. The survey looked at advertising on children's television over a 20-hour period. It found that 231 of the 598 advertisements were food advertisements. Of these, 192 were for sweet or fatty foods. There were no advertisements for healthy foods and the researcher deemed 339 of the 598 advertisements to be obesogenic in one form or another (such as for computer games and so on).[58]

Parental Influences

Research has identified that having an obese parent is a significant determinant for becoming overweight during childhood or adolescence.[59,60] An obvious implication from this research is a genetic predisposition to obesity. However, a shared family experience for food preferences, eating patterns and activity habits are more likely to be the dominant influences.[61]

Humans are born with an innate preference for sweet and salty foods and an aversion to sour and bitter tastes (as every herbalist knows), which can be altered by experience.[61] The strongest influence in shaping food preferences and habits from birth is the family, and particularly the parent who prepares the meals.[62] During the weaning phase children tend to reject new foods and it is recommended that from 8 to 15 repeated exposures to these foods are necessary before acceptance occurs.[63] (This lesson can be extended to herbal medicine compliance problems.) Children at risk of overweight tend to prefer foods that are high in fat, dislike vegetables and overeat.[64] This pattern is often seen in their parents and continues into adulthood.[61]

Studies demonstrate that children and adolescents who eat meals with their family are significantly less likely to be overweight and are more likely to have healthier eating habits.[65,66] It is thought that there are several reasons for this effect, including learning to eat at a slower pace and being sensitive to satiety clues, reduced consumption of energy-rich fast foods and, compared to those who do not eat regularly with the family, a higher consumption of fruit and vegetables.[66,67]

Portion Size and Energy Dense Foods

The incidence of overweight and obesity in the past few decades has been paralleled by an increase in portion size served in restaurants and fast food outlets.[68] This undoubtedly contributes to increased energy intake. It is also proposed that any internal satiety clues the child may feel when eating in restaurants could well be overridden by pressure from parents to "clean up the plate".[69]

It has been calculated that the average energy density of fast food menus is twice that of a recommended healthy diet for adults and 145% higher than traditional African diets.[70] Humans appear to have an innate inability to recognise foods with a high energy density and to appropriately downregulate their consumption in order to maintain energy balance.[70] However, this protective mechanism can be ignored with repeated exposure. In the US between 1977 and 1996 there was a three-fold increase in the proportion of food consumed from restaurants and fast food outlets by children.[71] This situation is no better in Australia, with a recent Australian survey of 3,841 adolescents reporting that 22% consumed fast food every day of the week.[72]

Along with fast food, the consumption of sugar-sweetened beverages has been implicated in childhood overweight. Several studies have linked the consumption of these beverages with increased obesity.[73,74] However, others have failed to establish a firm link.[75] It is unclear whether the consumption of fast food and sugar-sweetened beverages alone are causing the energy imbalance. It is more likely that the context in which it occurs is also important, such as sedentary behaviour.[61]

Sedentary Behaviour

Prospective, observational and intervention studies have consistently linked increased sedentary behaviours, particularly television viewing (TVV), and more recently the use of computers and game consoles, with an increased risk of obesity.[76,77,78] These associations prompted the American Academy of Pediatrics to propose a number of recommendations including:[79]

- Limiting total media time to no more that 1 to 2 hours of quality programming per day
- Removing televisions from children's bedrooms
- Discouraging TVV for children under 2 years of age and promoting talking, singing and reading together
- Encouraging alternative entertainment for children such as athletics, hobbies and creative play

It has been established that the TVV habits of children are directly influenced by parental habits, such that parents who watch excessive hours of television are more likely to have children who do the same.[80] It is thought that excessive TVV by children has four primary effects: it displaces physical activity, depresses metabolic rate, conveys poor quality dietary messages via advertisements and encourages the consumption of energy dense snack foods while watching television.[81,82]

Treatment of Overweight: Dietary and Lifestyle Considerations

The treatment of overweight/obesity seems an easy task: simply eat less and exercise more. However, it is unfortunately not as simple as that, given the above strong influences from an obesogenic environment. Patient and parent education is therefore a key element in the treatment plan. A recent weight-loss study in overweight children provides some clues to the important inclusions into an education package for parents and children.

Sixty overweight children were randomly assigned to receive either one of two interventions that also involved their parents. One group received a copy of a self-help book on weight loss for children, which was to be supervised by the parents. The other was an instructor-led intervention. Both interventions ran for 6 months. The instructor-led group received instructions on nutrition that included a coding system for specific foods. Foods were categorised as safe, caution or dangerous, according to energy density. The children were encouraged to use these categories in classroom exercises and written examinations. It also included weekly nutrition lessons focussed on teaching participants to make healthier food choices from the options available by reading labels and controlling portion sizes. In addition, parents were invited to attend monthly meetings to teach them how to adapt family meals and activities to facilitate healthy changes. The exercise programme consisted of two phases. The first phase of 6 weeks was aimed at increasing general physical fitness by a modified circuit-training regime of 40 minutes 4 days a week. The second phase was aimed at using the fitness gained in the first phase and applying it to various sporting (soccer, basketball, softball) and leisure activities (jumping rope, dance, kickboxing). A token economy was created where children received points for trying new fruit and vegetables, keeping their bodies moving during physical exercise and for meeting various goals. These points could then be exchanged for weekly prizes. The self-help book contained similar information, but was without the special programmes that involved and motivated both parents and children in the instructor-led group.

After 6 months children in the instructor-led intervention exhibited significantly reduced BMIs compared to the children in the self-help group. The average change in BMI was significantly different at both 3 and 6 months, with the instructor-led intervention showing greater decreases in weight. This has implications for the practitioner in that the family and child will need a great deal of support, and particularly education on healthy food choices and exercise programmes.[83]

Specific Behavioural Elements for Successful Weight Loss in Children

The emotional atmosphere of the meal is important, consequently a child's failure to eat should not cause unpleasantness and chastisement. Studies cited by Benton[84] have established that, in order to encourage the consumption of a particular food, it is counterproductive to complain if the food is not eaten, since this decreases the probability of that food being eaten in the future.

Siblings, peers and parents can act as role models to encourage the tasting of new foods. Studies have found that if a child observes the parent consistently consuming a food, whether it be good or bad, he or she will be encouraged to establish a preference for this food.[84,85] The child should be exposed to disliked food repeatedly in order to break down resistance. As previously mentioned, it may take 8 or more exposures to break down resistance and change rejection to acceptance.[84]

Offering the child a range of low energy dense foods allows him or her to balance energy intake. It has been observed that children can be taught to regulate their caloric intake and parents can help by talking to the child to ensure they are aware of body clues such as hunger and satiety.[84] Restricting access to particular foods increases rather than decreases the preference for and consumption of that food. Children are in need of guidance and eventually will make decisions for themselves, but when rigid guidelines are applied then the prescription has gone too far.[84]

Forcing a child to eat a certain food will decrease their liking of that food. The tendency to reject new foods, termed neophobia, is normal and should not be allowed to generate negativity.[84] Encouraging children to be aware of satiety clues and allowing these to define how much is eaten is important. If the parent wishes the plate to be cleared then the child should dictate the quantity placed on it or otherwise receive a series of small servings until no more is needed.[84]

Parents should be careful that high energy density foods are not used as rewards or treats. Offering one food as a reward for eating a less desirable one increases the preference for the reward food and decreases the preference for the less desirable food.[84] Research indicates that the size of a bowl or serving spoon can provide a visual bias that leads to overeating. It was observed that a large bowl and a large serving spoon led people to serve themselves 56.8% more ice cream than those given a smaller bowl and serving spoon, without them being aware of it.[86] Of note is the observation that Asian populations generally use small eating bowls and they do not experience the levels of overweight that impact western countries. Finally, and the most difficult of all for parents, is to be consistent in these guidelines.[85]

The Optimal Diet

Opinion is divided about what is considered to be the most appropriate diet. Diets range from a more scientific approach that incorporates meat and other animal products in conjunction with the zone, ketogenic and CSIRO diets to vegetarian diets based on harmony with universal principles, the best example of which is the macrobiotic diet. Most young children are natural vegetarians and will reject meat, chicken and fish. Hence diets based around incorporating more animal protein are likely to be difficult. Whatever the approach may be, it will undoubtedly be better in terms of weight loss than the one currently consumed. There are several common elements to all naturopathic diets, namely the elimination of all processed foods, the consumption of fresh seasonal organic fruit and vegetables and unprocessed whole grains and pulses. An important, and often overlooked, practice is correct chewing so that saliva is adequately mixed with food to begin the digestive process. This practice slows the act of eating and thereby facilitates a sense of fullness.

It might be useful to use an approach similar to the one known as the Stoplight Diet. This diet organises foods from the basic food groups into green, yellow and red categories. The classification is interpreted in much the same way as lights. Therefore the Stoplight Diet encourages the consumption of low calorie green light foods (fruits, vegetables) and moderate calorie yellow light foods (whole grains, meat) over high calorie red light foods (refined sweetened carbohydrates, carbonated beverages). However, no food is absolutely prohibited.[87] Studies using the Stoplight diet, along with parental education emphasising behavioural change, have proven to be quite effective in the long-term prevention and treatment of childhood obesity, compared to other programmes.[85,88] A consistent underlying message is that for change to occur the whole family must be involved. The child cannot be treated in isolation.

Herbal Support for Overweight/Obesity

Understandably, little clinical research has been conducted on the effect of herbal remedies on weight loss in children. However, adult studies are instructive. Herbal remedies often utilised for weight loss in adults such as Gymnema and Coleus may not be appropriate for many children, where the main mission is to move the child and family towards healthy eating and provide gentle herbal metabolic support. These herbs should be reserved for more stubborn cases. A protocol that incorporates a more a traditional approach seems more appropriate in milder cases. It is likely that, due to a poor diet and lack of exercise, the eliminative systems are clogged with stagnant waste and will need support. The lymphatic system is particularly prone to the effects of dietary lipids, as it is this system that transports the chylomicrons to the general circulation.[89] Therefore an important remedy in the herbal treatment of childhood overweight is blue flag, which is regarded as an antiobesity remedy in Ayurvedic medicine.[90] Blue flag offers several other important activities that can have a positive effect on a stagnant system. It has a mild laxative property, probably through its cholagogue action, that is further supported by diuretic and depurative actions.[91] It is thought that the antiobesity properties relate to central appetite suppressant effects and a catabolic effect on fat tissue, which is mobilised into the blood.[90] Fennel seeds also have a traditional reputation as an appetite suppressant.[90] There is at least some experimental support for this idea, albeit for the essential oil. The feeding of pigs with the essential oil of fennel blended into their feed resulted in a significant reduction in feed intake.[92] In recent years green tea and its primary constituent epigallocatechin gallate have received considerable attention as weight loss supplements. Numerous animal studies indicate increased thermogenesis and fat oxidation for epigallocatechin gallate and green tea extracts.[93,94] This is supported by several human studies that demonstrate increased thermogenesis and decreased body weight and visceral and total fat.[95] Globe artichoke, and specifically its primary constituent cynarin, are most noted for positive effects on the liver and gallbladder.[91] Interestingly, the administration of cynarin caused a significant reduction in body weight under double blind trial conditions.[90] These gentle herbs can be tried first in conjunction with appropriate dietary and lifestyle changes.

Example Formulations

An example liquid formulation is as follows:

Blue flag	1:2	35 mL
Fennel	1:2	30 mL
Globe artichoke	1:2	35 mL
	Total	100 mL

Dose: Calculate the standard dose according to the most appropriate guideline in Chapter 1, based on an adult dose of 5 mL. To be taken before meals with water 3 times a day.

As most environmental pollutants are lipophilic and are therefore stored most efficiently in fat cells, it may be wise to provide some support for the detoxification systems during weight loss. The following herbs may prove useful:

- Ginkgo to protect the nervous tissue
- St Mary's thistle (milk thistle) to protect the tissue of the liver, kidneys and possibly other tissues
- Turmeric to provide further liver support, but importantly to provide antioxidant activity in the lipid environment and to support hepatic detoxification
- Herbs mentioned in previous chapters that aid in mobilising persistent organic pollutants such as Schisandra and green tea. The green tea will also have the favourable metabolic effects noted previously

In more stubborn cases and for the older child, herbal tablets or capsules will be a useful alternative for weight management.

Key herbal formulations (examples provided in Appendix 1) which should be considered in weight management are *Coleus Forskohlii* tablets (adult dose 3 per day), Glucose Metabolism Support tablets (adult dose 1 before each meal) and finally Liver Detox

Assist tablets (adult dose 4 per day) to help the clearance of endocrine disruptors and environmental obesogens.

Calculate the child's tablet dose according to the most appropriate guideline in Chapter 1. For younger children the tablets can be crushed and mixed with honey or a suitable sweetener to improve compliance. See Appendix 1 for the suggested formulations for these tablets.

Type 1 Diabetes Mellitus

Type 1 diabetes mellitus (T1DM) is an autoimmune disease that occurs mainly in children and adolescents. T1DM is characterised by low or absent levels of endogenously-produced insulin and a consequent dependence on exogenous insulin to prevent the development of ketoacidosis, a life-threatening complication.[19]

Epidemiology and Pathogenesis

The incidence of T1DM has risen dramatically in recent years, with a 2- to 4-fold increase over the past 50 years, representing a rate of increase of 3% per year in children from 0 to 14 years.[96] Recent studies continue to report high annual rates of increase for T1DM, for example 2.8% in New South Wales, Australia[97] and 4.9% in Franche-Comte, France.[98] It is thought that changes of this magnitude over such a relatively short period of time cannot be due to fluctuations in genetic risk alone, and must involve environmental factors.[99] In support of this position, Finland and Estonia have populations with a similar genetic background. However, there is a 6-fold higher incidence of T1DM in Finland.[100]

The natural history of T1DM exhibits several stages. The first stage involves the onset of pancreatic β-cell autoimmunity with a progressive defect in insulin secretion. This is soon followed by the second stage of the onset of clinical diabetes.[19] Aggressive β-cell destruction may lead to disease manifestation within a few months for some, whereas in others the process may take years, sometimes even more than 10 years.[101] There are 4 autoantibodies that have been shown to predict overt T1DM. These are the classic islet cell antibodies, insulin autoantibodies and autoantibodies to an isoform of glutamic acid decarboxylase and to a tyrosine-related molecule.[102,103] Data suggest that a higher proportion of the population develops signs of β-cell autoimmunity (as evidenced by the presence of one or more of the implicated antibodies) than develops clinical T1DM.[101] However, it has been shown that the spreading of the humoral autoimmune response from one antigen to another and from one antibody to another can occur in a relatively short time.[104,105]

Long-term Complications

The prolonged survival of a child with T1DM as they grow to adulthood is dependent on the prevalence of the complications that follow poor glycaemic control.[19] These complications can be divided into three major categories: microvascular complications, specifically retinopathy and nephropathy; macrovascular complications, particularly accelerated coronary artery disease, cerebrovascular disease and peripheral vascular disease;

and finally neuropathies of both the peripheral and autonomic nervous systems, that can affect a variety of organs. Cataracts also occur more frequently.[19]

The risk of diabetic complications is so severe that 25% of T1DM patients will develop retinopathy after 5 years and 95% will have retinopathy after 15 to 20 years. Blindness is 25 times more common in adult diabetics. The insidious nature of T1DM means that 40% of newly diagnosed T1DM patients will have some degree of retinal vascular damage.[106] Diabetic nephropathy affects 20 to 30% of patients with T1DM 20 years after onset. Diabetes is the leading cause of kidney failure in adults, accounting for 44% of all new cases in 2002. It is the leading cause of renal disease in the US.[19] Adolescents with T1DM can show early signs of diabetic neuropathy and, 25 years after onset, 60-70% of diabetic patients have mild to severe forms of nervous system damage, resulting in somatic and autonomic neuropathy.[19]

All of these complications are a result of chronic hyperglycaemia, which disrupts the vascular endothelium causing a decrease in the production of trophic factors associated with endothelial and nerve cell growth. With time, microvascular cell death occurs causing glomerulosclerosis of the kidney and multifocal axonal degeneration of the peripheral nerves.[107]

The pathophysiology behind the above changes is complex and four hypotheses have been proposed:

- Increased polyol pathway flux. Under conditions of chronic hyperglycaemia, glucose is reduced to sorbitol by the enzyme aldose reductase and the cofactor NADPH, resulting in elevated sorbitol. Sorbitol is subsequently oxidised to fructose by sorbitol dehydrogenase with the concomitant reduction of NAD to NADPH. Hence sorbitol-induced oxidative stress is increased and there is a decrease in ATPase activity. All this results in osmotic vascular damage, decreased nitric oxide and increased free radical production[108]

- Increased advanced glycation end-product (AGE) formation. Glucose and other non-reducing sugars react with amino groups in proteins, complex lipids and nucleic acids to form Schiff base adducts. Subsequently these adducts form more stable AGEs, which induce intramolecular crosslinking in collagen, laminin and fibronectin. This results in altered function of endothelial cells, impacting permeability and elasticity. Reactive oxygen species are generated and changes in the expression of growth factors and cytokines are induced[107]

- Activation of protein kinase C (PKC). Hyperglycaemia enhances the activation of PKC by the synthesis of diacylglycerol (DAG). Both PKC and DAG are intracellular signalling molecules that regulate many vascular functions, including permeability, vasodilator nitric oxide release and growth factor expression[108]

- Increased hexosamine pathway flux. Increased glucose leads to increased fructose-6-phosphate. This enters the hexosamine pathway rather than glycolysis and as a result various transcription factors are increased[108]

Recently a unifying hypothesis has been proposed. The above pathways all seem to reflect a hyperglycaemia-induced process of overproduction of superoxide radicals by the mitochondrial electron-transport chain.[107] It could be that intracellular free radical activity induced by hyperglycaemia is at the centre of these pathways, leading to the chronic complications of diabetes.

Aetiology

Viral Infections and Vaccinations

It has long been speculated that viruses play a role in the aetiology of T1DM. The multiplicity of viruses and the problem of relating early viral infections with the later appearance of T1DM has made the research difficult. However it is known that Coxsackie virus, cytomegalovirus, rubella and mumps can infect human pancreatic β-cells.[19,99] Only congenital rubella infection is associated with T1DM later in life.[19] However, research has shown that newly-diagnosed children with T1DM have high titers of antibodies against a Coxsackie viral strain.[109] A large epidemiological study established a relationship between measles infection and later onset of T1DM in children living in Philadelphia.[110] Influenza has also been linked to cases of T1DM.[111]

Among the environmental factors suspected to have a diabetogenic effect, childhood vaccination is probably the most controversial. Vaccinations for mumps, Haemophilus influenza B and pertussis have been proposed as a risk factors for T1DM.[112,113,114] However, subsequent studies have failed to demonstrate a link.[115,116] The research discussed in Chapter 7 suggests that thimerosal, the mercury preservative found in many vaccines, could be implicated in vaccination responses. It is also thought that vaccination, in combination with other yet to be identified environmental factors, could promote an immune response that results in the destruction of pancreatic β-cells.[112]

Dietary Insulin and Other Proteins

It has recently been found that bovine insulin (BI) present in cows milk induces both a humoral and cellular immune response in infants.[117,118] Natural immunisation to BI, as reflected by antibodies to BI, is associated with, but not predictive of, the progression to T1DM in children. A recent infant study showed that human insulin in breast milk seems to be tolerogenic and may downregulate the IgG response to dietary BI. However, results for infants who developed β-cell autoimmunity suggest that breast milk insulin does not promote tolerance for this subgroup of children.[119]

Dietary gluten has been advocated as a risk factor for type 1 diabetes. Exposure to soy proteins and wheat gluten appears to increase the incidence of diabetes in rats[120] and nonobese diabetic mice.[121] Patients with T1DM are at a high risk of coeliac disease and the risk seems to be correlated with the duration of gluten exposure.[122] The gluten/T1DM link is suggested by the high prevalence of coeliac disease in patients with T1DM (1-8%) as compared to the rest of the general population (0.4-1.0%).[123] As many as 30% of newly-diagnosed children with T1DM have antibodies to tissue transglutaminase, an autoantigen in coeliac disease.[124] Antigliadin antibodies have been reported in infants newly-diagnosed with T1DM.[125] More recently, it was shown that cellular immune responses to gluten were enhanced in the peripheral blood mononuclear cells of T1DM patients.[126] Coeliac patients exposed to a gluten-containing diet had a significantly higher prevalence of anti-islet cell antibodies.[127]

The hypothesis that cows milk is a cause of T1DM is based on the concept that early consumption of cows milk might expose the immune system to a foreign protein that possesses immunological cross-reactivity with an antigen present on pancreatic beta-cells.[128] Researchers have demonstrated that antibodies against β-casein were significantly increased in T1DM patients, and these may cross-react with pancreatic β-cell antigens.[128] Epidemiological studies show a strong association between the intake of A1 milk, but not A2 milk (see Chapter 7), and the incidence of T1DM.[129,130,131] It has recently been demonstrated that T cell lines specific to bovine β-casein can be isolated from the peripheral blood of patients with T1DM and that these cell lines react to multiple and different sequences of the protein. In addition, the reactivity of these β-casein T cell lines suggests a cross-reactivity with beta-cell antigens.[132]

Gut Barrier Dysfunction and Inflammation

There are several indicators that increased gut permeability may contribute to T1DM. A number of studies have reported abnormally increased gut permeability in newly-diagnosed T1DM patients.[133,134,135] This human research is strongly supported by multiple animal studies that demonstrate the same results.[99] In all, the data suggest that gut inflammation, either induced or constitutive, is a feature of T1DM and is probably involved in the activation of autoimmunity, for possible reasons outlined in Chapter 4.

Herbal Treatment of T1DM

It is likely that by the time a child presents for herbal treatment of T1DM pancreatic β-cell destruction has progressed to the extent that little can be done in terms of protection and regeneration. However, several herbs have demonstrated an ability to regenerate pancreatic β-cells and a number have protective properties to protect against further destruction. Within the context of herbal treatment addressing the autoimmune factors, partial regeneration may be possible. At the very least, a better glycaemic control can be established, thereby stabilising insulin doses and protecting against the long-term consequences of T1DM.

Of the 3 or 4 significant hypoglycaemic herbs, Gymnema seems the most appropriate for T1DM. Gymnema (400 mg/day of Gymnema extract for 6 to 30 months) was clinically evaluated in 27 T1DM patients in an open-label, controlled trial. It demonstrated the ability to regenerate pancreatic β-cells, as evidenced by an increase in C-peptide.[136] Other significant outcomes from the trial were decreases in fasting blood glucose, glycosylated haemoglobin (HbA1c), cholesterol, triglycerides and free fatty acids, and above all reduced insulin requirements.[136] This putative effect of Gymnema in regenerating pancreatic β-cells has also been demonstrated in a diabetic animal model.[137] Hence Gymnema is likely to have more that just hypoglycaemic effects. Furthermore, a relatively recent animal study demonstrated that the aqueous extract of Gymnema exerted anti-inflammatory and antioxidant effects in various models of inflammation and free radical generation.[138] This activity could be significant, given the autoimmune/inflammatory nature of T1DM. Further herbal support can be provided by St Mary's thistle (milk thistle), as evidenced by an *in vitro* study using silymarin that demonstrated significant protection of pancreatic β-cells.[139]

Protection from the long-term consequences of T1DM is an important treatment priority. In the context of the research cited above concerning the role of free radicals in diabetes complications, it is interesting to note most of the herbs that have demonstrated an ability to protect against these complications have significant antioxidant properties.

Studies found that standardised extract of Ginkgo reduced the abnormal blood parameters seen in diabetic retinopathy. These included a reduction in lipid peroxidation, clotting factors and red blood cell deformities, plus improved blood viscosity and elasticity, resulting overall in improved retinal capillary blood flow.[140,141] A recently-published open study demonstrated that standardised extract of Ginkgo at 3 tablets per day (120 mg of extract) for 9 months in children and adolescents with long standing T1DM had a significant protective effect against the development of diabetic retinopathy.[142]

Gotu kola has a demonstrated ability to improve the venoarteriolar parameters consistent with preventing and treating diabetic neuropathy. A clinical study saw a significant reduction in resting blood flow and ankle swelling, as well as an increase in the venoarteriolar response.[143] Additionally, 6 months treatment with the total triterpenic fraction of gotu kola (60 mg twice daily) in patients with diabetic microangiopathy resulted in significant improvements in microcirculatory parameters.[144]

Of course the autoimmune aspects should be addressed if the issue of autoimmune damage to the pancreas is still current. See the case history for an example treatment. Additional herbs useful in the autoimmune context include Rehmannia, Bupleurum and Hemidesmus to balance the immune system and control inflammation.

An example liquid formulation is as follows:

Gymnema	1:1	30 mL
St Mary's (milk) thistle	1:1	30 mL
Ginkgo standardised extract	2:1	20 mL
Gotu kola	1:1	20 mL
	Total	100 mL

Dose: Calculate the standard dose according to the most appropriate guideline in Chapter 1 based on an adult dose of 5 mL. Take with water 3 times a day before meals.

For the older child or the younger one who will not take liquids, herbal tablets or capsules of appropriate quality will provide a useful alternative in T1DM management.

Key herbal formulations (examples provided in Appendix 1) which should be considered are Glucose Metabolism Support tablets (adult dose 1 before each meal) and Liver Protection Formula tablets (adult dose 3 per day). For preventing the long-term complications consider selecting from Gotu Kola Combination tablets (adult dose 4 per day), Herbal Antioxidant tablets (adult dose 2 per day), Bilberry tablets (adult dose 4 per day) and Ginkgo tablets (adult dose 4 per day). For the autoimmune aspects if relevant St John's Wort tablets (adult dose 4 per day) and Autoimmune Formula tablets (adult dose 4 per day) are indicated. In general, no more than 3 to 4 different formulations should be prescribed at the one time.

Calculate the child's tablet dose according to the most appropriate guideline in Chapter 1. For younger children the tablets can be crushed and mixed with honey or a suitable sweetener to improve compliance. See Appendix 1 for the suggested formulations for these tablets.

Case History

A 3-year-old asthmatic girl weighing 15 kg presented with her mother for herbal therapy. She had a flu-like illness in the previous 2 months and routine testing revealed high levels of blood sugar and ketones. Things stabilised but the paediatrician said that there was a 95% chance she would develop type 1 diabetes within 6 months. She was placed on a dairy-protein-free diet.

The herbal formulation prescribed was:

Echinacea root blend	1:2	40 mL
Gymnema	1:1	30 mL
St John's wort high in hypericin	1:2	15 mL
Thuja	1:5	10 mL
Astragalus	1:2	15 mL
	Total	110 mL

Dose: 5mL with water once a day

The Echinacea, Astragalus, Thuja and St John's wort were to control viral infections and balance immune function. Gymnema was included to protect and restore her pancreas.

The girl's asthma was initially unsettled but stabilised dramatically. There were occasional days when her fasting blood sugar readings spiked to abnormal levels in the first few months, but otherwise her readings were generally normal. Herbal treatment was continued for 2 years. For another 2 years after ceasing the herbal treatment all blood sugar readings were normal. Contact was then lost with the patient.

References

1   Ng PC. Arch Dis Child Fetal Neonatal Ed 2000; **82**(3): F250-F254
2   Seckl JR. *Eur J Endocrinol* 2004; **151**(3): U49-U62
3   Kapoor A, Dunn E, Kostaki A et al. *J Physiol* 2006; **572**(1): 31-44
4   Myatt L. *J Physiol* 2006; **572**(1): 25-30

5   Ohkawa T, Rohde W, Takeshita S et al. *Exp Clin Endocrinol* 1991; **98**(2): 123-129

6   Mastorakos G, Ilias I. *Ann NY Acad Sci* 2003; **997**: 136-149

7   White M. *IJCE* 2005; **20**(4): 4-7

8   Barker DJ. *Clin Sci* 1998; **95**(2): 115-128

9   McMillen C, Robinson JS. *Physiol Rev* 2003; **85**(2): 571-633

10 Barker DJ, Osmond C. *Lancet* 1986; **1**(8489): 1077-1081

11 De Boo HA, Harding JE. *Aust NZ J Obstet Gynaecol* 2006; **46**(1): 4-14

12 Sapolsky RM. *Why Zebras Don't Get Ulcers* 3rd Ed, Henry Holt & Co, New York, 2004.

13 Jones A, Godfrey KM, Wood P et al. *J Clin Endocrinol Metab* 2006; **91**(5): 1868-1871

14 Phillips DI. *J Intern Med* 2007; **261**(5): 453-460

15 Geis HK, Whittlesey SW, McDonald NB et al. *Child Adolesc Psychiatr Clin N Am* 1998; **7**(1): 73-85

16 Sood AB, Razdan A, Weller EB et al. *Curr Psychiatry Rep* 2006; **8**(2): 115-120

17 Chitkara DK, van Tilburg MA, Blois-Martin N et al. *Am J Gastroenterol* 2008 Jan 2 [Epub ahead of print]

18 Guillette LJ. *Environ Health Perspect* 2006; **114**(1): 9-12

19 Kleigman RM, Behrman RE, Jenson HB, Stanton BF. *Nelson Textbook of Pediatrics* 18th Ed, Saunders Elsevier, Philadelphia, 2007.

20 Colborn T. *Environ Health Perspect* 2004; **112**(9): 944-949

21 Solomon GM, Schettler T. *CMAJ* 2000; **163**(11): 1471-1476

22 Cooper RL, Kavlock RJ. *J Endocrinol* 1997; **157**(2): 159-166

23 Maervoet J, Vermeir G, Covaci A et al. *Environ Health Perspect* 2007; **115**(12): 1780-1786

24 Bernal J, Guadano-Ferraz A, Morte B. *Thyroid* 2003; **13**(11): 1005-1012

25 Bernal J. *Vitam Horm* 2005; **71**: 95-122

26 Koopman-Esseboom C, Morse DC, Weisglas-Kuperus N et al. *Pediatr Res* 1994; **36**(4): 468-473

27 Osius N, Karmaus W, Kruse H et al. *Environ Health Perspect* 1999; **107**(10): 843-849

28 Rogan WJ, Ragan NB. *Pediatrics* 2003; **112**(1): 247-252

29 Jacobson JL, Jacobson SW. *J Pediatr* 1990; **116**(1): 38-45

30 Stewart P, Darvill T, Lonky E et al. *Environ Res* 1999; **80**(Pt 2): S87-S96

31 Weiss RE, Stein MA, Trummer B et al. *J Pediatr* 1993; **123**(4): 539-545

32 Stein MA, Weiss RE. *Psychoneuroendocrinology* 2003; **28**(3): 304-316

33 Wise LA, Palmer JR, Hatch EE et al. *Environ Health Perspect* 2007; **115**(9): 1314-1319

34 McLachlan JA. *Endocrin Rev* 2001; **22**(3): 319-341

35 Crain DA, Guillette LJ, Rooney AA et al. *Environ Health Perspect* 1997; **105**(5): 528-533

36 Hayes TB, Case P, Chui S et al. *Environ Health Perspect* 2006; **114**(1): 40-50

37 Schell LM, Gallo MV, Denham M et al. *J Physiol Anthrop* 2006; **25**(1): 103-112

38 Denham M, Schell LM, Deane G et al. *Pediatrics* 2005; **115**(2): 127-134

39 Schoeters G, Den Hond E, Dhooge W et al. *Basci Clin Pharmacol Toxicol* 2008; **102**(2): 168-175

40 Blanck HM, Marcus M, Tolbert PE et al. *Epidemiology* 2000; **11**(6): 641-647

41 Vasiliu O, Muttineni J, Karmaus W. *Hum Reprod* 2004; **19**(7): 1506-1512

42 Colon I, Caro D, Bourdony CJ et al. *Environ Health Perspect* 2000; **108**(9): 895-900

43 Guo YL, Lambert GH, Hsu CC et al. *Int Arch Occup Environ Health* 2004; **77**(3): 153-158

44 Saiyed H, Dewan A, Bhatnagar V et al. *Environ Health Perspect* 2003; **111**(16): 1958-1962

45 Krugman SD, Dubowitz H. *Am Fam Physician* 2003; **68**(5): 879-884

46 Olsen EM, Petersen J, Skovgaard AM et al. *Arch Dis Child* 2007; **92**(2): 109-114

47 Wells J. *Pediatr Nurs* 2002; **14**(3): 37-42

48 Bone K. *The Ultimate Herbal Compendium,* Phytotherapy Press, Warwick, Qld, 2007.

49 Singhal V, Schwenk F, Kumar S. *Mayo Clin Proc* 2007; **82**(10): 1258-1264

50 Booth ML, Chey T, Wake M et al. *Am J Clin Nutri* 2003; **77**(1): 29-36

51 Waters EB, Baur LA. *MJA* 2003; **178**(9): 422-423

52 Ogden CL, Flegal KM, Carroll MD et al. *JAMA* 2002; **288**(14): 1728-1732

53 Hedley AA, Ogden CL, Johnson CL et al. *JAMA* 2004; **291**(23): 2847-2850

54 Must A, Strauss RS. *Int J Obesity* 1999; **23**(Suppl 2): S2-S11

55 Wang Y. *Pediatrics* 2002; **110**(5): 903-910

56 Miller J, Rosenbloom A, Silverstein J. *J Clin Endocrinol Metab* 2004; **89**(9): 4211-4218

57 Lobstein T, Baur L, Uauy R. *Obes Rev* 2004; **5**(1): 4-85

58 Lobstein T, Dibb S. *Obes Rev* 2005; **6**(3): 203-208

59 Whitaker RC, Wright JA. *NEJM* 1997; **337**(13): 869-873

60 Nader PR, O'Brien M, Houts R et al. *Pediatrics* 2006; **118**(3): 594-601

61 McCaffrey TA, Rennie KL, Wallace JMW et al. *Pediatrics* 2007; **20**(4): 89-94

62 Skinner JD, Carruth BR, Wendy B et al. *J Am Diet Assoc* 2002; **102**(11): 1638-1647

63 Carruth BR, Ziegler PJ, Gordon A et al. *J Am Diet Assoc* 2004; **104**(1): 57-64
64 Wardle J, Guthrie C, Sanderson S et al. *Int J Obes Metab Disord* 2001; **25**(7): 971-977
65 Taverus EM, Rifas-Shiman SL, Berkey CS et al. *Obes Res* 2005; **13**(5): 900-906
66 Gillman MW, Rifas-Shiman SL, Frazier AL et al. *Arch Fam Med* 2000; **9**(3): 235-240
67 Neumark-Sztainer D, Hannan PJ, Story M et al. *J Am Diet Assoc* 2003; **103**(3): 317-322
68 Nielsen SJ, Popkin BM. *JAMA* 2003; **289**(4): 450-454
69 McConahy KL, Smiciklas-Wright H, Birch LL et al. *J Pediatr* 2002; **140**(3): 340-347
70 Prentice AM, Jebb SA. *Obes Res* 2003; **4**(4): 187-194
71 St Onge MP, Keller KL, Heymsfield SB. *Am J Clin Nutr* 2003; **78**(6): 1068-1073
72 Savage GS, Ball K, Worsley A et al. *Asia Pac J Clin Nutr* 2007; **16**(4): 738-747
73 Berkey CS, Rockett HR, Field AE et al. *Obes Res* 2004; **12**(5): 778-788
74 Ludwig DS, Peterson KE, Gortmaker SL. *Lancet* 2001; **357**(9255): 505-508
75 O'Connor TM, Yang SJ, Nicklas TA. *Pediatrics* 2006; **118**(4): 1010-1018
76 Campbell KJ, Crawford DA, Ball K. *Int J Obes (Lond)* 2006; **8**(8): 1272-1280
77 Eisenmann JC, Bartee RT, Wang MQ. *Obes Res* 2002; **10**(5): 379-385
78 Doak CM, Visscher TL, Renders CM et al. *Obes Res* 2006; **7**(1): 111-136
79 American Academy of Pediatrics. *Pediatrics* 2001; **107**(2): 423-426
80 Yalcin S S, Tugrul B, Nacar N, et al. *Pediatr Int* 2002; **44**(6): 622-627
81 Ludwig DS, Gortmaker SL. *Lancet* 2004; **364**(4430): 226-227
82 Ebbeling CB, Pawlak DB, Ludwig DS. *Lancet* 2002; **360**(9331): 473-482
83 Johnston CA, Tyler C, Brian K et al. *Pediatrics* 2007; **120**(6): 1450-1457
84 Benton D. *Int J Obes* 2004: **28**(7): 858-869
85 Freedman M, Stern JS. *J Altern Comp Med* 2004; **10**(Suppl 1): S231-S244
86 Wansink B, van Ittersum K, Painter JE. *Am J Prev Med* 2006; **31**(3): 240-243
87 Drohan SH. *Pediatr Nurs* 2002; **28**(6): 599-610
88 Golan M, Crow S. *Obes Res* 2004; **12**(2): 357-361
89 Tortora GJ, Grabowsky SR. *Principles of Anatomy and Physiology* 10th Ed, John Wiley & Sons, New York, 2002.
90 Bone K. *Mod Phytother* 1995; **1**(2): 1-5
91 Bone K. *A Clinical Guide to Blending Liquid Herbs.* Churchill Livingstone, Edinburgh, 2000.
92 Schone F, Vetter A, Hartung H et al. *J Anim Physiol Nutr (Berl)* 2006; **90**(11-12): 500-510
93 Wolfram S, Raederstorff D, Wang Y et al. *Ann Nutr Metab* 2005; **49**(1): 54-63
94 Wolfram S, Wang Y, Thielecke F. *Mol Nutr Food Res* 2006; **50**(2): 176-187
95 Kovacs EMR, Mela DJ. *Obes Rev* 2006; **7**(1): 59-78
96 Gale EA. *Diabetes* 2002; **51**(12): 3353-3361
97 Taplin CE, Craig ME, Lloyd M et al. *MJA* 2005; **183**(5): 243-246
98 Mauny F, Grandmottet M, Lesradet C et al. *Eur J Epidemiol* 2005; **20**(4): 325-329
99 Lefebvre DE, Powell KL, Strom A et al. *Ann Rev Nutr* 2006; **26**(1): 175-202
100 Kondrashova A, Reunanen A, Romanov A et al. *Ann Med* 2005; **37**(1): 67-72
101 Virtanen SM, Knip M. *Am J Clin Nutr* 2003; **78**(6): 1053-1067
102 Bingley PJ, Bonifacio E, Williams AJK et al. *Diabetes* 1997; **46**(11): 1701-1710
103 LaGasse JM, Brantley MS, Leech NJ et al. *Diabetes Care* 2002; **25**(3): 505-511
104 Knip M. *Horm Res* 2002; **57**(1): 6-11
105 Kupila A, Muona P, Ponkainen M et al. *Diabetes* 2002; **51**(5): 646-651
106 Aiello LP et al. *Diabetes Care* 1998; **21**(1): 143-156
107 Brownlee M. *Nature* 2001; **414**(6865): 813-820
108 Wegewitz U, Gohring I, Spranger J. *Curr Pharml Des* 2005; **11**(18): 2311-2330
109 Frisk G, Tuverno T. *J Med Virol* 2004; **73**(3): 450-459
110 Lipman TH, Chang Y, Murphy KM. *Diabetes Care* 2002; **25**(11): 1969-1975
111 Sano H, Terasaki J, Tsutsumi C et al. *Diabetes Res Clin Pract* 2008; **79**(3): e8-9 [Epub 2008 Jan 4]
112 Wahlberg J, Fredriksson O, Vaarala O et al. *Ann NY Acad Sci* 2003; **1005**(1): 404-408
113 Ludvigsson J, Forsberg P. Fryden A et al. *Diabetes Res* 1988; **9**(4): 193-195
114 Classen JB. *Autoimmunity* 1996; **24**(3): 137-145
115 Hviid A, Stellfeld M, Wohlfahrt J et al. *NEJM* 2004; **350**(14): 1398-1404
116 Hviid A. *Expert Rev Vaccines* 2006; **5**(5): 641-649
117 Vaarala O, Knip M, Paronen J et al. *Diabetes* 1999; **48**(7): 1389-1394
118 Paronen J, Knip M, Savilahti E et al. *Diabetes* 2000; **49**(10): 1657-1665
119 Tiittanen M, Paronen J, Savilahti E et al. *Pediatr Allergy Immunol* 2006; **17**(7): 538-543
120 Scott FW, Clouthier HE, Kleeman R. *Diabetes* 1997; **46**(4): 589-598
121 Funda DP, Kaas A, Bock T et al. *Diabetes Metab Res Rev* 1999; **15**(5): 323-327

122 Auricchio R, Paparo F, Maglio M et al. *Diabetes* 2004; **53**(7): 1680-1683
123 Schuppan D, Hahn EG. *J Pediatr Endocrinol Metab* 2001; **14**(1): 595-605
124 Lampasona V, Bonfani R, Bazzigluppi E et al. *Diabetologia* 1999; **42**(10): 1195-1198
125 Catassi C, Guerrieri A, Bartolotta E et al. *Lancet* 1987; **2**(8551): 158
126 Klemetti P, Savilahti E, Ilonen J et al. *Scand J Immunol* 1998; **47**(1): 48-53
127 Verbeke S, Cruchet S, Gotteland M et al. *Rev Med Chil* 2004; **132**(8): 979-984
128 Cavallo MG, Fava D, Monetini L et al. *Lancet* 1996; **348**(9032): 926-928
129 Elliott RB, Harris DP, Hill JP et al. *Diabetologia* 1999; **42**(3): 292-296
130 McLachlan CN. *Med Hypotheses* 2001; **56**(2): 262-272
131 Laugesen M, Elliott R. *NZ Med J* 2003; **116**(1170): 1-19
132 Monetini L, Barone F, Stefanini L et al. *J Endocrinol* 2003; **176**(1): 143-150
133 Carratu R, Secondulfo M, de Magistris L et al. *J Pediatr Gastroenterol Nutr* 1999; **28**(3): 264-269
134 Secondulfo M, Iafusco D, Carratu R et al. *Dig Liver Dis* 2004; **36**(1): 35-45
135 Bosi E, Molteni L, Radaelli MG et al. *Diabetologia* 2006; **49**(12): 2824-2827
136 Shanmugasundaram ER, Rajeswari G, Baskaran K et al. *J Ethnopharmacol* 1990; **30**(3): 281-294
137 Shanmugasundaram ER, Gopinath KL, Radha Shammugasundaram K et al. *J Ethnopharmacol* 1990; **30**(3): 265-279
138 Diwan PV, Margaret I, Ramakrishna S. *Inflammopharmacol* 1995; **3**: 271-277
139 Matsuda T, Ferreri K, Todorov I et al. *Endocrinology* 2005; **146**(1): 175-185
140 Kudolo GB, Delaney D, Blodgett J. *Diabetes Res Clin Pract* 2005; **68**(1): 29-38
141 Huang SY, Jeng C, Kao SC et al. *Clin Nutr* 2004; **23**(4): 615-621
142 Bernardczyk-Meller J, Siwiec-Proscinska J, Stankiewicz W et al. *Klin Oczna* 2004; **106**(4-5): 569-571
143 Incandela L, Belcaro G, Cesarone MR et al. *Angiology* 2001; **52**(Suppl 2): S27-S31
144 Cesarone MR, Incandela L, De Sanctis MT et al. *Angiology* 2001; **52**(Suppl 2): S49-S54

Appendix 1: Example Tablet, Capsule and Preformulated Liquid Products

NAME	HERBS IN TABLET, CAPSULE OR 5 ML DOSE	AMOUNT
Allergy Support	*Albizia lebbek* (Albizia) extract equivalent to dry bark	800 mg
	Scutellaria baicalensis (Baical Skullcap) extract equivalent to dry root	800 mg
	Tanacetum parthenium (Feverfew) extract equivalent to dry herb	50 mg
Anxiety Support	*Piper methysticum* (Kava) aqueous extract equivalent to dry root containing kava lactones 50 mg	3.2 g
Autoimmune Formula	*Rehmannia glutinosa* (Rehmannia) extract equivalent to dry root	350 mg
	Bupleurum falcatum (Bupleurum) extract equivalent to dry root	700 mg
	Hemidesmus indicus (Hemidesmus) extract equivalent to dry root	500 mg
	Tanacetum parthenium (Feverfew) extract equivalent to dry herb	165 mg
Bilberry	*Vaccinium myrtillus* (Bilberry) extract equivalent to fresh fruit standardised to contain anthocyanosides 15 mg	6.0 g
Boswellia Combination	*Boswellia serrata* (Boswellia) extract equivalent to dry gum oleoresin standardised to contain boswellic acids 180 mg	1.2 g
	Curcuma longa (Turmeric) extract equivalent to dry rhizome standardised to contain curcuminoids 70.4 mg	2.0 g
	Apium graveolens (Celery) extract equivalent to dry fruit	1.0 g
	Zingiber officinale (Ginger) extract equivalent to dry rhizome	300 mg
Bowel Flora Complex	*Andrographis paniculata* (Andrographis) extract equivalent to dry herb containing andrographolide 10 mg	1.0 g
	Tabebuia avellanedae (Pau d'Arco) extract equivalent to dry stem bark	500 mg
	Anise (*Pimpinella anisum*) fruit essential oil	125 mg
	Oregano (*Origanum vulgare*) herb essential oil	75 mg
Cat's Claw Immune formula	*Uncaria tomentosa* (Cat's Claw) extract equivalent to dry inner stem bark	1.5 g
	Tabebuia avellanedae (Pau d'Arco) extract equivalent to dry inner stem bark	500 mg
	Echinacea purpurea (Echinacea) extract equivalent to dry root	500 mg
Chaste Tree	*Vitex agnus-castus* (Chaste Tree) extract equivalent to dry fruit	500 mg
Chronic Lung Support	*Curcuma longa* (Turmeric) extract equivalent to dry rhizome standardised to contain curcuminoids 38 mg	1.0 g
	Ginkgo biloba (Ginkgo) extract equivalent to dry leaf standardised to contain ginkgo flavonglycosides 4.8 mg	1.0 g
	Adhatoda vasica (Adhatoda) extract equivalent to dry leaf	750 mg
	Scutellaria baicalensis (Baical Skullcap) extract equivalent to dry root	500 mg
	Grindelia camporum (Grindelia) extract equivalent to dry herb	300 mg
	Foeniculum vulgare (Fennel) fruit/seed essential oil	5 m
Clear Lung Formula Liquid	*Glycyrrhiza glabra* (Licorice) extract equivalent to dry root	1.0 g
	Verbascum thapsus (Mullein) extract equivalent to dry leaf	625 mg
	Euphorbia hirta (Euphorbia) extract equivalent to dry herb	372.5 mg
	Grindelia camporum (Grindelia) extract equivalent to dry herb	372.5 mg
	Inula helenium (Elecampane) extract equivalent to dry root	372.5 mg
	Zingiber officinale (Ginger) extract equivalent to dry rhizome	250 mg
	Foeniculum vulgare (Fennel) fruit/seed essential oil	15 mcL

NAME	HERBS IN TABLET, CAPSULE OR 5 ML DOSE	AMOUNT
Clear Lung Formula Tablets	*Glycyrrhiza glabra* (Licorice) extract equivalent to dry root	500 mg
	Verbascum thapsus (Mullein) extract equivalent to dry leaf	470 mg
	Grindelia camporum (Grindelia) extract equivalent to dry herb	280 mg
	Euphorbia hirta (Euphorbia) extract equivalent to dry herb	280 mg
	Zingiber officinale (Ginger) extract equivalent to dry rhizome	180 mg
	Thymus vulgaris (Thyme) herb flowering essential oil	12 mg
	Foeniculum vulgare (Fennel) fruit/seed essential oil	12 mg
Coleus Forskohlii	*Coleus forskohlii* (Coleus) extract equivalent to dry root standardised to contain forskolin 18.7 mg	3.74 g
Dong Quai	*Angelica polymorpha* (*A. sinensis*, Dong Quai) extract equivalent to dry root	1.0 g
Echinacea Formula	*Echinacea angustifolia* (Echinacea) extract equivalent to dry root containing alkylamides 2.5 mg	600 mg
	Echinacea purpurea (Echinacea) extract equivalent to dry root containing alkylamides 2.5 mg	675 mg
Evening Primrose Oil capsule	*Oenothera biennis* (Evening Primrose) seed oil standardised to contain gamma-linolenic acid (GLA) 100 mg	1.0 g
Gastric Mucosal Support	*Glycyrrhiza glabra* (Licorice) extract equivalent to dry root containing glycyrrhizinic acid not more than 1%	3.42 g
	Matricaria recutita (Chamomile) extract equivalent to dry flower	600 mg
	Filipendula ulmaria (Meadowsweet) extract equivalent to dry herb	500 mg
	Matricaria recutita (Chamomile) flower essential oil	5 mg
Ginkgo	*Ginkgo biloba* (Ginkgo) extract equivalent to dry leaf standardised to contain ginkgo flavonglycosides 9.6 mg standardised to contain ginkgolides & bilobalide 2.4 mg	2.0 g
Glucose Metabolism Support	*Gymnema sylvestre* (Gymnema) extract equivalent to dry leaf standardised to contain gymnemic acids 100 mg	4.0 g
Golden Seal	*Hydrastis canadensis* (Golden Seal) extract equivalent to dry root & rhizome	500 mg
Gotu Kola Combination	*Vitis vinifera* (Grape Seed) extract equivalent to dry seed standardised to contain procyanidins 25.5 mg	3.6 g
	Centella asiatica (Gotu Kola) extract equivalent to dry herb standardised to contain triterpenes 50 mg	2.5 g
	Ginkgo biloba (Ginkgo) extract equivalent to dry leaf standardised to contain ginkgo flavonglycosides 4.8 mg standardised to contain ginkgolides and bilobalide 1.2 mg	1.0 g
Hawthorn	*Crataegus monogyna* (Hawthorn) extract equivalent to dry herb flowering top standardised to contain vitexin-2-rhamnoside 6.68 mg standardised to contain catechin polymers 15 mg	1.0 g
Herbal Antioxidant	*Vitis vinifera* (Grape) extract equivalent to dry seed standardised to contain procyanidins 42.5 mg	6.0 g
	Curcuma longa (Turmeric) extract equivalent to dry rhizome standardised to contain curcuminoids 70.4 mg	2.0 g
	Camellia sinensis (Green Tea) extract equivalent to dry leaf standardised to contain catechins 83.35 mg	1.0 g
	Rosmarinus officinalis (Rosemary) extract equivalent to dry leaf	1.0 g
Herbal Bowel Support	*Rhamnus purshianus* (Cascara) extract equivalent to dry stem bark	560 mg
	Taraxacum officinale (Dandelion) extract equivalent to dry root	375 mg
	Rumex crispus (Yellow Dock) extract equivalent to dry root	375 mg
	Anethum graveolens (Dill) extract equivalent to dry seed	375 mg
	Matricaria recutita (Chamomile) extract equivalent to dry flower	280 mg

NAME	HERBS IN TABLET, CAPSULE OR 5 ML DOSE	AMOUNT
Herbal Thyroid Support (large size)	*Fucus vesiculosus* (Bladderwrack) extract equivalent to dry herb containing iodine 600 mcg	1.05 g
	Bacopa monnieri (Bacopa) extract equivalent to dry herb standardised to contain bacosides calculated as bacoside A 25 mg	2.5 g
	Withania somnifera (Withania) extract equivalent to dry root	600 mg
Herbal Thyroid Support (small size)	*Fucus vesiculosus* (Bladderwrack) extract equivalent to dry herb containing iodine 250 mcg	437.5 mg
	Bacopa monnieri (Bacopa) extract equivalent to dry herb standardised to contain bacosides calculated as bacoside A 10 mg	1.0 g
	Withania somnifera (Withania) extract equivalent to dry root	250 mg
High Allicin Releasing Garlic	*Allium sativum* (Garlic) extract equivalent to bulb containing alliin 4.3 mg	1.04 g
	Allium sativum (Garlic) dry bulb powder containing alliin 1.4 mg	100 mg
High Potency Tribulus Leaf	*Tribulus terrestris* (Tribulus) extract equivalent to dry herb (aerial parts) standardised to contain a minimum of furostanol saponins as protodioscin 100 mg	2.83 g
High Potency Willow Bark Tablet	*Salix purpurea* (Willow) extract equivalent to dry stem bark standardised to contain salicin 60 mg	8.0 g
Immune/ Diaphoretic Liquid	*Achillea millefolium* (Yarrow) extract equivalent to dry herb	500 mg
	Echinacea angustifolia (Echinacea) extract equivalent to dry root	500 mg
	Glycyrrhiza glabra (Licorice) extract equivalent to dry root	500 mg
	Sambucus nigra (Elder) extract equivalent to dry flower	500 mg
	Tilia cordata (Lime Flowers) extract equivalent to dry flower	500 mg
	Zingiber officinale (Ginger) extract equivalent to dry rhizome	250 mg
Liver Detox Assist	*Silybum marianum* (St Mary's Thistle) extract equivalent to dry fruit standardised to contain flavanolignans calculated as silybin 24 mg	2.1 g
	Schizandra chinensis (Schisandra) extract equivalent to dry fruit	1.0 g
	Rosmarinus officinalis (Rosemary) extract equivalent to dry leaf	500 mg
Liver Protection Formula	*Silybum marianum* (St Mary's Thistle) extract equivalent to dry fruit standardised to contain flavanolignans calculated as silybin 168 mg	14.7 g
Liver/Biliary Tonic	*Silybum marianum* (St Mary's Thistle) extract equivalent to dry fruit standardised to contain flavanolignans calculated as silybin 80 mg	7.0 g
	Cynara scolymus (Globe Artichoke) extract equivalent to dry leaf	800 mg
	Taraxacum officinale (Dandelion) extract equivalent to dry root	400 mg
	Bupleurum falcatum (Bupleurum) extract equivalent to dry root	300 mg
	Chionanthus virginica (Fringe Tree) extract equivalent to dry root bark	160 mg
Long Term Immune Support	*Astragalus membranaceus* (Astragalus) extract equivalent to dry root	850 mg
	Eleutherococcus senticosus (Siberian Ginseng) extract equivalent to dry root standardised to contain eleutheroside E 600 mcg	750 mg
	Echinacea purpurea (Echinacea) extract equivalent to dry root	650 mg
Memory/Brain Tonic	*Bacopa monnieri* (Bacopa) extract equivalent to dry herb standardised to contain bacosides 37.5 mg	3.75 g
	Schizandra chinensis (Schisandra) extract equivalent to dry fruit	660 mg
	Eleutherococcus senticosus (Siberian Ginseng) extract equivalent to dry root standardised to contain eleutheroside E 400 mcg	500 mg
	Rosmarinus officinalis (Rosemary) herb top flowering essential oil	10 mg

NAME	HERBS IN TABLET, CAPSULE OR 5 ML DOSE	AMOUNT
Mushroom Immune Formula	*Ganoderma lucidum* (Reishi) extract equivalent to dry mushroom	6.6 g
	Lentinula edodes (Shiitake) extract equivalent to dry mushroom	800 mg
Nervous System Tonic	*Hypericum perforatum* (St John's Wort) extract equivalent to dry herb flowering top standardised to contain hypericin 413 mcg	750 mg
	Schizandra chinensis (Schisandra) extract equivalent to dry fruit	675 mg
	Turnera diffusa (Damiana) extract equivalent to dry leaf	625 mg
	Scutellaria lateriflora (Skullcap) extract equivalent to dry herb	500 mg
Sheep Sorrel Formula	*Arctium lappa* (Burdock) dry root powder	242 mg
	Rumex acetosella (Sheep Sorrel) dry herb powder	130 mg
	Ulmus rubra (Slippery Elm) dry stem bark powder	32 mg
	Rheum palmatum (Rhubarb) dry root powder	8 mg
Short Term Immune Support	*Andrographis paniculata* (Andrographis) extract equivalent to dry leaf standardised to contain andrographolide 50 mg	2.0 g
	Ocimum tenuiflorum (Holy Basil) extract equivalent to dry herb	500 mg
	Echinacea purpurea (Echinacea) extract equivalent to dry root	300 mg
	Echinacea angustifolia (Echinacea) extract equivalent to dry root	200 mg
	Ocimum tenuiflorum (Holy Basil) leaf essential oil	10 mg
Short Term Lower Respiratory Support Liquid	*Glycyrrhiza glabra* (Licorice) extract equivalent to dry root	1.0 g
	Asclepias tuberosa (Pleurisy Root) extract equivalent to dry root	500 mg
	Echinacea angustifolia (Echinacea) extract equivalent to dry root	500 mg
	Thymus vulgaris (Thyme) extract equivalent to dry leaf	500 mg
	Marrubium vulgare (White Horehound) extract equivalent to dry herb	250 mg
	Zingiber officinale (Ginger) extract equivalent to dry rhizome	250 mg
Short Term Lower Respiratory Support Tablet	*Glycyrrhiza glabra* (Licorice) extract equivalent to dry root	750 mg
	Asclepias tuberosa (Pleurisy Root) extract equivalent to dry root	375 mg
	Echinacea purpurea (Echinacea) extract equivalent to dry root	375 mg
	Marrubium vulgare (White Horehound) extract equivalent to dry herb	180 mg
	Zingiber officinale (Ginger) extract equivalent to dry rhizome	180 mg
	Thymus vulgaris (Thyme) herb flowering essential oil	10 mg
Skin/Elimination Support	*Galium aparine* (Clivers) extract equivalent to dry herb	360 mg
	Smilax ornata (Sarsaparilla) extract equivalent to dry root & rhizome	360 mg
	Berberis aquifolium (Oregon Grape) extract equivalent to dry root & rhizome	360 mg
	Arctium lappa (Burdock) extract equivalent to dry root	270 mg
	Rumex crispus (Yellow Dock) extract equivalent to dry root	270 mg
Sleep Support	*Valeriana edulis* (Mexican Valerian) equivalent to dry root & rhizome	1.0 g
Sleep/Anxiety Support	*Valeriana officinalis* (Valerian) extract equivalent to dry root & rhizome	700 mg
	Passiflora incarnata (Passionflower) extract equivalent to dry herb	500 mg
	Zizyphus spinosa (Zizyphus) extract equivalent to dry seed	900 mg
Slippery Elm	*Ulmus rubra* (Slippery Elm) stem bark powder	400 mg
Smooth Muscle Relaxant	*Corydalis ambigua* (Corydalis) extract equivalent to dry tuber	600 mg
	Zingiber officinale (Ginger) extract equivalent to dry rhizome	400 mg
	Rubus idaeus (Raspberry) extract equivalent to dry leaf	400 mg
	Dioscorea villosa (Wild Yam) extract equivalent to dry root & rhizome	400 mg
	Viburnum opulus (Cramp Bark) extract equivalent to dry stem bark	400 mg

NAME	HERBS IN TABLET, CAPSULE OR 5 ML DOSE	AMOUNT
St John's Wort	*Hypericum perforatum* (St John's Wort) extract equivalent to dry herb flowering top standardised to contain hypericin 990 mcg standardised to contain flavonoid glycosides 18 mg	1.8 g
Stress Adapt	*Eleutherococcus senticosus* (Siberian Ginseng) extract equivalent to dry root standardised to contain eleutheroside E 950 mcg	1.25 g
Stress Control	*Withania somnifera* (Withania) extract equivalent to dry root	950 mg
	Glycyrrhiza glabra (Licorice) extract equivalent to dry root	750 mg
	Scutellaria lateriflora (Skullcap) extract equivalent to dry herb	470 mg
	Panax ginseng (Korean Ginseng) extract equivalent to dry root standardised to contain ginsenosides calculated as Rg1 & Rb1 1.86 mg	100 mg
Upper Digestive Formula Tablet	*Silybum marianum* (St Mary's Thistle) extract equivalent to dry fruit	2.1 g
	Taraxacum officinale (Dandelion) extract equivalent to dry root	500 mg
	Citrus reticulata (Chen Pi) extract equivalent to dry fruit peel	500 mg
	Gentiana lutea (Gentian) extract equivalent to dry root	100 mg
	Zingiber officinale (Ginger) extract equivalent to dry rhizome	100 mg
	Citrus reticulata (Mandarin) fruit peel essential oil (cold pressed)	12.5 mg
	Matricaria recutita (Chamomile) flower essential oil	5 mg
	The coating of this tablet should contain a quantity of Gentian to provide a bitter taste as swallowed	
Upper Respiratory Tract Support	*Euphrasia officinalis* (Eyebright) extract equivalent to dry herb	650 mg
	Solidago virgaurea (Golden Rod) extract equivalent to dry herb	650 mg
	Echinacea purpurea (Echinacea) extract equivalent to dry root	370 mg
	Hydrastis canadensis (Golden Seal) extract equivalent to dry root and rhizome	125 mg
	Capsicum annuum (Cayenne) extract equivalent to dry fruit	10 mg
Urinary Tract Support	*Vaccinium macrocarpon* (Cranberry) juice concentrate equivalent to fresh fruit	2.5 g
	Crateva nurvala (Crataeva) extract equivalent to dry stem bark	1.0 g
	Arctostaphylos uva-ursi (Bearberry) extract equivalent to dry leaf	500 mg
	Barosma betulina (Buchu) leaf essential oil	12 mg
Wormwood Combination	*Artemisia absinthium* (Wormwood) extract equivalent to dry herb	100 mg
	Stemona sessilifolia (Stemona) extract equivalent to dry root	1g
	Juglans nigra (Green Hulls of Black Walnut) extract equivalent to dry fruit hull	100 mg
	Syzygium aromaticum (Clove) flower bud essential oil	20 mg

Appendix 2: Bibliography

Bone K. *A Clinical Guide to Blending Liquid Herbs. Herbal Formulations for the Individual Patient.* Churchill Livingstone, St Louis, 2003.

Bone K. *The Ultimate Herbal Compendium.* Phytotherapy Press, Warwick, 2007.

Braun L, Cohen M. *Herbs & Natural Supplements.* 2nd Ed, Churchill Livingstone, Edinburgh, 2007.

Christopher JR. *Childhood Diseases.* Christopher Publications, Utah, 1978.

Ellingwood F, Lloyd JU. *American Materia Medica, Therapeutics and Pharmacognosy.* 11th Edn. Naturopathic Medical Series: Botanical Volume 2. First published 1898, reprinted Eclectic Medical Publications, Portland, 1983.

Felter HW, Lloyd JU. *King's American Dispensatory.* 18th Edn, 3rd revision, Volumes 1 and 2. First published 1905, reprinted Eclectic Medical Publications, Portland, 1983.

Kasper DL, Fauci AS, Longo DL, Braunwald E, Hauser SL, Jameson JL. *Harrison's Principles of Internal Medicine.* 16th Ed, McGraw-Hill, New York, 2005.

Kliegman RM, Behrman RE, Jenson HB, Stanton BF. *Nelson Textbook of Pediatrics.* 2nd Ed, Saunders Elsevier, Philadelphia, 2007.

McIntyre A. *Herbal Treatment of Children. Western and Ayurvedic Perspectives.* Elsevier, Edinburgh, 2005.

Mills S, Bone K (eds). *The Essential Guide to Herbal Safety.* Churchill Livingstone, St Louis, 2005.

Mills S, Bone K. *Principles and Practice of Phytotherapy: Modern Herbal Medicine.* Churchill Livingstone, Edinburgh, 2000.

Schilcher H. *Phytotherapy in Paediatrics.* Medpharm, Stuttgart, 1997.

Weiss RF, Fintelmann V. *Herbal Medicine.* 2nd Ed, Thieme, Stuttgart, 2000.

Wood M. *The Practice of Traditional Western Herbalism.* North Atlantic Books, Berkeley, 2004.

Herb Index

A

aconite 8
Adhatoda 105, 107, 136
Adhatoda vasica 105
Albizia 53, 64, 65, 77, 91, 95, 136, 180
Albizia lebbeck 53, 105
Allergy Support tablets 65, 100, 180
Allium cepa 105
Althaea officinalis 105
American ginseng 135
Andrographis 10, 29, 37, 76, 81, 82, 87, 88, 90, 95, 105, 136, 164, 166, 180
Andrographis paniculata 105
Angelica 37, 57, 65, 190
anise 76
Arnica 10
Asparagus officinalis 152
asparagus root 152, 153
Astragalus 10, 37, 81, 87, 95, 101, 166, 203
Autoimmune Formula tablets 145, 175, 181, 203

B

Bacopa 10, 119, 122, 132, 133, 136, 137, 138, 145, 146, 147
Baical skullcap 53, 64, 65, 77, 91, 95, 100, 106, 107, 108, 136, 180, 181
balmony 39, 58
Baptisia 43, 58, 87, 88, 89, 168
barberry 10, 28, 58
bayberry 101
bearberry 10, 153, 158
belladonna 8, 89
bilberry fruit 10, 29
Bilberry tablets 203
bitter orange 38, 58, 170
bitter orange oil 170
bittersweet 10
black cohosh 10, 42
blackcurrant seed oil 23, 58, 178
black haw 10
black tea 28, 58
black walnut hulls 10, 66, 67, 70
bladderwrack 10
blue cohosh 10
blue flag 11, 196, 197
boldo 11
borage oil 23, 58, 178
Boswellia 11, 105, 108, 145
Boswellia Combination tablets 145
buchu 11, 37, 153, 158, 159
buchu essential oil 158
bugleweed 11
Bupleurum 11, 105, 145, 173, 174, 180, 202

burdock 11, 39, 87, 174, 180
butcher's broom 11
butternut 71, 72

C

Calendula 11, 21, 22, 23, 41, 42, 44, 64, 88, 89, 91, 92, 96, 97, 136, 145, 146, 147, 166, 167, 168, 169, 174
Californian poppy 11
Camellia sinensis 168
cascara 11, 71
cat's claw 11, 28, 39, 43, 66, 68
cayenne 37, 57, 86, 91, 95, 100
celery seed 11
chamomile 4, 11, 21, 24, 25, 26, 27, 42, 56, 57, 61, 62, 64, 65, 68, 71, 72, 81, 82, 83, 84, 91, 92, 95, 96, 119, 122, 123, 136, 145, 146, 147, 179, 180
chaparral 11
chaste tree 11, 174
Chaste Tree tablets 175
Chelone glabra 39
chen pi 38, 57, 58, 61, 62, 64, 65, 136
chickweed 11, 24, 39, 181
Chinese skullcap 64, 65, 77, 91, 95, 100, 106, 107, 108, 136, 180, 181
Chronic Lung Support tablets 108
cinnamon 37, 57, 58, 61, 62, 64, 76, 82, 84, 190
Citrus aurantium 170
Citrus reticulata 57
Clear Lung Formula tablets 108
clivers 11, 87, 95, 96
clove oil 67, 87
Codonopsis 11
Coleus 57, 76, 105, 196, 197
Coleus Forskohlii tablets 197
corn silk 11, 153, 156
couch grass 12, 153
cramp bark 12, 61, 62, 155
cranberry 12, 158
cranesbill 12, 28, 29, 58, 66, 67, 70, 168
Crataeva 12, 153, 156, 158

D

Damiana 12
dandelion 36, 58, 65, 71, 72, 153, 163, 190
dandelion leaf 153
dandelion root 36, 58, 65, 71, 72, 190
devil's claw 12
dill seed oil 25, 58
dong quai 12